Advance Praise for
Real Food for Pregnancy

"Real Food For Pregnancy should find its way into every medical school and prenatal clinic. Lily Nichols' first book, *Real Food for Gestational Diabetes*, is a staple in my teaching here at West Virginia University and has shifted how many in our department view nutrition. Her second book is encyclopedic; it's amazingly well-referenced and more in-depth than many textbooks. If mothers embrace Lily's advice, the next generation will hopefully suffer less obesity and diabetes."

—Mark Cucuzzella, MD, FAAFP, Professor at West Virginia University School of Medicine

"Finally, a book about nutrition in pregnancy that won't put you to sleep, and might, in fact, make your mouth water! No sign of the 'Pregnancy Police' here, as Lily brings together a straight-talking combination of 'sauce and science.' As a midwife, this book will be on my must-read list for every pregnant person I know."

—Tracy Donegan, Midwife & Founder of GentleBirth

"Real Food for Pregnancy should be considered essential reading for any woman who is currently pregnant or planning conception in the near future. I have not found a similar text with the breadth and depth of discussion on prenatal nutrition. What sets *Real Food for Pregnancy* apart is how it logically explains the current scientific evidence that is disrupting modern nutrition science and pushing conventional dogma into a new direction. Lily Nichols' meticulously cited text provides not only a quick read but also plenty of details and references for those who wish to dig further. This book may very well serve as the tipping point leading to a sea change in nutrition science and medical care. I will be recommending it to my patients within my busy high-risk obstetrics practice."

—Amit Bhavsar, MD, Board certified Obstetrician-Gynecologist practicing outside of Austin, TX

"Lily Nichols has written a must-read for any woman or health professional interested in prenatal nutrition. During my first pregnancy I felt like I spent hours upon hours trying to research all of the information that is summed up beautifully in *Real Food for Pregnancy*. Lily questions conventional wisdom and offers new and practical, science-based recommendations to support optimal health for both mom and baby. I hope this book will inspire change in current prenatal nutrition guidelines."

—Shannon Weston, MPH, RD, LD, CDE, Houston, TX

"*Real Food for Pregnancy* is replacing my Prenatal/Maternal Nutrition textbook. The information meets every pregnant woman's needs and provides evidence-based "real food" solutions."

—Rochelle Anzaldo, RD for an OB clinic in Bakersfield, California

"Lily Nichols is like the Michael Pollan of prenatal nutrition. *Real Food for Pregnancy* is an enlightening and informative read that focuses on the quality of food rather than calories. Having worked with Lily, it's refreshing to hear from a dietitian I trust, who values research, truth, and real world application."

—Brittany Maughan, RD, Knoxville, TN

"As a practicing CNM (midwife) for almost 30 years, I am thrilled to have found Lily's writing and expertise. *Real Food for Pregnancy* is one that we'll keep in stock at our clinic and will teach from during our early pregnancy classes. I really enjoyed the descriptions of the vitamins and minerals and how to get them from food. In my experience, too many people believe that prenatal vitamins will solve all of their problems or will guarantee the health of the baby."

—Cheryl Heitkamp, APRN, CNM, President of Willow Midwives in Minneapolis, MN

"I was recently pregnant for the first time (I unfortunately had a miscarriage) and this is exactly the book I had been searching for. *Real Food for Pregnancy* was a difficult book for me to read, in the best possible way. As a longtime vegetarian, it made me confront many of my food choices and preferences head on and acknowledge that they are not even close to optimal for pregnancy. Despite my internal conflict, I walked away from reading this book feeling incredibly empowered. While reading it I wrote down many questions, only to find that Lily devoted an entire chapter to answering my exact question later in the book. Lily provides all the tools pregnant women need to start optimizing their diets immediately. She lays out the science and interprets it into a series of actionable items that each woman can choose to do or not to do, depending on her specific needs."

—Anna Gajewski, MPH, Research Coordinator, Managua, Nicaragua

"*Real Food for Pregnancy* covers a lot of ground. From debunking some of the way-too-common misconceptions about dietary fat, to the importance of micronutrients and where to find them in real food, to lab testing, to the eye-opening section on toxins, there is so much information packed into this book. I especially liked the discussion of food aversions and cravings; it's a curse for so many women, and I love how Lily encourages healthy choices and also some leeway at the same time. There is so much "lazy information" given out to save on time and costs of educating women; this book offers more detailed and proactive guidance than you'll find anywhere else. I want to give a copy to every single OBGYN office I see."

—Katie Miller, RDN, Gilbert, AZ

As a dietitian specializing in pregnancy and gestational diabetes, I consider *Real Food for Pregnancy* (along with Lily's previous book, *Real Food for Gestational Diabetes*), my go-to resource for research-backed nutrition information. I've had my doubts about the standard nutrition recommendations for pregnancy, but never had the time (nor patience) to dig through the research to the depth that I'd like. Not only did Lily do all the work for me (and you), she did it in a way that is easy to read and understand by anyone. Being in the field, I thought I had a pretty solid understanding of prenatal nutrition, but reading this book was a humbling experience. This is an extremely comprehensive book that I would highly recommend to healthcare providers, as well as ALL women, regardless of their stage of pregnancy (including those who are just in the planning stage). I have full trust in all of Lily's work and I am so glad she is sharing even more of her wisdom and expertise with us in this book. I'm already looking forward to reading it again."

—Katrina Yoder, RD, CDE, San Luis Obispo, CA

"I have read numerous books on nutrition and *Real Food for Pregnancy* is simply incredible. I always tell my patients that I don't practice out of popular books. Lily Nichols' book seems to fit in a different category as it is really of textbook quality; it could be called an easy reading version of an encyclopedia of nutrition. Lily is meticulously thorough in combining current scientific understanding with the wisdom of the past. Nutritional demands are undoubtedly most intense during pregnancy, and *Real Food for Pregnancy* offers crucial insight into the importance of eating a nutrient dense diet during this time."

—John Madany, MD, Dillon, MT

"This amazing book is long overdue. As a midwife, I am relieved to finally be able to recommend a one-stop resource for proactive nutritional guidance. It's reader-friendly and well-organized with loads of information, but at the same time not overwhelming. The information is based on solid research but also from the experience of a professional with a long history of success working with expectant and postpartum mothers. Lily Nichols' common sense approach is both accessible and effective. *Real Food for Pregnancy is great* for expecting parents and professionals alike, who wish to get up-to-date on the best ways to minimize complications and use nutrition for the best pregnancy outcomes."

—Elke Saunders, CPM, Anchorage, Alaska

"I highly recommend *Real Food for Pregnancy* and will be making it "required reading" for all future mothers in my nutrition practice."

—Diana Rodgers, RD, LDN, NTP, Author of *The Homegrown Paleo Cookbook*

REAL FOOD
for
PREGNANCY

Real Food for Pregnancy
Copyright © 2018, Lily Nichols
Foreword © 2018, Melissa Powell
First edition.
Printed in USA.

www.realfoodforpregnancy.com

ISBN-13 (print): 978-0-9862950-4-1
ISBN-13 (ebook): 978-0-9862950-5-8

Cover design and graphics: Lily Nichols
Cover photography: Jessica Beacom
Copyediting: Dana Nichols

Table of Contents

Foreword

The book you're holding in your hands is powerful. The way you nourish yourself during pregnancy quite literally shapes your baby's health, and not just in early infancy, but for the rest of his or her life. The foods you eat, the supplements you take, the way you move your body, the toxins you are exposed to (or not), and the way you handle stress, can leave a direct—and *lasting*—mark on your baby's DNA, and thus his or her risk for health problems later in life.

Lily and I live in very different regions of the United States. When a friend of mine moved to my area, she was literally warned by her pediatrician about the higher risk of obesity that comes with living in the South. While this may seem extreme, the rising rates of chronic disease, especially in children, point to the truth in that warning.

As a nutrition professor, I teach courses specifically on maternal and child nutrition. My goal is to use current prenatal nutrition guidelines and scientific literature to guide students' understanding of the complex nature of this field. I take the responsibility of shaping the minds of future dietitians very seriously. Ultimately, they will be the ones guiding the food choices of countless individuals, including pregnant women, throughout their careers.

There is often a gap between new research and public policy—sometimes a very wide gap—and my goal is to help bridge the two for my students. After learning about Lily and her expertise in the nutritional management of gestational diabetes, I started using her book, *Real Food for Gestational Diabetes*, as required reading in my courses. It taught my students about a common pregnancy complication, yes, but more importantly, it helped them think critically about many other aspects of prenatal nutrition that have gone unchallenged for decades.

I trust Lily because her practice stems from her academics, research, and clinical work. Moreover, she doesn't accept nutrition policies at face value before rigorously researching all sides. In *Real Food for Pregnancy*, she examines the latest research, putting into question many tenets that are central to conventional prenatal nutrition guidelines.

Why does this matter to you? Well, if you've done any reading on prenatal nutrition thus far, you've probably found conflicting advice on topics such as: which foods to avoid, how much protein, fat, or carbohydrate you need, and which supplements to take. As Lily masterfully unpacks in the coming chapters, a lot of the advice you've been given is well-meaning, but frankly, outdated or not evidenced-based. In this book, you'll get clear answers on what to eat and why, with research to back up every recommendation. Drawing from traditional diets and cultural food practices, you'll also learn the history of nourishing foods for pregnancy.

This book goes way beyond food, however, covering a wide range of topics including: exercise during pregnancy, common complaints (how to naturally manage nausea, constipation, high blood pressure, etc.), specific lab tests to guide your food and lifestyle choices, how and why to avoid common toxins while pregnant, and a whole section on postpartum recovery. Several controversial topics get a much-needed review, such as screening methods for gestational diabetes (including alternatives to the glucola), the safety of ketosis and low-carbohydrate diets, how diet quality affects the nutrient-density of breast milk, the latest research on alcohol consumption in pregnancy, and much more.

This thoroughly researched book is likely to become a coveted resource for dietetics educators, students, and healthcare providers. More importantly, though, its readability and practicality will make it a valuable reference manual for pregnant women. Real food and healthy lifestyle choices support your body in the midst of one of life's most beautiful mysteries—where cells build organs that grow organ systems that develop into a human body—giving us the next generation. In many faiths, including my own, this is truly holy ground.

Depending on your familiarity with real food, some of the advice in this book may take time to wrap your mind around. If embracing full-fat dairy products (like grass-fed butter), eating eggs *with the yolks,* or making bone broth from scratch seems out-of-the-box for you, I would encourage you to try one new practice at a time. The meal plans and recipes, along with the mindful eating suggestions, will help you find your sweet spot. This way of eating can be both delicious and sustainable.

As you'll see firsthand in the pages ahead, *Real Food for Pregnancy* also infuses joy into eating during pregnancy. By putting into perspective the warnings about food poisoning, you'll learn that you can *safely* enjoy many conventionally forbidden foods, like fish and sunny-side-up eggs (provided you take a few food safety precautions). By debunking myths surrounding salt and fat, you'll actually *enjoy* the food you're eating, while helping to stave off pregnancy complications (believe it or not). Finally, you'll learn that you can relax more around food. Obsessive portion control and calorie counting are *not* on the menu; instead, mindful eating takes its place. Simply put, you have permission to eat delicious food and in quantities that leave you full and satisfied. The nutrition habits that Lily will guide you in developing during your pregnancy will be a gift that you give to your baby, your family, and yourself both now and for years to come.

Melissa Powell, MEd, RDN
University of Tennessee at Chattanooga
December 2017

Introduction

"Maternal nutrition plays a critical role in fetal growth and development."
- Dr. Guoyao Wu, Texas A&M University

The message that a mother's nutrient intake during pregnancy affects the development of her baby is well accepted across multiple nutrition philosophies and among traditional cultures. Even if this is the first nutrition book you've ever picked up, I'm sure you agree as well.

You might be wondering why I bothered to write a book about prenatal nutrition if everyone agrees on this basic principle. Well, outside of a few select nutrients, there's actually more disagreement than there is consensus on this subject. Digging into the details of conventional prenatal nutrition guidelines—and comparing them to both scientific research and the wisdom from ancestral diets of traditional cultures—uncovers many discrepancies, which is why I've written this book.

Before I go any further, allow me to define a few terms that I will reference frequently. Conventional nutrition refers to dietary advice based on the U.S. government's nutrition policies. These dietary guidelines formed the basis of the notorious food pyramid. Although the food pyramid was officially replaced with a plate, the overall message has remained virtually unchanged for decades: eat less meat, limit saturated fat, and eat more grains. Ancestral diets and those of traditional cultures refer to the dietary practices of people who lived several hundred years ago and beyond (although there are still some isolated populations that live this way). Since this was before the advent of mass-produced food and industrialization, the focus was on real food, obtained locally and eaten in its natural, unprocessed form. I will use the terms ancestral diets, ancestral nutrition, foods from traditional cultures, and real food interchangeably.

Although both conventional nutrition and traditional cultures have their similarities—for one, they generally tend to emphasize the importance of fresh produce—they most certainly have their differences. Conventional prenatal guidelines discourage the consumption of fatty meat and organ meats, suggest limiting seafood intake (no more than 12 oz per week, they say), direct you to choose only low-fat dairy products, and contend that you need a high intake of carbohydrates (45-65% of calories) to ensure the health of your baby.

In stark contrast, traditional cultures consumed animals "nose-to-tail," prized the fattiest cuts of meat, went out of their way to obtain seafood (even in landlocked areas), never skimmed the fat off of their milk (if they were a milk-drinking community in the first place), and did not consume anywhere near the level of carbohydrates currently recommended. Plus, refined carbohydrates—like white flour and white sugar—didn't even exist until the last century or two. Conventional prenatal nutrition guidelines only specify making "half of your grains whole." Flip that around and what they're essentially saying is that it's perfectly acceptable to eat half of your grains in the form of refined cereal and white bread.

So who's right: conventional nutrition or traditional cultures? As I started to meticulously pick apart the scientific literature, I came to surprising, and rather disappointing, conclusions. As a dietitian, I would expect better from our public policies.

In short, current research finds that the nutrients most commonly lacking in a prenatal diet—like vitamins A, B12, B6, zinc, iron, DHA, iodine and choline—are found in the very foods you're told to limit by conventional prenatal nutrition guidelines. Plus, the more carbohydrates you eat—especially refined carbohydrates—the fewer micronutrients your diet contains (meaning vitamins and minerals), and the higher your chances of developing pregnancy complications.

Though some may shrug their shoulders and think "Well, that's why a prenatal vitamin is recommended," I'm sorry to say that most prenatal vitamins contain nowhere near the levels of nutrients required to ensure a healthy pregnancy and many lack key nutrients entirely (such as iodine and choline). In addition, some prenatals contain poorly utilized forms of nutrients (like folic acid instead of L-methylfolate). A high-quality prenatal vitamin can serve as an insurance policy of sorts, but there really is no replacement for a nutrient-dense diet of real food.

Although I've always had an interest in prenatal nutrition, I didn't come to fully appreciate its importance until I witnessed the effects of suboptimal nutrition on pregnancy outcomes firsthand. It was working both clinically and at the public policy level on gestational diabetes, the type of diabetes that either first develops or is first recognized during pregnancy, that really piqued my interest. Upwards of 18% of pregnant women face this diagnosis, and when not well managed, it can leave a lasting impact on their children's health. In fact, babies born to women with gestational diabetes face a 6-fold higher risk of developing type 2 diabetes by the time they are 13 years old.[1] Between 2001 and 2009, there was a more than 30% increase in the prevalence of type 2 diabetes among children, and the rates are only projected to increase.[2] These statistics are frightening and highlight just how important a mother's nutrition and blood sugar levels are to her baby. The epidemic of childhood diabetes and obesity we're currently witnessing is not only due to poor food choices or inactivity during childhood, but also to inadequate nutrition and metabolic problems they have been exposed to *in utero*.

The striking difference between conventional prenatal nutrition and a real food or ancestral approach was made especially clear in my clinical gestational diabetes work. It was in this role that I was able to put conventional nutrition advice to the test alongside my "real food approach" and see how it impacted both blood sugar levels and pregnancy outcomes.

The results were nothing short of astounding. Using my real food approach, we were able to cut in *half* the number of women who required insulin or medication to manage their blood sugar. We also had excellent outcomes: healthier moms who didn't struggle with hunger or excessive weight gain; who had far lower rates of preeclampsia; and who had healthy babies who were born at a normal weight and with normal blood sugar levels. It was amazing to witness the impact that real food had on pregnancy outcomes. It wasn't effective just because my approach was lower in carbohydrates, but because it contained exponentially higher levels of nutrients than the conventional gestational diabetes diet.

I was encouraged to write my first book, *Real Food for Gestational Diabetes,* to get the message out to other moms, dietitians, and healthcare providers, and within a few months, it became (and remains, at the time of writing this) the bestselling gestational diabetes book on the market. I'm heartened to regularly receive messages from mothers, even those who have had gestational diabetes in previous pregnancies, who share stories of their smooth pregnancies and healthy babies as a result of their efforts in following my approach.

I started getting asked to write a book on general prenatal nutrition shortly after the release of my first book. Midwives and doctors who had seen the positive impact on gestational diabetes wanted to have a resource for their non-diabetic clients. They also wanted my take (or really, a summary of the research) on other topics related to pregnancy, like supplements, exposure to toxins, the validity of typical "foods to avoid" lists and more.

Initially, I resisted, figuring there were already plenty of books on the market on this topic. But, I've come to find there really *aren't*—at least none with the level of evidence-based information that we so desperately need in order to finally shift the most outdated prenatal nutrition advice. Most of what I've come across either shares conventional guidelines or offers their personal opinion, without citing sources for their information, nor studies to back their claims.

The last straw was when a colleague came to me with several questions about prenatal nutrition based on what she had read in the *Academy of Nutrition and Dietetics'* policy paper on pregnancy nutrition entitled "Nutrition and Lifestyle for a Healthy Pregnancy Outcome." In case you're not familiar, the *Academy of Nutrition and Dietetics* (formerly known as the *American Dietetics Association)* is the professional organization that governs the practice of registered dietitians and influences nutrition public policies in the United States. My jaw nearly dropped to the floor as I read through this policy paper. While I didn't disagree with *everything,* there were some obvious oversights and it was clear that *now* was time for me to write this book.

Among the most disappointing things in this document was the sample meal plan. It was the epitome of prenatal nutrition gone wrong. Breakfast was nearly devoid of protein and fat (only oatmeal, strawberries and *low-fat* milk). The quantity of carbohydrates was through the roof (over 300 grams). And there was absolutely nothing satisfying about the afternoon snack of crackers and carrots. There was no red meat, no eggs (unless you count the tiny amount in *low-fat* mayonnaise), and certainly no organ meats. Just about the only thing I was relieved to see was salmon served at dinner, though it was accompanied by plain steamed broccoli, white rice, and *more* low-fat milk (and there was no mention of the importance of choosing wild-caught vs. farm-raised salmon). This was the polar opposite of a sample meal plan I might share with a client. I was hungry just reading it.

I couldn't fathom, given all that I know about the food sources of tricky nutrients, like choline and vitamin A, how this diet could ever meet a pregnant woman's needs. I decided to compare a nutrient analysis of their sample meal plan to one of my own.

The results confirmed my suspicions. Each meal plan had equivalent calories, but the nutrient-density was a different story. Of the micronutrients I analyzed, my meal plan came out on top for 19 of them. Specifically, my meal plan had approximately triple the quantities of vitamin B12, double the quantities of vitamins A and E, 55% more zinc, 37% more iron, and nearly 70% more choline. It was also higher in brain-boosting omega-3 fats and had a more favorable ratio of omega-3 to omega-6 fats. It was particularly worrying to see that the *Academy of Nutrition and Dietetics'* meal plan had very little preformed vitamin A, known as retinol, since animal fats were extremely limited.

Needless to say, I respectfully disagree with the conventional prenatal nutrition guidelines and I cannot, in good conscience, recommend their sample meal plan to pregnant women. Depriving a mother's growing baby of key nutrients needed for things like brain development goes against the "first, do no harm" principle that's central to ethical medical care across the globe. It often takes decades for research to make it into practice—and for old policies to be significantly reformed—so it's not surprising that we have found ourselves in this situation. But, we can do better.

Real Food for Pregnancy Sample Meal Plan	Conventional Nutrition Sample Meal Plan
Breakfast: Crustless spinach quiche Pork breakfast sausages (pasture-raised) Banana	**Breakfast:** Oatmeal Low-fat milk Strawberries
Morning Snack: Apple + almond butter	**Morning Snack:** Trail mix (almonds + mixed dried fruit)
Lunch: Homemade chicken & vegetable soup Lentils (mixed into soup) Arugula salad Lemon-herb dressing Parmesan cheese	**Lunch:** Turkey sandwich (whole wheat bread, turkey, light mayonnaise) Salad (lettuce, tomato, kidney bean salad, French dressing) Banana Low-fat milk
Afternoon snack: Sardines packed in olive oil Brown rice crackers	**Afternoon snack:** Carrot slices Whole wheat crackers
Dinner: Grass-fed beef meatloaf Roasted Brussels sprouts Roasted red potatoes	**Dinner:** Coleslaw (cabbage, pineapple, light mayonnaise) Grilled salmon (w/ oil) Broccoli stalks, steamed White rice Low-fat milk
Evening Snack: Greek yogurt (full-fat) + vanilla extract Chia seeds	**Evening snack:** Air-popped popcorn
Dessert: Raspberries + homemade whipped cream	**Dessert:** Frozen vanilla yogurt, low fat

My goal with *Real Food for Pregnancy* is to not only take prenatal nutrition advice out of the dark ages, but to give you an easy-to-follow guide for making the best food and lifestyle choices during pregnancy. At the time I began writing, my son was less than a year old, so it was easy for me to think back to all the questions I had during pregnancy and address them head-on.

Real Food for Pregnancy	Conventional Nutrition	Nutrient Comparison
Total calories 2,329	Total calories 2,302	Nutrients Higher in Real Food for Pregnancy

Macronutrients
Carbohydrate: 156 g 26%
  Fiber: 41 g
Protein: 140 g 24%
Fat: 134 g 51%
	Macronutrients
	Carbohydrate: 319 g 54%
	  Fiber: 43 g
	Protein: 109 g 19%
	Fat: 72 g 28%	

Essential Fatty Acids Omega-3s: 3.3 g Omega-3-to-6 ratio: 3.2:1	**Essential Fatty Acids** Omega-3s: 2.9 g Omega-3-to-6 ratio: 4.3:1	Omega-3: 114%

Vitamins
Vitamin A: 13,935 mcg
  Retinol: 2,492 mcg
Vitamin C: 194 mg
Vitamin D: 18 mcg
Vitamin E: 18 mg
Vitamin B1: 1.5 mg
Vitamin B2: 3.1 mg
Vitamin B3: 32 mg
Vitamin B6: 3.0 mg
Vitamin B12: 23 mcg
Folate: 609 mcg
Choline: 633 mg
	Vitamins
	Vitamin A: 6,753 mcg
	  Retinol: 83 mcg
	Vitamin C: 171 mg
	Vitamin D: 16 mcg
	Vitamin E: 9.3 mg
	Vitamin B1: 1.5 mg
	Vitamin B2: 2.0 mg
	Vitamin B3: 25 mg
	Vitamin B6: 2.6 mg
	Vitamin B12: 8.1 mcg
	Folate: 518 mcg
	Choline: 374 mg
		Vitamins
		Vitamin A: 206%
		  Retinol: 3002%
		Vitamin C: 113%
		Vitamin D: 112%
		Vitamin E: 193%
		
		Vitamin B2: 155%
		Vitamin B3: 128%
		Vitamin B-6: 115%
		Vitamin B-12: 284%
		Folate: 118%
		Choline: 169%

Minerals Calcium: 1,462 mg Copper: 4,700 mcg Iron: 20.5 mg Magnesium: 482 mg Potassium: 4,522 mg Selenium: 131 mcg Zinc: 17 mg	**Minerals** Calcium: 1,394 mg Copper: 1,200 mcg Iron: 15 mg Magnesium: 433 mg Potassium: 4,027 mg Selenium: 126 mcg Zinc: 11 mg	**Minerals** Calcium: 105% Copper: 392% Iron: 137% Magnesium: 111% Potassium: 112% Selenium: 104% Zinc: 155%

If you knew that eating the right foods *now* could prevent your baby from developing diabetes or struggling with obesity or having chronic skin rashes later in life, would you eat differently? Most women answer with an enthusiastic "*Yes!*" as they want nothing but the best for their children. In my practice, pregnant women are the most motivated clients I encounter.

Sadly, if you follow conventional prenatal nutrition advice, you're almost guaranteed to be eating a *nutrient-deficient* diet, not a *nutrient-dense* one.

It doesn't have to be that way. I questioned the status quo, so you don't have to question yourself when making food and lifestyle choices during pregnancy. This book is the missing prenatal nutrition education that proactive pregnant women and their healthcare providers have been searching for to no avail. I will break down the complicated science to give you the most evidence-based guide on prenatal nutrition available. Every chapter is meticulously cited, so much so that my husband jokes that I have written a textbook. I wouldn't go that far, but as a self-confessed nutrition nerd, I want you to know that I'm not "making this stuff up." I believe every woman should have access to the most accurate information available, whether or not she's a researcher or a nutritionist. Multiple chapters have over 100 citations apiece, so you can go back to the medical journals, if you're so inclined, and read the primary research yourself.

With pregnancy, there are no guarantees, but there are things you can do to ensure it is as easy as possible, and that your baby gets everything he or she needs to develop optimally. The primary focus of this book is nutrition, however, there are also chapters on related topics such as prenatal exercise, chemicals and toxins to limit, stress management, and how to navigate the postpartum phase and breastfeeding. In other words, I cover a lot more than food.

This book is geared towards women who are already pregnant; however, because your health *pre*-pregnancy impacts your health *during* pregnancy, this advice is equally appropriate if you are trying to conceive. There's no wrong time to embrace real food and optimize your health; it simply becomes exponentially more important when you're creating and growing a new life.

Chapter 1:

Why You Should Have a Real Food Pregnancy

"Whilst good nutrition is important at all life stages, it is increasingly recognised that the nutritional environment and individual experiences before birth and in early infancy is of particular importance for their later metabolic health, and that exposure to an inappropriate nutritional supply during critical windows of development can predispose an individual to obesity and type 2 diabetes later in life. By extension, the diet consumed by pregnant and breastfeeding women is a key determinant of metabolic health."
- Dr. Beverly Muhlhausler, University of Adelaide

There's something miraculous about pregnancy. The fact that we have the power to literally *grow a new human* is still mind-boggling to me. When I was pregnant, I remember being keenly aware that all sorts of complex processes (both known and unknown in the scientific literature) were going on inside my body every second of every day. And I didn't even need to consciously think about it; my body just *knew* what it was doing. It knew to create five fingers on each hand, where to place fingernails, where to grow hair, where the heart went, where each and every blood vessel should go, and on and on.

Sometimes this line of thinking—the idea that your body will take care of all the needs of fetal development without your input—is extrapolated to mean that you have *no* control over the trajectory of your pregnancy or the future health of your baby. Your body will just "do what it's gonna do" and all you can do is hope you were dealt a good hand of cards and pass along good genes.

But that's only partly true.

Allow me to share a quick metaphor. Anyone who has ever had a garden understands that when you plant a tomato seed, you can expect a tomato plant to grow (not a pea vine or a broccoli plant). The seed has the blueprints, and even if you're not a very good gardener, that seed will grow given the bare essentials: some soil, water, and light. However, what separates a novice from a master gardener is their attention to optimal conditions. They have learned that amending the soil with nutrient-dense and microbe-rich compost will provide the plant with more of the raw materials for growth. They understand that there's a sweet spot in the amount of water and light that helps a tomato plant not just survive, but *thrive*. Ultimately, they know that with a little TLC, they will have a healthier plant with vibrant green leaves and plentiful, delicious tomatoes.

This same line of thinking applies to pregnancy. Simply put, humans are wired to reproduce successfully. Even when conditions aren't optimal, your body will do everything in its power to follow the blueprints and carry your precious baby to term. If that weren't the case, there would be no way we'd have so many humans on the planet despite all sorts of common interferences, like malnutrition and toxin exposure. The problem is that chronic diseases are on the rise, especially among children, and a number of researchers have linked the development of things like heart disease, hormonal imbalance, diabetes, and obesity to exposures in utero. Unfortunately, it takes decades for this type of research to make it into clinical practice and public policies. That's why you have to *really* search to connect the dots—and that's exactly what I did while writing this book

Don't get me wrong, there are a lot of things in pregnancy that are out of your control (your genetics, your age, your family history of disease, just to name a few). But, the things that *are* within your control—your diet, exercise, sleep habits, the way you handle stress, your exposure to toxins, and more—can have significant effects on your pregnancy and may leave a permanent imprint on your baby's health. It's called "fetal programming," a decades old hypothesis (now well-studied and well-accepted in scientific research) which proposes that inadequate nutrition during pregnancy can impair the development of your baby and lead to lifelong metabolic changes that increase the risk of diseases, like heart disease, diabetes, high blood pressure, and the risk of obesity.[1]

Though most of us view our genetics as a solid blueprint, researchers have found that genes can be turned on or off by certain exposures in utero, such as levels of nutrients, a mom's blood sugar and insulin levels, exercise habits, stress hormones, toxins, and much more. That means that even if you think you have "bad genes," you have the ability to minimize the impact of these on your baby with optimal nutrition and informed lifestyle choices. On the flipside, even if you have "good genes," they could be turned off to some degree if your diet and lifestyle aren't healthy.

When it comes to *your* experience of pregnancy, you have the power to lower your chances of developing gestational diabetes, preeclampsia, delivering prematurely, becoming anemic, and gaining too much or too little weight during your pregnancy, all by the way you live your life. How empowering is that?

Ask any pregnant woman and she'll tell you the most important thing to her is to have a healthy baby and an easy pregnancy, so NOW is the time to do everything in your power to "stack the deck" in your favor.

Why Real Food?

When I first ventured into the world of prenatal nutrition, I was shocked by how little is actually known about fetal development. Researchers are still piecing together what exactly is happening and when. Believe it or not, we're still uncovering which nutrients are needed, in what amounts, and at which stage in pregnancy. Even the recommended dietary allowances (RDAs), which tell you how much of each nutrient you require on a daily basis, are best guesses.[2] Until we have better information (and perhaps we never will), we need another plan.

One option is to look at the diets of traditional cultures who have long histories of having healthy babies and to learn from them. The work of Dr. Weston Price, a dentist and nutrition researcher from the early 1900s, found that traditional cultures prized certain nutrient-dense foods during the preconception and prenatal period.[3] Dr. Price traveled the globe and investigated the dietary practices of numerous cultures, the nutrient-density of their foods, and their overall health. The groups studied included the Swiss, Gaelics, Eskimos, Malay tribes, Maori of New Zealand, Native Americans in Canada and the U.S., tribes in Eastern and Central Africa, Pacific Islanders (Polynesians and Melanesians), Australian Aborigines, South Americans of the Amazon basin, and ancient civilizations and their descendants in Peru. He found remarkable differences in the nutrient content of traditional foods compared to imported foods.

He also found that the health of these populations was a direct reflection of what they ate, noting that people who followed their ancestral diet remained disease-free and had robustly healthy children. In contrast, relatives who incorporated modern foods into their diet suffered more health problems, as did their children. Tooth decay, narrow palate, crooked teeth, deformities (like club feet and neural tube defects), poor immune health (higher rates of infectious diseases, like tuberculosis), psychological problems, and numerous other health problems were more prevalent in children of people who ate more "foods of modern commerce," like sugar and refined grains, and less of their traditional foods. What struck me most about his work was that the negative consequences of a bad diet affected more than just their children, but also their *children's* children.

Dr. Price's observations have been replicated in animal studies and it's now more widely accepted that exposure to positive influences like a nutrient-dense diet and exercise have beneficial effects on pregnancy outcomes, while exposure to toxins, stress, and processed foods have the opposite effect.[4,5,6,7,8] There's currently a whole field of research devoted to the study of what's called "epigenetics," or how your genes (or your children's genes) are affected by your lifestyle choices and other exposures.[9]

It was from reading Price's research (and learning which foods were most prized in these cultures) that I began to question what I had been previously taught about prenatal nutrition in my conventional dietetics training. How could a low-fat diet be acceptable if it means the richest food sources of vitamin A, choline, iron, and zinc are limited? Traditional cultures did the exact opposite. Conventional nutrition heavily advocates for fortified foods in pregnancy—like cereal fortified with folic acid and iron—while frequently ignoring foods that are naturally good sources of those same nutrients. In fact, consumption of certain nutrient-dense foods, like liver and full-fat dairy, are commonly discouraged. How did traditional cultures ensure they had healthy pregnancies when fortified foods didn't exist?

Modern nutrition research tends to isolate and study single nutrients instead of whole foods, resulting in a lot of attention given to prenatal vitamins or individual supplements. That approach—often called "nutritionism"—has never made much sense to me. Why not, instead, take the information we've learned from modern science and apply it to real food?

In other words, let's figure out which foods are naturally rich sources of the most important nutrients for fetal development instead of swallowing a bunch of pills. **After all, nutrients work synergistically. Nature is not stupid. And a supplement is rarely superior to what's available in real, whole foods.**

That's why my real food approach is to reverse engineer the perfect prenatal diet. We can take what we've learned from single-nutrient studies and combine it with what we know from traditional cultures.

The result? We have the best of both modern nutrition science and ancestral wisdom to help you "grow a healthy baby." In the coming chapters, you'll learn which foods, nutrients, and lifestyle habits to embrace *and why*—and which ones to avoid—so you can be assured that you're doing everything within your power to have a healthy pregnancy. Like I said before, let's "stack the deck" in your favor.

Real Food for Pregnancy

Chapter 2:

Real Food Nutrition for Pregnancy

"The biological importance of maternal nutrition is well-established. Not only is it the sole way for the fetus to receive the required nutrients but it also affects the maternal metabolic adjustment capacity to the hormones secreted by the placenta that affect the metabolism of all nutrients.
Nutrition during early development is associated with the offspring's growth, organ development, body composition and body functions. It also exerts long-term effects on health, morbidity and mortality risks in adulthood, as well as on the development of neural functions and behavior, a phenomenon called 'metabolic programming.'"
- Dr. Irene P Tzanetakou, European University Cyprus

Think for a moment about the nutrition advice you've heard about pregnancy. Most women turn to their doctors for advice, but aren't aware that the majority of them receive very little education on the matter (only 25% of accredited U.S. medical schools require a dedicated nutrition course).[1] If you walked away with the message to "just take a prenatal vitamin and avoid alcohol" and thought there must be more to it than that, let me assure you: You can do more—*a lot more*—to stay healthy during pregnancy.

In this chapter, I'll introduce some of the basic concepts of a well-balanced *real food* prenatal diet. For those of you who are nutrition-savvy, know that I'll be starting with the basics and working my way to more complex topics both here and in later sections. That means starting with some definitions and categorizing things, so we can make sense of it all later.

By now you understand there are benefits to eating "real food for pregnancy," but you might be wondering what that actually entails. So before we move on, let's define real food.

What is Real Food?

Everyone has their own definition of real food, but for the purpose of this book, here's my take:

- Real food is as close to its source as possible and grown or raised in conditions that maximize nutrient density. For example, fresh vegetables that are in-season, eaten soon after harvest, and grown without the use of pesticides are going to be more nutritious than the canned version.
- Real food is minimally processed, so it appears just like you would find it in nature. Beyond the above vegetable example, think about dairy products. Cows are naturally meant to graze on grass and their milk naturally contains fat. So, from a real food perspective, full-fat dairy from grass-fed cows is nutritionally superior to low-fat dairy from cows that are fed grains and raised in confinement.
- Real food often doesn't have a label (like fresh vegetables or meat), but when it does, it is made with simple ingredients and no additives. Of course, some purists would argue that "real foods don't have labels," but in this busy, modern world, you're probably going to be buying a fair amount of food with labels and that's okay. When buying packaged foods, always check the ingredients. If it reads like a list of chemicals, it isn't real food.

In a nutshell, real food is made with simple ingredients that are as close to nature as possible and not processed in a way that removes nutrients.

At minimum, a well-balanced real food diet for pregnancy includes vegetables, fruit, meat, poultry, fish and seafood, nuts, seeds, legumes and plenty of healthy fats. Most women benefit from the inclusion of dairy products, but they are not required. And, if they agree with your body, your real food diet may also include whole grains.

I'll be delving into *why* some of these foods are essential during pregnancy based on the specific nutrients they contain in the next chapter, but for now, let's take a broad view of prenatal nutrition and clear up some misconceptions.

Should I "Eat for Two?"

The concept of "eating for two" isn't necessarily bad, but it's misinterpreted almost universally. It implies that you need to eat double the quantity of food while pregnant.

In reality, your body does not need *that* many more calories to grow a healthy baby. Conventional wisdom suggests that calorie needs start to increase around the end of the first trimester, after which your body needs approximately 300 extra calories per day for the baby. However, research on pregnant women from across the globe shows that this number is simply an estimate. In fact, some women's energy needs go up as little as 70 extra calories per day.[2] That said, if we assume 300 calories is a ballpark figure, that's the equivalent of adding an extra snack to your day, not double portions at every meal. As one scientist puts it, "the old saying that a "pregnant woman needs to eat for two," is an overstatement, and should be modified to "a pregnant woman needs to eat for 1.1.""[3] What *does* increase significantly is your need for certain nutrients, such as vitamin A, folate, vitamin B12, choline, iron, iodine, and many others.[4]

Instead of using "eating for two" to defend excessive portions or extra junk food, let it serve as a gentle reminder that your baby is relying on *you* for nourishment. Treat it as an incentive to optimize the nutrient density of your diet, meaning every bite of food that crosses your lips is packed with nutrition. Think *quality* over *quantity*.

The better you nourish yourself, the better you will nourish your growing baby. That starts with understanding what it means to eat a balanced diet.

Macronutrients

A *macro*nutrient is something that gives you energy, while *micro*nutrients are the vitamins and minerals that your body needs for other functions. Optimal prenatal nutrition requires that you get enough energy from a good balance of the three major macronutrients: carbohydrates, fat, and protein.

All real foods contain a blend of the three macronutrients, with a few exceptions containing only one or two of them. For example, sweet potatoes are primarily made of carbohydrates with a teeny tiny amount of protein and almost no fat. On the other hand, eggs are mostly protein and fat with no carbohydrates. Many dairy products, like full-fat milk and yogurt, contain a mix of all three macronutrients.

I find it's helpful to understand the macronutrients and their effects on the body, as well as some of their major food sources, so you can plan out a way of eating that will work best for your individual needs.

Modern nutritional science is uncovering that some macronutrients can be over- or under-done and cause problems during pregnancy. As you may have guessed, there's no one-size-fits-all here. You might benefit from a low-carb diet, while another woman who's very physically active may need a little more. We'll talk more about customizing your prenatal diet later on.

In my experience having worked one-on-one with hundreds of pregnant women, I've observed that it's quite common (and easy) for women to over-consume carbohydrates, but rarely do I observe women over-consuming protein or fat.

I believe this is primarily due to outdated nutrition guidelines that have demonized fatty foods and spurred the food industry to create oodles of low-fat (in other words, *high-carb*) processed foods. These refined carbohydrates (found in foods like bread, cereal, pasta and crackers) are often "staple" foods, yet they offer little in terms of nutrition. For that reason, I like to talk about carbohydrates first when explaining prenatal nutrition needs.

Before I jump in, let me say this: When I was first studying nutrition in college, I remember feeling like it was pointless and reductionist to try to categorize foods by macronutrients. *("Food is so much more than grams of carbs or fat or protein!" I would argue.)* But, after working clinically for many years and seeing how common it is for people to eat imbalanced meals, I realized there *is* a time and a place to think in term of macronutrients. It can help you plan out well-balanced meals without needing to rely on a strict meal plan and can help you visualize what that looks like on a plate. I'm digging into the details to ultimately make your life easier, I promise.

Carbohydrates

Carbohydrates are found in a wide variety of foods, both healthy and unhealthy. They naturally occur in almost all plant foods, but are most concentrated in grains, root vegetables, fruit, legumes, and certain dairy products (and any processed foods made with these ingredients).

Carbohydrates are like long chains of sugar all linked together. When digested, your body breaks them down into individual chain links of sugar to be absorbed. Once the sugar is absorbed, your blood sugar level goes up.

In fact, carbohydrates are the *only* macronutrient that significantly raises your blood sugar.

Most women assume this is only important to be aware of if you have a health condition that requires you to watch your blood sugar, like gestational diabetes. However, research is showing that even mild elevations in blood sugar during pregnancy can affect your baby. For example, researchers at Stanford University have shown that elevated blood sugar (far below the diagnostic threshold for gestational diabetes) is linked to a significantly higher risk of congenital heart defects.[5] In a different study, high insulin levels (your body's response to high blood sugar) in early pregnancy were linked to a significantly higher risk of neural tube defects.[6] That's frightening considering most of us are unaware of our blood sugar or insulin levels. A 2015 analysis in the *Journal of the American Medical Association* found that 49% to 52% of adults in the United States have either diabetes or prediabetes, many of whom remain undiagnosed, and the rates continue to rise at an alarming rate.[7]

For this reason, I believe it's wise for *all* women to be proactive about their blood sugar balance during pregnancy, and to understand how food is related.

Aside from its effect on blood sugar, excessive carbohydrate intake (particularly refined carbohydrates like juice, soda, and white flour products) increases your risk of gaining too much weight during pregnancy and makes it more likely that your baby will grow unhealthily large (called macrosomia).[8,9] In fact, women who eat more refined carbohydrates have an average pregnancy weight gain 18 pounds higher than women who eat mainly unprocessed carbohydrates—and their babies are significantly larger and have a higher percent body fat.[10] A separate study suggests that this effect persists into childhood, with bodyweight remaining elevated at ages 2, 3, and 4 among children of mothers who consumed a high-carb diet while pregnant.[11] It doesn't stop there, however. Researchers suggests that a child's metabolism can be *permanently* affected by a mother's diet and by excessive weight gain during pregnancy.[12]

A high carbohydrate diet during pregnancy is also linked to higher chances of developing gestational diabetes, preeclampsia (or high blood pressure during pregnancy), gall bladder disease in pregnancy (gallstones), and of your baby having metabolic problems later in life (like diabetes and heart disease).[13,14,15] Excessive maternal carbohydrate intake has been linked to impaired lung development for baby and higher likelihood of catching life-threatening respiratory viral infections in childhood.[16]

This does not mean *all* carbohydrates need to be eliminated from your diet, just that their intake should be carefully balanced with other foods to minimize spikes in blood sugar. It's also wise to choose the most nutrient-dense carbohydrates (those found in whole foods) while avoiding processed, refined carbohydrates.

With that in mind, when learning about what combinations of food work best for your body, you'll want to know which foods contain the most carbohydrates (don't worry—I'll explain how these foods fit into your diet later in this section).

Main Sources of Carbohydrates:

- Grains: whole grains, refined grains, and anything made with flour (e.g., pasta, bread, tortillas, pancakes, crackers, cereals, granola, etc.)
- Starchy vegetables: potatoes, sweet potatoes/yams, winter squash, green peas, corn
- Legumes: beans, lentils, split peas
- Fruit
- Milk and yogurt (these contain lactose or "milk sugar")

If you're nutrition savvy, you may notice that some of the above foods are also good sources of protein and wonder why I'm listing them alongside bread and pasta. Well, although legumes, milk, and yogurt all contain protein, they also contain a significant amount of carbohydrates and therefore raise your blood sugar. They are, however, a wise carbohydrate choice compared to breads, crackers, pasta, and cereals *because* of their protein content. Legumes are also rich in fiber, which slows how quickly the carbohydrates found within them are digested. Higher-fiber and higher-protein foods slow the rise in blood sugar, which is why you may hear them described as having a "low glycemic index."

When it comes to dairy products, you'll notice only milk and yogurt are included in the above list. That's because they contain a significant amount of lactose ("milk sugar") and thus count as a source of carbohydrates. Aside from sweetened dairy products, like chocolate milk or ice cream, many other dairy products are not a significant source of carbohydrates, such as cheese, butter, heavy cream, and plain Greek yogurt (which is strained to remove most of the lactose-rich whey).

The above list does not include *all* sources of carbohydrates in the diet, just the ones with the highest concentrations compared to other whole foods. A low-carbohydrate diet is not a *zero* carbohydrate diet. Carbohydrates are found in many other real foods, but in smaller proportions relative to other nutrients (like nuts, seeds, and non-starchy vegetables). However, these foods have a very low glycemic index, because much of the carbohydrate they contain is in the form of fiber and, in the case of nuts and seeds, also provide fat and protein. These foods can generally be eaten freely without worrying about your blood sugar levels.

Some processed foods are very concentrated in carbohydrates and are best limited or avoided completely (more on that in Chapter 4). In my personal experience, women achieve the best blood sugar levels and maximize their nutrient intake by getting most of their carbohydrates from non-starchy foods. Researchers confirm that women who get their carbohydrates primarily from real foods with a low glycemic index have significantly higher micronutrient intake. In contrast, women who eat more starch, even in the form of "complex carbohydrates" like whole grains, have lower vitamin and mineral intakes, likely because they displace more nutrient-dense foods.[17]

How many carbohydrates should you eat?

Welcome to one of the most hotly-debated topics in prenatal nutrition. Conventional prenatal nutrition guidelines contend that carbohydrates should make up the bulk of your diet, providing 45-65% of calories.[18] That equates to roughly 250-420 grams of carbohydrates per day for the average pregnant woman who eats 2,200-2,600 calories per day. Interestingly, higher levels of obesity have been observed among infants and children exposed to this level of carbohydrate intake (52% of calories) in utero, even among healthy weight mothers eating within or below their estimated calorie needs.[19] Conventional guidelines also warn against eating fewer than the minimum cut-off of 175 grams per day.

If you are familiar with my book, *Real Food for Gestational Diabetes,* you'll know that I'm the first dietitian to openly advocate for—and provide substantial scientific evidence that supports—a lower-carbohydrate, low-glycemic diet during pregnancy. If you've been told you "need more carbohydrates because you are pregnant" or that your "placenta and baby require carbohydrates to grow" or that "ketones are dangerous," you haven't heard the full story. In fact, there is no evidence to support a minimum carbohydrate intake of 175 grams per day. (For more on ketones, see Chapter 9. For a full analysis of the research and controversy surrounding conventional carbohydrate recommendations and ketosis in pregnancy, see Chapter 11 of my book, *Real Food for Gestational Diabetes.*)

Despite the exceedingly high levels of carbohydrates pushed on pregnant women, most traditional cultures consume far less. A 2011 study estimated carbohydrate intake in 229 modern hunter-gatherer populations worldwide and determined that average carbohydrate intake is approximately 16-22% of calories.[20] In other words, *half* or *one-quarter* of the levels suggested in conventional prenatal nutrition guidelines. It's worth mentioning that traditional intake of carbohydrates varies based on proximity to the equator, so people residing in warmer climates eat more (29-34%), while those living in colder climates, as expected, eat a lot fewer carbohydrates (3-15%).[21] Even after accounting for regional differences, conventional carbohydrate recommendations are considerably higher than what hunter-gatherers eat, including those who live in tropical climates with an abundance of fruit.

In addition, ancestral foods tend to be less "carbohydrate dense," meaning they have a lot more vitamins, minerals, fiber, fat, and protein than modern foods.[22] If we take a close look at the required nutrients for optimal fetal development, we see fairly low concentrations of these micronutrients in high-carbohydrate foods, even "healthy" whole grains. When you start to reverse engineer a well-balanced prenatal diet, you'll see there's simply not much room for high-carbohydrate foods without greatly exceeding calorie needs or missing out on important micronutrients. Conventional advice to eat 9-11 servings of bread, rice, cereal, and pasta every day is seriously flawed.

In my years of clinical experience, I've observed that most women benefit from a carbohydrate intake *significantly lower* than the standard 45-65% of calories (250-420 grams) and find my average client thrives on roughly 90-150 grams of carbohydrates per day (this is reflected in the sample meal plans in this book). When you do the math, this fits right into the ancestral carbohydrate intake observed in hunter-gatherers in the aforementioned study.

There will be some who can tolerate more, and some who need fewer, carbohydrates (something that's true for virtually every nutrient). I'll be honest, I'm not one to nitpick numbers, but I know it's important to run through them for context. With the exception of those with gestational diabetes or other complications, I simply encourage you to prioritize the most nutrient-dense, low-glycemic sources of carbohydrates, like non-starchy vegetables, Greek yogurt, nuts, seeds, legumes, and berries. There's still room for more carbohydrate-dense foods, like sweet potatoes, fruit, and whole grains, but treat them as a small side dish or snack rather than the bulk of your meals. You'll see exactly how this looks in "real world" terms in the meal plans included in Chapter 5.

For example, instead of planning meals that center around pasta or rice, aim for your protein option and vegetables to take center stage. If your hunger, activity levels, and blood sugar allow, add in more high-carbohydrate foods. If you're unsure how many carbohydrates you're eating or where they are found in your diet, you can do a short-term experiment and log your food intake in a meal-tracking app. You might be surprised at how easy it is to accidentally eat a high-carbohydrate diet when you thought you were eating low-carb. Testing your blood sugar after eating is one of the best ways to find your "sweet spot" for carbs if you really want to get specific (see the Home Glucose Monitoring section in Chapter 9).

> **NOTE:** For all you first trimester mamas coping with nausea and food aversions, know that it's both normal and OK to eat more carbohydrates during this phase. If that's you, head over to Chapter 7 for more information on why this happens and how to cope.

The Bottom Line: Both modern nutrition science and ancestral diets suggest that a moderately low-carbohydrate diet optimizes micronutrient intake and pregnancy outcomes. In other words, carbohydrate needs are lower than conventional prenatal nutrition guidelines. Opt for unprocessed, low-glycemic carbohydrates.

Protein

Proteins are quite literally the building blocks of human life. Every cell in your body contains protein and you require the amino acids in protein to build new cells. As you can imagine, there are a lot of new cells being created during pregnancy, making protein an absolute necessity to supply your growing baby (and your growing uterus and other tissues) with the raw materials to carry out the job effectively.

Just as carbohydrates are made of smaller components (sugars), proteins are made of individual amino acids. There are 20 standard amino acids, all with different functions in your body. Some protein foods contain a mix of all of them (we call these complete proteins), while others contain only a selection (incomplete proteins). Foods of animal origin or "animal foods"—such as meat, fish, eggs, and dairy—are complete proteins. Plant foods—such as beans/legumes, nuts, and seeds—are incomplete proteins.

Eating a wide selection of protein sources is a wise choice, however there's more to the story than just "eat enough complete protein." Certain amino acids become increasingly important during pregnancy due to a shift in nutrient needs. For example, requirements for an amino acid called glycine increase so much during pregnancy that many women don't receive enough. Normally this amino acid is not considered "essential," meaning that if you don't consume much, your body can produce it from other amino acids. But during pregnancy, glycine becomes "conditionally essential," meaning you must consume it directly for an optimally healthy pregnancy.[23] This amino acid is involved in the formation of fetal DNA, internal organs, connective tissue, bones, blood vessels, skin, and joints (and is absolutely required to fuel your growing uterus, placenta, and stretching skin). I cover the primary food sources of glycine, which are animal foods, in the next chapter. The low concentration of glycine in plant foods is one of several reasons that a vegetarian diet can be problematic during pregnancy, as I outline in Chapter 3.

How much protein do you need?

When it comes to the amount of protein you need, there are two sides to the story. On one hand, inadequate protein intake during pregnancy may increase a child's risk for developing heart disease, high blood pressure, and diabetes later in life.[24,25] Low protein intake is also tied to low birthweight in infants.[26,27] This is particularly true if consumption of meat and dairy protein is low during late pregnancy.[28]

On the other hand, animal studies have shown that excessive protein intake in pregnancy also carries risks, often similar to the problems caused by receiving too little.[29] However, it's worth noting that protein intake in some of these rat studies would equate to a (human) woman consuming approximately 240 grams of protein per day or more, which is double or triple the protein intake I typically observe in clinical practice.[30] Suffice to say, you have to *really* work hard to eat too much protein.

Conventional nutrition guidelines suggest an estimated average protein requirement of 0.88 g/kg, or about 60 g of protein per day for a 150 lb woman. However, this recommendation is not as evidence-based as we would hope, as it relies primarily on data from nonpregnant adults. In fact, only a single protein requirement study of pregnant women was considered when setting this recommendation.[31]

Recent advances in the way we quantify protein requirements has allowed researchers to take a more critical look into protein needs in pregnancy, and perhaps not surprising, past estimates are due for an update. According to one very well-designed study, the first ever to directly estimate protein requirements at various stages of pregnancy, current dietary guidelines considerably *underestimate* protein requirements. Actual protein needs are 39% higher in early pregnancy (defined as less than 20 weeks by this study) and 73% higher in late pregnancy (after 31 weeks) when compared to current estimated average requirements.[32] This puts optimal protein intake at or above 100 g per day for an average weight woman in her third trimester (1.22 g/kg in early pregnancy and 1.52 g/kg in late pregnancy). The take home message from this research is that your body's demand for protein 'increases steadily as pregnancy progresses."

You may be reassured to hear that average protein intake from healthy pregnant women tends to fall right in line with what was found in this study.[33] Assuming you have access to plenty of food, you'll likely eat the right amount of protein if you just listen to your body and eat mindfully. I'll share more about mindful eating later in this chapter.

Given that protein needs will vary depending on the stage of pregnancy, it can be helpful to set some general goals. In the first half of pregnancy, aim for a minimum of 80 g of protein per day. In the second half of pregnancy, aim for a minimum of 100 g of protein per day. If you're a larger person or are very physically active, you may want to aim a little higher.

Protein foods are naturally very filling and help to stabilize blood sugar levels, both preventing it from going too high or too low. This is helpful to keep in mind if you find yourself with low energy, imbalanced blood sugar, frequent hunger pangs, food cravings (especially for sugar) or headaches. These are common signs that you might not be getting enough protein. If you are facing nausea or food aversions, you may find that eating small amounts of protein every time you eat, whether it's a snack or a meal, can help. Do the best that you can given how you feel and be sure to read more about nausea and food aversions in Chapter 7, as I have several other strategies for you.

Below are some high-protein foods. For reference, one ounce of meat or one egg provides about 7 g of protein.

Main Sources of Protein:

- Beef, lamb, pork, bison, venison, etc. (ideally from pasture-raised animals)
- Chicken, turkey, duck, and other poultry (ideally from pasture-raised birds)
- Fish & seafood (ideally wild-caught)
- Sausage & bacon (ideally from pasture-raised animals)
- Organ meats (liver, heart, kidney, tongue, etc.)
- Homemade bone broth or stock (or powdered gelatin or collagen protein)
- Eggs (ideally from pasture-raised hens)
- Cheese (ideally from grass-fed or pasture-raised animals)
- Yogurt (Greek yogurt is especially high in protein and low in carbohydrates)
- Nuts: Almonds, pecans, peanuts, walnuts, hazelnuts, pumpkin seeds, sunflower seeds, cashews, etc.
- Nut butter, such as peanut butter or almond butter
- Beans, peas, lentils and other legumes (also a source of carbohydrates)

Strive to include a variety of protein-rich foods in your diet. This ensures you get a good balance of amino acids and other key vitamins and minerals. For example, fish and seafood are the richest sources of omega-3 fats, by far. Red meat is exceptionally high in iron (particularly organ meats), whereas dairy sources of protein contain almost none. Bone broth and slow-cooked cuts of meat contain high amounts of glycine, whereas muscle meats contain much less (and plant proteins contain very small amounts). Organ meats, like liver and kidney, contain up to 200 times the levels of vitamin B12 than muscle meats, like steak or chicken breast. Plant proteins contain *zero* vitamin B12.

In addition to variety, aiming for the best quality proteins is especially important during pregnancy. For example, beef from grass-fed cows contains two to four-fold more omega-3 fats, seven-fold more beta-carotene, and twice the levels of vitamin E compared to grain-fed cows.[34] Grass-fed and pasture-raised animals also tend to be exposed to fewer antibiotics, pesticides, and toxins, which ultimately lowers your exposure (and your baby's) as well.[35]

The Bottom Line: Protein needs go up during pregnancy and are considerably higher than conventional prenatal nutrition guidelines. Quality and variety are important considerations.

Fat

You've likely heard that fat should be limited in your diet during pregnancy, however this advice doesn't stand up to scientific scrutiny or, in my opinion, to common sense. You may have noticed while reading the above section that most of the protein foods listed are also naturally a source of fat. This is by design. Real food sources of protein tend to come with fat unless they are processed to remove it (such as protein powders, skinless chicken, and skim milk).

Your body's need for fat-soluble vitamins and other nutrients found in high-fat foods goes up during pregnancy. For example, requirements for choline and vitamin A, both found in high concentrations in liver and egg yolks, rise significantly in pregnancy. Were you to avoid these foods due to their fat (or cholesterol) content, your diet would be lower—perhaps even deficient—in these nutrients. Already, 94% of women don't consume enough choline and fully one-third of pregnant women don't consume enough vitamin A.[36,37] In women who do not consume liver, 70% don't meet the recommended dietary allowance (RDA) for vitamin A.[38] Choline intake directly affects your baby's brain development, with effects on memory and learning that can impact them even as adults.[39] Low choline intake is also a risk factor for neural tube defects.[40] Inadequate vitamin A intake raises the risk for birth defects, improper lung and liver development, low birth weight and other complications.[41] In other words, serious problems can occur if you don't eat *enough* fatty foods.

If you've been told to limit your intake of fat or cholesterol while pregnant, you might be surprised to hear that scientific evidence from studies conducted on *humans* is lacking. These claims arise primarily from rat studies that enrich rat chow with more fat, usually in the form of refined soybean oil, and then measure pregnancy outcomes. However, the *quality* of fat consumed is equally important to the *quantity*.[42] The majority of rat studies which find high-fat diets are detrimental to pregnancy outcomes are really saying that diets high in *omega-6 fats* are detrimental to pregnancy outcomes (we'll talk more about omega-6 fats below). I know of only one study on pregnant rats that took the *quality* of fat into consideration. Typically, rat studies using soybean oil-enriched diets find adverse effects, including excessive weight gain, high blood sugar levels, and elevated markers of inflammation. In this study, researchers compared rats fed a high-fat diet using a combination of coconut oil, walnut oil, and fish oil to the typical soybean oil-based diet. The mice fed the healthy combination of oils gained significantly less weight and had a lower percent body fat compared to those fed soybean oil, despite eating the same number of calories.[43] They also tended to have better blood sugar and insulin levels as well as healthier liver function. In other words, *quality counts*. A diet high in soybean oil (laden with inflammatory omega-6 fats) is an entirely different story than one with a combination of fats that provides a balance of saturated, monounsaturated, and omega-3 fats and with low levels of omega-6 fats. The next time someone tells you that "fat is bad for pregnant moms," know that there's a lot more to the story.

Consider that your baby's brain, which is approximately 60% fat, is being formed *from scratch* during pregnancy.[44] There are high demands for cholesterol, choline, omega-3 fats, and a variety of fat-soluble nutrients at this time. As one researcher puts it, "Because the brain is predominantly made of fat, almost all of its structures and functions have a crucial dependency upon essential fatty acids, which we get directly from our food."[45] Cholesterol itself plays a key role in the development of your baby, is required for hormone synthesis (in you and baby), and is a part of every cell in your (and your baby's) body.[46] We know that essential fatty acid levels in baby mirror the levels in mom, which should give even more incentive to eat wisely.[47]

One type of omega-3 fat, called DHA, is especially important at this time, as it plays a fundamental role in brain and vision development. As we'll explore in later sections, DHA is found primarily in fatty fish and seafood, grass-fed meat, and pasture-raised eggs. On the other hand, another type of fat, called omega-6, is linked to abnormal fetal brain development and anxiety in later life when mothers consume too much during pregnancy.[48] Studies show that consuming too many oils rich in omega-6 (like corn, soy, cottonseed, and safflower oil) inhibits the synthesis of DHA.[49] This may explain why infants of women with a high omega-6 to omega-3 ratio in their diets are twice as likely to experience developmental delays.[50] For additional information on the harmful effects of vegetable oils, as well as man-made trans fats, see Chapter 4.

Unfortunately, most of us consume far too much omega-6 fat now that vegetable oils (perhaps more accurately called "processed seed oils"), have taken the place of traditional fats in our diets. Humans once consumed a diet with a ratio of omega-6 to omega-3 of close to 1:1; now it's as high as 30:1.[51] One of the best ways to shift the balance is to avoid cooking with vegetable oils or using products made with them, like commercial salad dressing and fried foods. If you scroll through vintage cook books, you'll see butter, heavy cream, lard (pork fat), and tallow (beef fat) used quite frequently. Drippings and fat that rendered from cooked meat was saved for later use, or turned into rich gravies. In contrast, most modern recipes specifically tell you to drain the pan of any fat and replace it with so-called "healthier" vegetable oil before you proceed with cooking the rest of the dish. This advice is a nutritional—and culinary—travesty.

It probably goes counter to everything you've been told about what constitutes a "healthy fat," but lard and butter are far better choices than vegetable oil. Because I received my formal training in nutrition from a conventional dietetics program, it took me a long time to accept that animal fats might actually be healthy. After analyzing a great deal of research (presented here and in Chapter 3), I recognized that many of the key nutrients for a successful pregnancy were found in high-fat animal foods. Suddenly, it all clicked. These foods contain fat for a reason, and discarding the fat goes counter to the dietary practices of virtually all traditional cultures.[52] Instead of blindly following advice to "eat lean meats and low-fat dairy," we should be doing the opposite: ensuring that the food we eat comes with the fat it is naturally meant to contain. That means eating chicken with the skin, full-fat dairy, eggs with the yolks, and not trimming the fat off of that juicy grass-fed steak.

The key is to prioritize high-quality animal foods whenever your budget allows, since the types of fats found in meat, eggs, and dairy reflect what those animals have eaten themselves. For example, animals that have been grass-fed (instead of grain-fed) have more omega-3 and less omega-6 in their meat.[53] Eggs from pasture-raised hens are also more nutritious compared to conventionally-raised hens, as I detail in the next chapter. Luckily, the flavor of grass-fed and pasture-raised animal foods is so much better that your taste buds will make the transition a no-brainer.

Another reason to embrace fat is the research on dairy products and fertility. I always find it interesting to read through conventional prenatal nutrition policies and see *low-fat* dairy recommended. There's strong evidence showing that eating high-fat dairy improves fertility—while eating low-fat dairy contributes to infertility—so I struggle to understand why that would suddenly shift when a woman gets pregnant.[54] The nutrients that help you *get* pregnant help you *stay* pregnant. In fact, among women who have become

Real Food for Pregnancy

pregnant through IVF, the chances of having a live birth are highest among women who consume the most dairy products and, specifically, the most dairy fat.[55]

Many women find themselves especially drawn to higher fat foods in the third trimester. This makes sense given that fat is naturally energy-dense and filling. When your belly is being compressed by your baby and you have less room for food at mealtimes, it's natural to want to "fill up on less." Plus, when it comes to maintaining energy and blood sugar levels, fat is king. Fat does not raise your blood sugar or insulin levels and instead supplies a consistent, slow burning stream of energy. Last, but not least, fat tastes good. If your instincts tell you to consume more fat, I believe there's a good reason for it.

Given that fat almost always accompanies protein in real food, I often don't bother to separate them out. But, for clarity, I've singled out some healthy high-fat foods below.

Main Sources of Fat:

- Animal fat: lard (pork fat), tallow (beef fat), duck fat, chicken skin, etc. (from pasture-raised/grass-fed animals, of course)
- Dairy fat: butter, ghee (clarified butter), heavy cream, sour cream, cream cheese, etc. (from pasture-raised/grass-fed animals)
- Plant fat: olives, coconuts, avocados, nuts, seeds, and any unprocessed oils derived from these foods. (Choose "extra virgin" oils. Plant oils are easily damaged with heat, so avoid cooking at high temperatures, with the exception of coconut or palm oils, which are naturally high in heat-stable saturated fat. Also, be sure to purchase oils packaged in dark glass bottles, *not clear plastic,* since these delicate fats can even be damaged by exposure to light.)
  - Avoid processed vegetables oils/seed oils that are high in omega-6 fats such as: corn oil, soybean oil, peanut oil, canola oil, safflower oil, and cottonseed oil. Also, avoid any oils that have been "partially hydrogenated," as these are a source of man-made trans fats. (See Chapter 4 for a full explanation.)

It can be scary to embrace eating fat if you've been told to avoid it for your whole life. It took me *three full years* of reading through the research to get the confidence to use butter again and to liberally cook with fat. No matter how many good studies have cleared saturated fat of its unfounded "artery clogging" nickname (and there are many), it can still take some time to get comfortable eating them.[56,57,58,59]

Ideally, aim to include a source of fat at each meal and snack. This is especially important when eating vegetables, since many of the nutrients and antioxidants found in vegetables are better absorbed by your body when eaten with fat.[60] Don't be shy about putting butter on your green beans or using full-fat salad dressing.

You've probably noticed that I haven't put a number on the amount of fat to eat in a day. That's intentional. Haven't we all spent enough of our lives obsessing over fat? The ultimate gram amount or percentage of fat that's right for you will depend on your intake of carbohydrates and protein. Essentially, as long as you meet your minimum protein requirements and do not over-consume carbohydrates, you can trust your body to eat enough fat. The section on mindful eating later in this chapter will be invaluable to you.

The Bottom Line: Fats from unprocessed real foods, including meat and dairy, are an important source of nutrients during pregnancy. The only fats that should be limited are those high in omega-6 fats, such as vegetable oils, and man-made trans fats.

Vegetables

Finally, it's worth giving a little shout out to vegetables. These nutritional powerhouses are not particularly high in protein and fat, however they aren't nearly carb-heavy enough for me to categorize them with the carbohydrates. They are worthy of their own category altogether.

Aside from a select few high-carbohydrate vegetables (like potatoes), most vegetables have little effect on your blood sugar due to their high fiber content (fiber does not get converted into sugar in large quantities). As a whole, these are referred to as non-starchy vegetables and they should make up the bulk of your vegetable intake.

Fiber from vegetables is especially helpful during pregnancy. It helps slow down how quickly your body breaks down other carbohydrates and converts them into sugar, it acts as fuel to your intestinal bacteria (probiotics), and it helps prevent constipation.

Aim to include vegetables with each meal with the goal of filling half of your plate with them. I suggest eating non-starchy vegetables to satiety (that feeling of having enough to be satisfied, but not overstuffed), without worrying about an exact portion size. Below is a select list of non-starchy vegetables.

As mentioned in the previous section, many nutrients and antioxidants found in vegetables are better absorbed when eaten with some fat, so you should feel good, *not* guilty, about making them taste good.

Also, aim for as much variety as you can, not only to maximize your nutrient intake, but because your growing baby's preferences for healthy foods are partly formed in utero.[61] Yes, your baby can "taste" what you're eating via your amniotic fluid. This early exposure to healthy foods helps set the stage for a non-picky eater once your child transitions to solid food.

Non-Starchy Vegetables:

- Artichoke
- Asparagus
- Bell pepper
- Broccoli
- Brussels sprouts
- Cabbage
- Cactus (nopal)
- Cauliflower
- Celery
- Chayote squash
- Cucumber
- Eggplant
- Garlic
- Greens: beet, collard, dandelion, mustard, spinach, kale, chard, turnip greens, spinach, watercress, bok choy, arugula, etc.
- Tomatillo
- Tomato
- Green beans
- Kohlrabi
- Leek
- Lettuce: endive, escarole, iceberg, romaine, "baby" greens, etc.
- Mushroom
- Okra
- Onion (all types)
- Radish
- Rutabaga
- Summer squash
- Zucchini
- Turnip
- Beet*
- Carrot*
- Jicama*

- Parsnip*
- Snap peas, snow peas*
- Spaghetti squash*

*Moderately-starchy vegetables: These vegetables have up to 15g net carbs per cup. Unless you struggle with high blood sugar *after* you've reduced your intake of added sugars and refined carbohydrates, there's no need to limit your intake of these vegetables.

The Bottom Line: Vegetables are an important source of vitamins, minerals, fiber, and antioxidants. Eat them liberally.

Fluids

When you're pregnant, your fluid needs go up. Your baby is literally swimming in amniotic fluid inside your uterus and your blood volume increases significantly starting in the first trimester. Water is essential for maintaining good circulation, which brings nutrients to your baby and removes waste products.

At a cellular level, water provides shape and structure to every cell in your body, helps regulate body temperature, aids in the digestion and absorption of nutrients, helps transport oxygen to your cells, and is a major component of mucus and other lubricating fluids.[62] Staying hydrated can help prevent constipation, hemorrhoids, muscle cramps, headaches, bladder infections, and many other discomforts.[63]

The Institute of Medicine recommends pregnant women drink about 100 oz of fluids per day. Keep in mind that fluids from all sources count, meaning you can count your cup of tea and bowl of soup toward your total fluids for the day. A good way to gauge whether you are getting enough fluids is to watch the color of your urine. It should be clear or a very pale yellow when you're well hydrated. A list of recommended beverages is included in Chapter 5.

The Bottom Line: Your body requires more fluids while pregnant; aim for 100 oz per day.

Salt

With an increase in fluid levels in your body comes the need for more electrolytes. Electrolytes are necessary for keeping your energy levels up (they are required to keep your heart beating normally, after all), and may help prevent common annoyances like headaches and leg cramps. This means that getting enough minerals in your diet, *including salt*, is very important. The best type of salt to consume is unrefined sea salt, as this contains not only sodium, but trace minerals as well. Other forms of salt, such as kosher salt and table salt, have been heat-treated and purified, which removes trace minerals.

Although salt often gets a bad rap, it is vital to the normal function of your body, especially during pregnancy. As one researcher notes, "In pregnancy, dietary salt intake seems to facilitate the numerous physiological changes that must occur to support the growth and development of the placenta and fetus."[64] The sodium and chloride it contains are key for electrolyte balance (to keep your cells talking to one another), helping to maintain the correct plasma volume in your bloodstream (to regulate fluid levels), and facilitating neural signaling (so you can think straight and move your muscles on command). Salt also supports normal stomach acid levels by supplying chloride (stomach acid is hydro*chloric* acid). Adequate stomach acid is necessary for the absorption of minerals and vitamin B12, protein digestion, and killing off pathogenic bacteria before food leaves your stomach. In addition, salt plays an important role in food preservation, preventing unfriendly organisms from growing in food that could make you sick.[65]

It's no coincidence that cravings for salty pickles and olives are so common in pregnancy, but you've probably been told to avoid salt during pregnancy to keep your blood pressure from going up. However, this is not evidence-based advice. For most people, salt does *not* have an impact on blood pressure. In fact, according to researchers from the University of Virginia School of Medicine, only about 25% of the population is salt-sensitive (meaning only a quarter of us will see our blood pressure go up from eating salt). Plus, 15% of the population will have *elevated* blood pressure on a *low-salt* diet.[66] A low-salt diet has also *not* been proven to help prevent or control preeclampsia (high blood pressure that occurs in pregnancy), despite continual assertions to the contrary.[67] For more on managing high blood pressure and preeclampsia, see Chapter 7.

Cutting back severely on salt can have serious consequences. Aside from the already mentioned functions, salt is important to your baby's development. As one researcher explains, "Salt is one of the integral components for normal growth of fetuses. Salt restriction during pregnancy is connected to intrauterine growth restriction or death, low birth weight, organ underdevelopment and dysfunction in adulthood probably through gene-mediated mechanisms."[68] It is also "well reported that during critical developmental periods, salt restriction might affect fetal hormonal, vascular, and renal systems to regulate fluid homeostasis in the fetus."[69] In addition, research has shown that low salt intake can worsen blood sugar and insulin resistance, both of which are undesirable during pregnancy.[70] **To put it simply, salt is your friend—not your enemy—when you're pregnant.**

Does this mean you get a free pass to eat lots of salty processed food? Of course not, though the actual *salt* in the processed food isn't my concern—it's all the other stuff in it that's problematic. The take-home message is that consuming enough salt in the context of a *real food* diet is important. Keep the (sea) salt shaker on the table, salt your food as you cook, and enjoy pickles and sauerkraut. Let your taste buds guide your salt intake. Salt naturally brings out the flavors in many foods, especially vegetables. If you've never been a fan of bitter vegetables, like kale or arugula, salt may be the missing ingredient.

If you happen to be salt-sensitive, meaning your blood pressure goes up when you eat salt, you may benefit from a *slightly* lower salt diet. However, keep in mind that one of the key drivers of salt sensitivity is over-consumption of a type of sugar called fructose.[71] Before you drastically reduce your salt intake, it would be wise to cut out sugary beverages and other sources of fructose (especially high-fructose corn syrup). Furthermore, high blood pressure and high blood *sugar* tend to go hand in hand, hence lower-carbohydrate diets tend to reduce the severity of high blood pressure.[72] In other words, ditching the processed carbohydrates and added sugars may allow you the freedom to have a little more salt in your diet.

The Bottom Line: Salt is an essential nutrient and should not be limited during pregnancy. Use sea salt to taste.

How to Combine Foods

A lot of pregnant women struggle with cravings and intense hunger (that need to eat *immediately*). Both of these can be a side-effect of having an imbalanced intake of macronutrients at meals and snacks. Fortunately, now that we've covered the basics about diet composition, planning well-balanced meals and snacks will be easier.

Let's start with a simple example: an apple.

If you eat that apple by itself, your blood sugar will go up and it will do so fairly rapidly because apples are high in carbohydrates and have very little fat or protein.

Now, take that same apple, but this time eat it with a small handful of almonds. Your blood sugar will still go up, because there are carbohydrates in the apple, *but* your blood sugar might not go up *as high* or go up *as quickly* because the fat and protein in the almonds will slow down how fast those carbohydrates are digested into sugar and absorbed.

I like to think of eating the apple by itself as eating "naked carbohydrates." When you "dress it up" by matching it with another food that contains fat and protein, your body responds completely differently (in a good way). When your blood sugar doesn't spike, it also doesn't crash. That means you stay full for longer and have fewer sugar cravings.

This same approach works when planning meals as well.

The Plate Method

The Plate Method is a great way to visually plan out your meals without strictly measuring portions. There are many versions of the Plate Method out there, but this is my preferred breakdown. Aim for half of your plate to be non-starchy vegetables, one quarter of your plate to be proteins and fats, and the remaining one quarter to be carbohydrates. Take a close look at the carbohydrate section of the plate; it includes grains, beans/legumes, starchy vegetables, milk/yogurt, and fruit.

Meal breakdown (general guide):

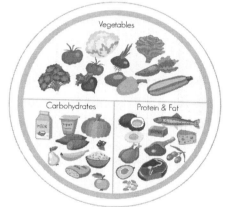

- 2 cups+ vegetables (with some fat, like butter or olive oil)
- 3-4 oz of protein (with naturally-occurring fat, like the skin on chicken)
- ½ to 1 cup of starchy or carbohydrate-rich whole foods*

* Some women thrive on a lower-carbohydrate diet and do better with smaller portions of carbohydrates at meals (or none at all), while others can handle larger portions. See Chapter 5 for more specific advice on fine tuning your diet.

Unlike most dietitians, I shy away from providing strict portion measurements unless there's a clear reason. For example, if you're gaining weight more rapidly than expected, if your blood sugar is high, or if you're concerned you are undereating, you might want to track your meals for a week or two—and potentially work with your healthcare provider or a real food dietitian/nutritionist—to see where to make adjustments.

Mindful Eating

Some women feel nervous about eating this way without having strict guidance on portions or calories. One of the most effective and natural ways to ensure you're getting the right amount of food for your body is to apply mindful eating techniques. Mindful eating means listening to the signals your body sends you about food and honoring what it has to say. It means eating when you're hungry and stopping when your body has had enough.

Many times we eat on autopilot, since we've become disconnected from our body's inner cues or perhaps because we're responding only to external cues. Sometimes that means we eat everything on our plate regardless of how full we feel (the "clean your plate" trap). Or we eat simply because everyone around us is eating, even when our body is not hungry for more food. On the other hand, you might feel tempted to restrict your food due to fears of getting "huge" with this pregnancy and begin to avoid eating even when you're hungry. None of the above is healthy. **When you ignore your hunger cues, you tend to ignore your fullness cues as well.** So mindlessly overeating or consciously undereating are equally unhealthy and unsustainable.

Luckily, our bodies are incredible teachers and they are always communicating with us. It takes practice to tune into these cues; but I promise, over time, you'll learn to trust your body. To begin eating more mindfully, try the following Hunger Awareness Exercise.

Hunger Awareness Exercise

Before each meal or snack, calmly check in with how your body is feeling. Do you have any sensations of hunger? Is there a gnawing feeling in your stomach? If so, is it mild or intense? Are you hungry for a small amount of food or do you want a whole meal? How are your energy levels? What kinds of foods are you craving: sweet, salty, or something else? (This only needs to take 15-30 seconds.)

In the middle of your meal or snack, check in again. Are you starting to feel full? What sensations is your body sending you? Are the flavors and textures of this food satisfying or would you prefer to stop and eat something else? How quickly are you eating: slow, moderate, or fast? Ask these questions without judgement. No answer is right or wrong.

Towards the end of your meal or snack, do a final check in. What would your body say if it could talk? Would it ask for more? Would it tell you to stop eating? Would it tell you that there's absolutely, positively no more room

Real Food for Pregnancy

for food? How did your body respond to the speed at which you were eating? Again, ask these questions without judgement. No answer is right or wrong.

You might start to notice patterns in the way you eat. Maybe you rush through meals, or you feel driven to clean your plate even when you're full. Maybe you have anxiety while you eat because you're nervous that your stomach might be upset afterwards. There can be any number of feelings that come up.

Learn to listen to your body without judgement and get curious about how small tweaks can affect how you feel when you eat. Treat it as one big (ongoing) experiment.

Practicing mindful eating can help you learn to eat until you no longer feel hungry and also avoid feeling uncomfortably full. That's the sweet spot to aim for each time you eat. You won't always accomplish this, but if you can do this more often than not, you're well on your way.

Some people feel that mindful eating doesn't provide enough structure or "rules" around food, however mindful eating doesn't mean throwing nutritional common sense to the curb. Part of listening to your body is recognizing when your food choices don't leave you feeling well and making a *mindful* choice to opt for a more nutritionally balanced option the next time you eat. Your body deserves nourishing foods *and* you deserve to enjoy your food. There is a place for these two things to coexist. In fact, research has shown that women who practice mindful eating during pregnancy tend to eat a more nutritious diet overall and consume less junk food.[73] Don't underestimate the power of listening to your body, as it can affect both the quantity *and quality* of the food you eat.

Meal Timing & Spacing

When you're pregnant, you'll probably notice some changes in your appetite from early pregnancy all the way until the day you deliver. From food aversions and nausea that often hit in the first trimester, to the struggle of heartburn or early fullness that hits towards the end, you may feel best when you eat smaller meals and a few snacks per day, even if you were not a "snacker" before pregnancy.

There are no set-in-stone rules, so if you feel best eating three "square" meals and no snacks, more power to you. However, for most women, eating small meals and snacks has three benefits:

1. You never get too hungry (this stabilizes your blood sugar and energy levels)
2. You don't have to eat huge portions at meals
3. Your baby gets a consistent supply of nutrients throughout the day

Smaller meals are also helpful if you're managing common pregnancy complaints like nausea or vomiting, heartburn, reflux, or feeling full quickly.

Tips for Getting Started

If this is all new and overwhelming, don't worry. What seems challenging today will become second nature a few weeks from now.

Start by looking at your meals and applying the Plate Method:

> Do you have a good balance of macronutrients at your meals?
> Are you consuming vegetables with most of your meals (with some fat)?
> Are you pairing your carbohydrates with enough protein?
> Are you eating enough healthy fats, including animal fats?

Make it a priority to include more real food in your diet and minimize your intake of processed and sugary foods.

Next, become mindful of your hunger and fullness cues. Notice how your body feels before, during, after, and between meals. This is your chance to get really curious about how food affects your body and to play around with what works and what doesn't work *for you*. This is a process of self-discovery. Think of it like an experiment rather than a final exam.

You'll be learning as you go, taking notes, and adjusting day to day. When you learn what *doesn't* work for you, you learn what *does*. Pregnancy is a time where your body is constantly in flux, so be open to your hunger levels, portions, and eating times shifting from week to week.

In the next chapter, we'll take a closer look at which foods are especially helpful at building a healthy baby.

Chapter 3:

Foods That Build a Healthy Baby

"Pregnancy tends to markedly widen the nutritional gap. The decrease in the nutritional adequacy of observed diets of women of childbearing age cannot be solved by a simple increase in energy intake, as recommended in some countries… but to qualitative changes in the diet."
- Dr. Clélia Bianchi, Université Paris-Saclay

M any women intuitively feel that they should be eating certain foods to nourish their growing baby. Indeed, traditional cultures from around the globe had unique foods that were prized before, during, and after pregnancy. In our modern culture, we've lost the connection with these traditions and focus instead on individual nutrients. But focusing on one little piece rather than the whole food from which it is sourced ignores many other nutrients, known and unknown, something that's been referred to as "nutritionism."

So, in this chapter, we will focus primarily on the *food*. The foods I review here have a long history of use in many cultures, but modern nutrition science is just beginning to reveal *why* these foods serve such an important role in our health. I will point out which nutrients are abundant in these foods, how they support your overall health and the development of your baby, and the consequences of deficiency. I'll also spend some time looking at the challenges of meeting prenatal nutritional needs if your diet does not include these foods (such as a strict vegetarian diet).

Ideally, you'll be able to use this information to consciously and intelligently modify your meals to meet all of your nutrient needs *and* satisfy your taste buds. After all, enjoying what you're eating is part of nourishing yourself and your baby.

Eggs

Eggs are an incredible superfood, especially during pregnancy. Not only are they a convenient source of protein, but they are excellent sources of many vitamins and minerals commonly lacking in a prenatal diet.

To start, egg yolks are rich in choline. Choline is a relative of the B-vitamins that didn't gain much attention until the last two decades. In fact, the first recommended intakes for choline were issued in 1998. It turns out that choline has some of the same beneficial effects on a developing baby as folate, including fostering normal brain development and preventing neural tube defects.[1] Choline can also permanently change, in a *good* way, the genetic expression of your growing baby.[2]

According to one researcher, "When rat pups receive choline supplements (*in utero* or during the second week of life), their brain function is changed, resulting in lifelong memory enhancement. This change in memory function appears to be due to changes in the development of the memory center (hippocampus) in the brain. These changes are so important that investigators can pick out the groups of animals whose mothers had extra choline even when these animals are elderly. Thus, memory function in the aged is, in part, determined by what mother ate."[3]

Unfortunately, most women only consume a fraction of the choline they need, partly because food sources are limited or perhaps because they've been scared away from eating egg yolks. In fact, it's estimated that fully 94% of women do not meet the recommended intake of 450 mg of choline per day.[4]

Egg yolks and liver have, by far, the highest concentrations of choline compared to any other foods. Just two eggs (with the yolks!) meets about half of a pregnant woman's daily choline needs. That's why eggs are frequently included in the sample meals in this book.

Eggs are one of the few non-seafood sources of DHA, a key omega-3 fat that is linked to higher IQs in infants.[5] Choline works synergistically with the omega-3 fat, DHA, enhancing how much DHA is incorporated into cells.[6] In rat studies, combined supplementation of choline alongside DHA improves brain development more than supplementing with either one in isolation.[7] It's no accident that eggs are rich in both nutrients. Egg yolks also boast high amounts of folate, B-vitamins, antioxidants (including lutein and zeaxanthin, which are crucial to eye and vision development), and trace minerals (notably, iodine and selenium).

Real Food for Pregnancy

When it comes to eggs, quality counts. Eggs from chickens raised on pasture (meaning outdoors, in grass, pecking at insects and enjoying the sunlight) are particularly healthy and more nutrient-dense than conventionally-produced eggs.

Nutrient-density of eggs from pasture-raised chickens compared to commercially-raised hens:[8]

- Vitamin A content is 30% higher, which is clearly visible from the rich, orange color of the yolks. The more fresh greens, grasses, and bugs a chicken eats, the higher the vitamin A levels.
- Vitamin E content is *double* that from commercially-raised hens.
- Omega-3 content is 2.5x higher than eggs from commercially-raised hens.
- Omega-6 fats are found in lower levels, which is favorable, since these fats tend to cause inflammation. Eggs from pastured chickens have less than half the ratio of omega-6 to omega-3 fatty acids compared to commercially-raised hens.
- Vitamin D content is 3-6x higher, due to regular sun exposure.

I should mention that all of the nutrients discussed above are found in the egg yolk, so do eat the *whole* egg, otherwise you miss out on many of the benefits. There's a reason an egg comes with a yolk, after all.

When you analyze macronutrients, eggs contain only fat and protein (no carbohydrates), so they don't raise your blood sugar. This makes eggs a perfect breakfast option if you often have food cravings, feel very hungry in the morning, struggle with low energy, or find yourself gaining weight faster than you expected.

Researchers investigating people's responses to different types of breakfast have found that, compared to a bagel, those who eat eggs naturally eat less throughout the day, have fewer cravings, and experience fewer spikes in blood sugar and insulin.[9] Eggs are full of nutrients, they keep you satisfied, and they stabilize your energy levels. They are a win-win-win.

If you're nervous to eat eggs because you are worried about cholesterol, know that recent research has disproven the theory that dietary cholesterol increases the risk of heart disease.[10,11,12,13] And often, the opposite is true. It turns out that excessive dietary carbohydrates are more closely linked to high blood lipids than dietary cholesterol (or saturated fat).[14] Besides, our brains *need* cholesterol. In fact, 25% of the cholesterol in our bodies is found in the brain where it plays a crucial role in normal neural function. If you want to provide the raw materials to help your baby develop a healthy brain, you should absolutely be consuming cholesterol.

Some women have been told to avoid eggs (especially if the yolks remain runny after cooking) because they can cause food poisoning. Food safety concerns over eggs have been overstated again and again, especially to pregnant women. According to a 2012 analysis from the Centers for Disease Control and Prevention, food poisoning due to eggs accounts for only 2% of all food poisoning reports nationwide.[15] It turns out that you're 8x more likely to get food poisoning from fresh produce than from eggs.[16] Yet, you never hear health officials warning pregnant moms to avoid apples and spinach. Sourcing your eggs from pasture-raised, organic chickens is one of the best ways to reduce the risk of food poisoning, since organic farms have a 7-fold lower rate of *Salmonella* infection compared to commercial producers.[17] This is likely due to the chickens being raised outside of a confined barn and having a more varied diet, both of which protect against the spread of disease. Even eggs from conventional farms are very unlikely to contain *Salmonella*, with estimates ranging from 1 in 12,000 to 1 in 30,000.[18] So, put the worries about cholesterol and *Salmonella* to rest and know that the nutritional benefits of eating eggs—*with the yolks*—are worth making them a regular part of your diet.

From a food safety *and* nutritional perspective, it's ideal to consume eggs from pasture-raised chickens. Check with local farmers or at health food stores. If you cannot find or afford pasture-raised, know that eggs from all sources are *still* a very good source of nutrition and are absolutely worth including in your diet.

One of the questions I commonly get is from people who are allergic to eggs: "What can I do if I can't eat eggs?" If you cannot consume eggs due to a food allergy, sensitivity, or other factors, most of the nutrients in eggs can be found in sufficient quantities in other foods in an omnivorous diet (one that includes both animals and plants). The most likely exception is choline. Egg-eaters consume roughly double the amount of choline compared to those who do not eat eggs.[19] If eggs are off the menu, I encourage you to consider a choline supplement and/or to consume liver on a more regular basis. Choline is discussed in more detail in the section on vegetarian diets later in this chapter.

Liver

Many people have described liver as nature's multivitamin, a well-deserved nickname, if you ask me. Aside from eggs, liver is the only other major dietary source of choline. It also happens to be rich in almost every other vitamin and mineral that modern nutrition science has identified so far.

Liver is the single richest source of iron, a mineral that protects against maternal anemia and numerous other health problems. The iron found in liver (and animal foods, in general), called heme iron, is very well absorbed and does not carry the annoying side effect of constipation common to iron supplements. Low iron status during pregnancy is a risk factor for preeclampsia, hypothyroidism, and preterm birth. It also directly affects the iron status of your baby—low levels are associated with impaired brain development and stunted growth.[20] In one study, infants of moms who were iron-deficient during pregnancy showed delayed cognitive development when examined at 10 weeks and 9 months of age.[21]

Liver is also one of the richest food sources of folate and vitamin B12, both key to maintaining healthy red blood cells and fostering healthy brain development in your baby. Folate is best known for its role in preventing birth defects. Most women seek this vitamin from supplements (in the synthetic form known as folic acid), but few know that the folate obtained from food is far superior. Due to a common genetic variation in an enzyme called MTHFR, up to 60% of the population is unable (or less able) to use the synthetic folic acid that's commonly found in supplements or added to fortified foods.[22] Eating liver ensures you obtain the form of folate that your body can fully utilize, no matter your genetics. (You can ask your healthcare provider about genetic testing to determine your MTHFR status; see Chapter 9. If you have the MTHFR mutation, see Chapter 6 for specific instructions on choosing a prenatal vitamin.)

Ounce per ounce, liver contains up to 200x more vitamin B12 than muscle meat does, such as chicken breast or steak. The importance of vitamin B12 is commonly overlooked during pregnancy; however, inadequate maternal vitamin B12 increases the risk of neural tube defects and miscarriage.[23] An in-depth analysis of over 11,000 pregnant women from 11 countries strongly tied vitamin B12 deficiency to a higher risk of preterm delivery.[24] Although a diet that doesn't contain liver can technically meet the recommended dietary allowance (RDA) for vitamin B12, researchers have shown that the current RDA is inadequate to maintain optimal B12 levels in the body. In fact, they now estimate that the true need for B12 is *triple* the current RDA.[25] Suffice to say, it's wise to err on the higher end of B12 intake.

Liver is also incredibly rich in fat-soluble vitamins, including vitamins A, D, E, and K; all nutrients that are difficult to obtain otherwise. Many of you reading this may have been specifically warned to *not* consume liver during pregnancy, precisely because it is rich in vitamin A. This has sparked controversy over the years, mostly because old studies linked high-dose *synthetic* supplemental vitamin A to birth defects. However, we now know that naturally occurring vitamin A does *not* exert this toxicity, particularly when consumed with adequate vitamin D and vitamin K2, nutrients that are also found in abundance in liver.[26] This illustrates perfectly why obtaining nutrients from food is far safer than getting them from supplements.

As one researcher points out, "Liver and supplements are *not* of equivalent teratogenic potential [risk of causing birth defects]. Advice to pregnant women on the consumption of liver based on the reported teratogenicity of vitamin A supplements should be reconsidered."[27]

Ongoing concerns over vitamin A toxicity from liver consumption are perplexing, considering that deficiency is fairly common in pregnant women. One study found that one-third of pregnant women were borderline deficient, despite having access to plenty of vitamin A-rich foods.[28] This essential nutrient is widely recognized for its role in normal growth and development during pregnancy, including the developing lungs, kidneys, heart, eyes, and other organs. Even the National Institutes of Health states, "pregnant women need extra vitamin A for fetal growth and tissue maintenance and for supporting their own metabolism."[29] Certainly, an excessive amount of any nutrient is problematic, and since vitamin A is fat-soluble, it does raise the risk of toxicity. However, given what we know about deficiency and the safety of food-sourced vitamin A, this does not defend the recommendation to avoid liver, our most valuable food source of the vitamin.

In fact, avoidance of liver is a known risk factor for inadequate vitamin A intake. In a Dutch study of over 1,700 women, those who ate liver almost always consumed adequate vitamin A, while an astonishing 70% of women who avoided liver failed to meet the RDA.[30] This study is important, because it highlights a huge oversight in conventional prenatal nutrition policy. It's generally assumed that vitamin A deficiency is something that is only common in developing countries with limited access to food, but this study is from one of the wealthiest countries in the world. In this case, it's not a matter of access to (nor the affordability of) nutritious foods, it's that women are being actively steered away from them.

This quote perfectly illustrates the disconnect between research and nutrition policy (and explains the confusion that pregnant women face when making food choices): "Pregnant women or those considering becoming pregnant are generally advised to avoid the intake of vitamin-A rich liver and liver foods, based upon unsupported scientific findings."[31]

Nonetheless, the "safer" alternative to consuming liver—say conventional nutrition authorities—is to just eat *plant* sources of vitamin A. Unfortunately, this is not great advice, since plant sources of vitamin A are not equivalent to animal sources. Plant sources, such as sweet potatoes, carrots, and kale contain carotenoids (provitamin A) as opposed to true, preformed vitamin A (retinol). Although our bodies can *theoretically* convert provitamin A into true vitamin A (retinol), the conversion rate is highly variable person to person, and is partly influenced by genetics.[32] The most commonly discussed carotenoid, beta carotene, is up to 28 times less potent than retinol.[33] And paradoxically, the more beta-carotene you eat, the *less* you convert to vitamin A.[34] That means you indeed need *some* dietary sources of preformed vitamin A—from liver or other animal foods—to ensure you get enough for yourself and your growing baby. Loading up on carrots won't cut it.

To meet your vitamin A needs, consuming just a few ounces of liver once or twice a week is sufficient along with the carotenes from vegetables, and the other dietary sources of vitamin A (grass-fed butter, animal fats from pasture-raised animals, egg yolks, etc.). In one sheep farming community in South Africa, where almost all residents consume liver an average of 2.3 times per month, the rates of vitamin A deficiency are extremely low—only 6% of children and *none* of the adults tested deficient. In contrast, the national rate of vitamin A deficiency in the rest of South Africa, where liver consumption is less frequent, is nearly 64%.[35] Overall, the benefits far outweigh the risks when it comes to eating liver. (The one exception is polar bear liver, which is unique in that it *does* have excessive amounts of vitamin A for most people.[36] Unless you plan on an Arctic expedition, this is probably a moot point.)

If the idea of eating liver is new, foreign, or downright repulsive, you're not alone. Organ meats were once a staple in our diets, but most of us haven't grown up eating them. If you're not used to eating liver or dislike the taste, it can easily be "hidden" in recipes that use ground meat. Go to the Recipe Appendix to see how I use liver in Beanless Beef Chili, Grass-fed Beef Meatloaf, Low-Carb Shepherd's Pie, Twice Baked Spaghetti Squash with Meatballs, and Grass-fed Beef Liver Pate. In addition, you might try chicken liver, as it has a more mild taste compared to beef liver.

When buying liver, remember that source matters. This organ is designed to filter toxins and store nutrients, so ideally, seek liver from healthy, pasture-raised animals. Unlike a fancy steak, liver is a very inexpensive cut of meat, so go out of your way to buy the best quality you can find. If you're especially averse to the taste, you can purchase desiccated liver from grass-fed cows in capsule form and take it as a supplement.

Meat on the Bone, Slow-Cooked Meat, and Bone Broth

Whether you're talking beef, pork, poultry, or wild game, meat is an incredibly important source of nutrition when pregnant. It contains complete protein, minerals, B-vitamins, fat-soluble vitamins, and several other nutrients that can be difficult to match in other foods.

Animal foods provide the most readily absorbed forms of iron and zinc.[37] This explains why vegetarians are more at risk for deficiency in both of these minerals.[38,39] The consequences of iron deficiency in pregnancy include maternal anemia, miscarriage, premature delivery, impaired thyroid function, and problems with fetal brain development. Zinc deficiency is linked to miscarriage, preterm delivery, fetal growth restriction, stillbirth, and neural tube defects.[40]

Meat is also rich in vitamin B6, a nutrient that 40% of women of childbearing age in the United States are deficient in, and yet deficiency is tied to miscarriage, preterm birth, low birth weight, and low APGAR scores at birth.[41,42] In addition, animal foods are the only food sources of vitamin B12, the importance of which was reviewed in the section on liver. There are many other micronutrients that are found in abundance in meat, but either lacking or poorly absorbed from other foods, which makes meat necessary for optimal prenatal nutrition. Given all the nutrients found in meat, it's probably no surprise that low intake of animal protein in late pregnancy is linked to lower birthweight in infants.[43]

But the benefits of meat go beyond protein, vitamins, and minerals. Specific cuts of meat and preparation methods can provide even more nutritional benefits, hence why I specify these foods in the title of this section.

Chances are your grandmother knew how to make soup from scratch, but now most of us grab a can or carton of "broth" at the store instead. Homemade broths made from bones are not just a way to save money on food, but a valuable source of nutrients otherwise lacking in our diets. Traditional cultures didn't eat boneless, skinless chicken breasts and throw out the rest of the animal. They ate the organs, the fat, and they used any tough cuts of meat, bones and skin to make soup.

Modern research is showing us that this practice is something we should return to. The bones, skin, and connective tissues of animals are rich in protein, gelatin, collagen, glycine, and minerals. Bones contain more minerals per ounce than any other body tissue. When you simmer a big pot of bone broth, some of these minerals leach into the broth, making it a source of calcium, magnesium, iron, zinc, potassium, and many trace minerals. Think of it as an electrolyte beverage—like savory Gatorade.

Bone broth and slow-cooked meats also provide gelatin and collagen, the two richest sources of an important amino acid called glycine. Glycine is commonly glossed over in conventional nutrition because it's "conditionally essential," meaning the body can make plenty of it from other amino acids. However, pregnancy is a special case where the body requires additional glycine from the diet. Researchers have found that "the demand for glycine during pregnancy may already exceed the capacity for its synthesis, making it conditionally *indispensable.*"[44]

Glycine is needed for the synthesis of fetal DNA and collagen, among other functions. It's particularly important to include enough glycine in your diet in later pregnancy when your baby is gaining weight rapidly. Your baby's developing bones, connective tissues, organs, and skin need glycine in the highest amounts at this stage. One study points out, "As pregnancy advances, the endogenous production of glycine [meaning, what your body produces from other amino acids] may be insufficient to satisfy the increasing demands."[45]

In addition, *your* body is depending on glycine just as much as your baby is in order to support your growing uterus, breasts, and stretching skin. In fact, your uterus contains 800% more collagen at the end of your pregnancy compared to pre-pregnancy.[46] It's possible, though certainly not guaranteed, that adequate dietary glycine may help prevent stretch marks, given that collagen is one-third glycine by weight.[47]

Glycine, however, is not abundant in lean meats, skinless poultry, dairy products, or vegetarian sources of protein. Moreover, eating exclusively from the above foods for your protein needs may provide excessive methionine, an amino acid that reduces glycine stores and may be toxic in large quantities.[17] Excess methionine has been linked to high homocysteine (a marker of inflammation), neural tube defects, preeclampsia, spontaneous abortion, and premature delivery.[48] As one researcher explains, "Diets with an inappropriate balance of methionine can adversely affect both short-term reproductive function and the long-term physiology of the offspring. The catabolism [in other words, breakdown] of unused methionine increases the demand for glycine and may cause a deficiency."[49]

The most reliable food sources of glycine include bone broth, slow-cooked tough cuts of meat (think pot roast or pulled pork), skin-on and bone-in poultry (like chicken wings, thighs, or whole roasted chicken), pork rinds, bacon, and sausage or ground meat (as these are often made from tougher cuts). Another option is to add pure gelatin powder or collagen powder to other foods, as these are naturally very rich in glycine (not the pre-sweetened kind of gelatin, of course!).

Consequences of inadequate glycine intake in pregnancy have been demonstrated in animal studies. Few studies are done on humans that purposefully restrict intake of essential nutrients during pregnancy for obvious ethical reasons, but these studies are still performed on lab rats.

When rats are fed a diet low in protein, their offspring develop cardiovascular problems and high blood pressure. However, when low protein diets are supplemented with glycine, these effects are not seen. Researchers comment, "The availability of glycine appears to be of critical importance for normal cardiovascular development."[50] This may be due to glycine's interconnected role in folate metabolism.[51] Or that glycine is required for the production of elastin, a structural protein that allows your blood vessels to expand and contract.

Glycine is also protective against oxidative stress, a hallmark of preeclampsia, and has been shown to reduce blood pressure and blood sugar in studies.[52] Women with preeclampsia excrete less glycine in their urine, suggesting increased demands for glycine and/or depleted maternal stores.[53] In addition, "poor glycine status has been suggested in preterm infants."[54]

We also know that choline and glycine are related in their functions in the body—both are involved in methylation, a process that ensures that your baby's genes develop properly.[55] In other words, your baby's optimal development is dependent upon your consumption of these two nutrients. Choline may be converted into glycine if the diet is not sufficient. Of course, that assumes a mom is also obtaining enough choline, a nutrient that most women don't even have on their radar.

Another benefit of glycine is that it's required for the production of glutathione, one of the body's most powerful detoxification enzymes which helps to naturally detoxify chemicals we encounter on a daily basis. Chemical exposure is a risk factor for a variety of birth defects and pregnancy complications, so nutrients that improve your ability to detoxify harmful chemicals are worth your attention.[56] I explore the risks associated with toxin exposure in Chapter 10.

Clearly the amount of glycine in your prenatal diet is crucial. From the creation of your baby's DNA and cardiovascular system to the needs of your growing uterus, its role in maintaining a healthy pregnancy cannot be overstated. You can feel good about eating nourishing soups, pulled pork, and pot roasts, knowing that you're giving your baby the raw materials to develop just as nature intended.

As with all animal foods, source your meat and bones from pasture-raised and grass-fed animals whenever possible. They are often more expensive, but one way to offset the cost is to purchase tougher cuts of meat (which are both less expensive *and* higher in glycine), as opposed to fancier cuts, like steak. I actually *prefer* these cuts because they are more flavorful and easier to make (you can't ruin pulled pork, but pork chops take some finesse). As consumer demand rises, more grocery stores are carrying pasture-raised and

Real Food for Pregnancy

grass-fed meat. Stock your freezer when meat goes on sale. Also be sure to talk to your local butcher—some will give away soup bones or sell them for a very low price. Another option is to purchase direct from a farmer, such as a cow share or pig share, which brings the cost-per-pound down significantly.

If purchasing grass-fed is cost-prohibitive, no matter how creative you get, know that conventionally-raised animal food is *still* nutritious. You will still be providing your baby with key nutrients that would likely otherwise be lacking from your diet if it did not contain meat.

Vegetables, Especially Leafy Greens

This may be the most obvious of the foods to emphasize when you're expecting. Green, leafy vegetables are nutritional powerhouses that are concentrated in vitamins, minerals, and antioxidants. Researchers have identified 45 different flavonoids (a type of antioxidant) in kale alone.

Greens are one of the most abundant sources of folate, which makes sense considering that folate derives from the word "foliage," meaning leaves (the other two major sources are liver and legumes). They also contain vitamin C, beta-carotene, fiber, many B-vitamins, and trace minerals. Vitamin C works together with amino acids and other nutrients to maintain normal collagen production, which is important for your baby's growth and to support *your* tissues (like your growing uterus and the skin on your belly).

Greens have high amounts of vitamin K1, which plays a crucial role in normal blood clotting, something that can lower your risk of postpartum hemorrhage (excessive blood loss at birth). Leafy greens are also high in two nutrients that help prevent or ease the severity of morning sickness in some women: vitamin B6 and magnesium. Lastly, they are a source of potassium, a key electrolyte that helps you maintain normal blood pressure and prevents swelling.

Keep in mind that the nutrients in all vegetables, especially the antioxidants and fat-soluble vitamins, are best absorbed when you eat them with some fat, so don't be shy about eating grass-fed butter, coconut oil, olive oil, avocado, nuts, or other healthy fats alongside your vegetables.[57]

Certain nutrients are better preserved when vegetables are raw (like vitamin C), while some are enhanced when vegetables are cooked (like beta-carotene).[58] For that reason, I recommend eating a combination of cooked and raw vegetables. Ideally, purchase organically-grown vegetables to minimize exposure to pesticide residues.[59] Buying vegetables from local farmers is a great way to ensure your produce is picked at its peak, in both flavor and nutrition, and gives you the opportunity to ask about growing practices, such as the use of pesticides and other chemicals. In many areas, buying from local farmers and purchasing in-season is less expensive. If you do not have access to—or cannot afford—organic or local vegetables, know that it's still better to eat conventionally-grown vegetables than to go without.

Salmon, Fatty Fish, and Other Seafood

With increased awareness about mercury and other contaminants in fish, some women have been told not to consume fish while pregnant or to limit it to less than 12 oz per week. The fear is that mercury is a neurotoxin and could harm brain development, so the logic follows that limiting seafood consumption should limit mercury exposure and protect your baby.

Unfortunately, this information is a little misguided. While there *are* certain fish that are very high in mercury and should be avoided (namely swordfish, king mackerel, tilefish, and shark; tuna should be limited to <6 oz per week), many other types of fish are perfectly safe to eat while pregnant, even if they contain small amounts of mercury. Here's why: fish also contains high amounts of selenium, a mineral that readily binds with mercury and prevents it from exerting toxic effects in the human body.[60]

In one of the best designed studies on maternal fish consumption and neurodevelopment with nearly 12,000 mother-infant pairs, consumption of *more than* 12 oz per week was strongly linked to higher childhood IQ and communication skills. In fact, the *worst* cognitive outcomes were among children whose mothers consumed *no seafood* during pregnancy. These children were more likely to have problems with fine motor skills, social development, and communication skills.[61] Even though mercury intake was higher in the fish-eating mothers, the nutritional benefits (and presence of selenium to bind mercury) seemed to offset the exposure.

Still, it doesn't hurt to be aware of the types of fish and seafood that contain high or low levels of mercury. It sounds too simplistic to be accurate, but the size of fish is the best predictor of mercury levels.[62] Larger species of fish, who have both lived longer and eaten more smaller fish/seafood, tend to have higher concentrations of mercury. For example, sockeye salmon (which weigh <15 pounds and live for ~7 years) is generally a better choice than albacore tuna (which weigh up to 130 pounds and live for ~13 years). Hopefully, these little known facts about fish size—and selenium—will lessen some fears about mercury.

Cold water fish are especially beneficial to consume while pregnant thanks to high levels of the brain-boosting omega-3 fat, DHA. Fatty fish such as salmon, herring, and sardines (plus fish eggs or "roe") provide the most concentrated sources of dietary DHA and are also low in mercury. I'll explore exactly how and why DHA is important to consume directly from your diet (or supplements) in Chapter 6.

Aside from DHA, fatty fish and seafood are among the few foods rich in vitamin D, a nutrient that most pregnant women are deficient in.[63] Seafood also contains many trace minerals, including iodine, zinc, and selenium. Iodine needs are increased by 50% during pregnancy and deficiency is common.[64] Iodine is necessary for normal thyroid function in both mother and fetus, and is essential to healthy brain development.

According to the *Journal of the American Medical Association*, "Iodine deficiency remains the leading cause of preventable intellectual disability worldwide."[65] Consuming seafood—in particular, seaweed, scallops, cod, shrimp, sardines, and salmon—is a great way to meet iodine needs.

When it comes to quality, seek wild-caught fish whenever possible, since farmed fish is often contaminated with PCBs, dioxins, and other unwanted chemicals.[66] Farmed fish may also contain antibiotic-resistant bacteria thanks to the heavy use of antibiotics in aquaculture.[67,68] This can pose a risk for hard-to-treat infections, which could be especially dangerous while pregnant. With few exceptions, wild-caught fish is almost always higher in DHA compared to farm-raised fish.[69]

Full-Fat and Fermented Dairy Products

First, let me state that I do not believe that everyone needs to consume dairy products to obtain calcium, but if you can tolerate them, they offer many benefits. In addition to calcium, dairy is a good source of protein, fat-soluble vitamins (A, D, E, and K), certain B vitamins, probiotics, and iodine.

I'd like to specifically discuss vitamin K2, a nutrient found in dairy products that is otherwise not widely available in our diets. This vitamin is different from the other major type of vitamin K, called vitamin K1, which we find in plants. Vitamin K2 functions along with vitamins A and D to support normal mineral metabolism in the body, primarily by directing minerals to be incorporated into the right places—the bones and teeth—rather than soft tissues. As you can imagine, your baby's skeleton is being formed in utero, so these vitamins in combination with calcium and other minerals are the ideal nutrient matrix to form strong bones. Vitamin K2 is also important for *your* bone health. During pregnancy, if your intake of nutrients is too low, your body can "borrow" from your own tissues. In other words, you can become depleted in nutrients over the course of a pregnancy, and may develop health problems as a result. One such problem is maternal osteoporosis, or weak bones, which most assume is a sign of calcium deficiency. However, this condition has been reversed with vitamin K2 supplementation.[70]

The positive effects of vitamin K2 aren't just limited to bone health. One side benefit is that vitamin K2 may also increase insulin sensitivity, meaning that getting enough of this nutrient could help you maintain normal blood sugar.[71] If you can recall from the previous chapter, maintaining normal blood sugar is important for every pregnant woman, whether she has gestational diabetes or not.

Dairy products are also a significant source of iodine, thanks to the common use of iodine supplements for dairy cows to improve fertility and the use of iodine as a disinfectant prior to milking. Among women who do not consume seafood, dairy products (and eggs) are the most important contributors to iodine intake.[72]

Just like any food, quality counts. Sourcing your dairy products from farmers who raise their cows on pasture (grass-fed) means the milk has higher levels of fat-soluble vitamins and lower levels of pesticide residues (because they're not munching on conventionally-grown corn and soy). Dairy products labeled "organic" are the next best option, although these animals do not necessarily consume grass, just organic feed (you'd need to talk to the farmer to know for sure). If you can find dairy products that are both grass-fed *and* certified organic, fantastic. Of course, you only benefit from the fat-soluble vitamins if you eat the fat, so seek out full-fat dairy products.

I also recommend including some fermented dairy, such as yogurt, kefir, and aged cheese. Fermented dairy products contain more vitamin K2 since levels of the vitamin increase through bacterial fermentation. These bacteria, known as probiotics, are beneficial in their own right. In fact, maternal intake of fermented milk products has been shown to reduce the development of eczema and allergic rhinitis (also known as hay fever) in infants.[73] Regular consumption of fermented dairy may also reduce the risk of preterm delivery.[74]

If you are lactose intolerant, you may be able to eat butter, cream, full-fat Greek yogurt, and aged cheese without discomfort, since these are lower in lactose. It's unclear why, but some women report being able to tolerate dairy in pregnancy even if they were not able to do so before becoming pregnant. Alas, if that's not you, I'll discuss alternative sources of probiotics, calcium, vitamin D, and other nutrients in Chapter 6.

Real Food for Pregnancy

The Challenge of a Vegetarian Diet During Pregnancy

As you may have noticed, the foods reviewed in this section are of animal origin with the exception of vegetables. Traditional cultures revered these so-called "fertility foods" for good reason; they are rich sources of the nutrients required to support baby's development, mom's health during pregnancy, and her ability to heal from birth and produce nutrient-rich breast milk. Research on modern hunter-gatherer populations worldwide estimates that animal foods provide between 55-65% of calories in their diets.[75] This echoes the findings of Dr. Weston Price, who was unable to find an indigenous population that ate an entirely plant-based diet in his documentation of traditional diets across the globe in the early 1900s.[76] Attempting to match the nutrients found in an omnivorous diet with one that's solely plant-based is a nutritional dilemma. Supplementation only goes so far. Not all nutrients found in animal foods are available in supplemental form, nor are they as easily absorbed or provided in the synergistic quantities found in whole foods. I'm frequently asked for my take on vegetarian diets during pregnancy, which is why I've chosen to include an in-depth discussion on the matter.

In short, the following nutrients are challenging to obtain in a vegetarian diet: vitamin B12, choline, glycine, preformed vitamin A (retinol), vitamin K2, DHA, iron, and zinc. If you follow a strictly vegan diet, meaning you consume absolutely *no* animal foods—no meat, poultry, fish, dairy, or eggs— some of these nutrients may be impossible to obtain from your diet. For the purposes of this discussion, any reference to vegetarian diet is one that avoids animal foods with the exception of dairy and eggs (lacto-ovo vegetarian). The following section details the reasons a vegetarian diet may not be optimal for pregnancy—for you or your baby.

Vitamin B12

Vitamin B12 plays a crucial role in fetal development and is only found in animal foods. Vitamin B12 is required for a process called methylation, which is involved in gene expression, cell differentiation, and organ formation.[77] As you might infer, methylation is absolutely essential to normal fetal development. Without enough vitamin B12, the risk of miscarriage, neural tube defects, and preterm delivery go up.[78,79] On average, 62% of vegetarian pregnant women are deficient in vitamin B12 while deficiency is uncommon in omnivorous women.[80]

One study measured blood levels of vitamin B12 along with markers of vitamin B12 status, including homocysteine, in the first, second, and third trimesters among women eating a vegetarian diet (that included eggs and dairy), a low-meat diet (<10.5 oz of meat per week), or an omnivorous diet.[81] The combination of low serum vitamin B12 and high homocysteine is considered particularly detrimental, as it may limit the availability of folate and impair myelin synthesis, both of which are crucial for nervous system development.[82] This pattern was observed in 22% of vegetarians, in 10% of low-meat eaters, and in 3% of omnivores. In other words, even vegetarian women who can theoretically get B12 from their diet (from eggs and dairy) or those not eating *enough* meat are at risk for vitamin B12 deficiency. What's interesting about this study is that the RDA for vitamin B12 was met (by diet alone) in 60% of vegetarians, 94% of low-meat eaters, and 100% of omnivorous women, and yet deficiency was still relatively common. This study and others have pointed out that the RDA for vitamin B12 is set too low. As already mentioned in this chapter, the latest research suggests that the current RDA underestimates the need of this vitamin during pregnancy by approximately 3-fold.[83] This means that relying on an occasional meal with eggs or dairy, taking a typical prenatal vitamin (which provides "100% of the RDA" for B12), or even eating foods fortified with vitamin B12, is unlikely to be enough. Inclusion of enough animal foods and/or an additional vitamin B12 supplement would be needed.

Vitamin B12 deficiency is problematic *during* pregnancy, but also presents a major challenge *after* pregnancy for women who breastfeed. That's because mothers who are deficient produce breast milk that's also deficient in vitamin B12. There are numerous case studies in the medical literature of severe infant vitamin B12 deficiency and the resulting developmental delays, stunted growth, and motor problems—some of which are *irreversible*—among exclusively breastfed infants of vegetarian or vegan mothers.[84] When considering what constitutes an optimal prenatal diet, we need to take into consideration the nutrients that are required for your baby's development in utero *and* outside of the womb. Truly, a diet that meets your nutrient needs during pregnancy should also ensure you have enough nutrients to make breast milk with sufficient nutrients for your baby's growth. Prior to about 150 years ago, infant formula didn't even exist (the first one was formulated in 1865). In other words, breastfeeding was not a choice until relatively recently; it was imperative for infant survival. This may explain why traditional cultures placed such a heavy emphasis on foods of animal origin prior to, during, and after pregnancy. For a more detailed discussion on breastfeeding nutrition, see Chapter 12.

Some vegetarian and even vegan women, whose dietary choices are for ethical reasons, make an exception to eat oysters to obtain vitamin B12, as they do not have a central nervous system and purportedly do not feel pain.[85]

Real Food for Pregnancy

Oysters are incredibly rich in vitamin B12, with 1 oz providing more than the RDA. Other foods high in B12 are discussed earlier in this chapter.

Choline

Choline is required for fetal brain development, placental function, helps prevent neural tube defects, and shares many of the same nutritional benefits of folate.[86] As we have already covered, the two major sources of choline in the diet are egg yolks and liver. If you eat a vegetarian diet that includes eggs, you may be able to obtain enough choline, but a woman who eats a vegan diet may not. Egg-eaters have, on average, double the intake of choline compared to those who avoid eggs.[87] During pregnancy, you need a minimum of 450 mg of choline per day. An egg (with the yolk) provides 115 mg and 1 oz of beef liver provides 119 mg. The richest vegetarian sources of choline include certain cruciferous vegetables, legumes, and certain nuts. Still, they are far less concentrated sources of choline compared to animal foods and it would be challenging to eat 450 mg from these foods alone. For reference, ½ cup of cooked pinto beans, Brussels sprouts, or broccoli provides ~30 mg, ½ cup quinoa or yogurt provides 20 mg, 2 Tbsp of peanut butter provides 20 mg, and ¼ cup of almonds provides 18 mg. Soy is also a source of choline (½ cup of tofu provides 35 mg), however I discourage heavy consumption of soy, especially during pregnancy, for reasons outlined in Chapter 4. The alternative is a choline supplement, such as choline bitartrate or sunflower lecithin.

Keep in mind that while 450 mg is the current target for choline, newer research notes that "choline intakes that exceed dietary recommendations during pregnancy may improve maternal and child health outcomes."[88] Studies that supplemented pregnant women with 930 mg of choline per day have shown beneficial effects on fetal development and placental function.[89,90] This level of intake is specifically beneficial to brain development. A recent well-designed study tested the effect of a prenatal diet containing 480 mg per day compared to 930 mg per day on infant brain development. Infants were tested at 4, 7, 10, and 13 months of age and reaction time was significantly faster at all time periods for infants born to mothers in the 930 mg/day choline group.[91] In other words, it's smart to aim high for choline. For women who have the common genetic mutation known as MTHFR—which affects up to 60% of the population—choline needs may be substantially higher than the current recommended level.[92] This makes a vegetarian or egg-free diet for women with MTHFR mutations especially risky.

Glycine

Glycine is the most abundant amino acid in collagen and, in turn, collagen is the most abundant protein in the human body. Glycine is a "conditionally essential" amino acid during pregnancy, meaning you must obtain it *through your diet* to provide enough to support the growth of your baby's skeleton, teeth, internal organs, hair, skin, and nails. Plus, it is necessary to support your own stretching skin, growing uterus, placenta, and to help your circulatory system adapt to the demands of pregnancy. Glycine also plays a key role in methylation, much like folate, choline, and vitamin B12.

In general, plant foods are low in glycine. I reviewed the top 1,000 food sources of glycine and all except a handful are animal foods. I'm not sure it's possible to obtain enough glycine on a vegetarian diet during pregnancy as demands are so high, but researchers have yet to define the exact amount required in the diet. Studies have shown that non-pregnant vegetarians frequently have urine markers of glycine deficiency.[93] Likewise, a "high proportion of pregnant women exhibit markers of glycine insufficiency."[94] It stands to reason that the combination of a diet lacking in glycine (vegetarian) plus a metabolic state that exponentially increases glycine needs (pregnancy) is not wise. We know that "the fetus requires disproportionately large amounts of glycine both for structural development and as a metabolic precursor."[95] And even outside of pregnancy, "glycine is a semi-essential amino acid" that, when lacking in the diet, may impair collagen formation, which is key for bone, skin, and dental health.[96]

Though there is no official RDA for glycine, researchers estimate the minimum amount of glycine needed in the diet (for non-pregnant adults) is 10 g per day (that's 10,000 mg).[97] This need is likely higher during pregnancy. Of the top 1,000 food sources of glycine, the major plant sources I noted are (in order of most to least glycine): sesame seed flour, spirulina algae, sunflower seed flour, pumpkin seeds, nori (a type of seaweed), watercress, beans, and spinach. Again, be aware that the relative concentration of glycine in plants is very low compared to animal sources. For example, pork rinds, which are very high in glycine have 6,760 mg per 2 oz compared to only 1,940 mg in 2 oz of sesame seed flour, 1,760 mg in 2 oz of dried spirulina powder (that's about ½ cup), 280 mg in a ½ cup of black beans, and 60 mg in ½ cup cooked spinach. You'd really have to go out of your way to obtain enough glycine from solely plant-based foods. Dairy and eggs are not particularly rich sources of glycine compared to other animal foods, since glycine is a structural amino acid found mostly in connective tissue, skin, and bones. This means both vegetarians and vegans are unlikely to consume enough.

Vitamin A

Vitamin A helps regulate gene expression and fetal growth with specific roles in the development of the heart, eyes, ears, limbs, and immune system.[98] Lack of vitamin A can lead to serious malformations, including improperly formed craniofacial structures, limbs, and internal organs.[99] Most of us have been taught that plant foods are a good source of vitamin A, but it's important to recognize that plants don't contain true *preformed* vitamin A (retinol); rather, they contain provitamin A (carotenoids). This means your body must convert carotenoids into retinol, however, this conversion rate is quite low in many individuals. You might think you can just eat a lot of sweet potatoes and carrots to flood your system with provitamin A, but that's unlikely to help. The more beta-carotene you eat, the *less* you convert to vitamin A.[100] Simply put, you *need* to eat preformed vitamin A from either animal sources, such as full-fat dairy or eggs, or supplement to ensure you get enough. Women who eat a vegan diet would not obtain *any* preformed vitamin A unless they supplement. At the same time, supplements of preformed vitamin A can be risky if taken in large quantities (increase the risk of certain birth defects), but this is not observed with the vitamin A from animal foods. See the section on liver found earlier in this chapter for a deeper discussion on this topic.

Vitamin K2

Vitamin K2 is essential to proper bone mineralization, meaning your baby's skeleton requires it to develop properly. In short, vitamin K2 ensures that calcium accumulates in bone tissue rather than soft tissue. In the field of nutrition, it is a relatively newly investigated vitamin—in fact, the first official database of vitamin K2 levels in foods wasn't published until 2006.[101] Food sources of vitamin K2 are fatty animal foods (such as full-fat dairy, eggs, and liver), and certain fermented foods. One of the richest sources of vitamin K2 is a fermented soybean product called natto, but it's rarely consumed outside of Asia (believe me, it's an acquired taste and texture!). The source of K2 in natto is the bacteria used to ferment the soybeans, not the soy itself. It's important to note that vitamin K1, which is found in leafy greens and plant foods—while important for other reasons, like blood clotting—does not affect bone mineralization and cannot be converted into vitamin K2 in your body in sufficient quantities.[102] It is possible to obtain enough vitamin K2 on a vegetarian diet if you regularly consume natto, egg yolks, cheese, and full-fat fermented dairy products. Hard cheeses that have undergone a long fermentation time, like parmesan, cheddar, and gouda, tend to have higher levels of vitamin K2 than soft, mild cheeses. Strict vegans who do not consume natto require a supplement and yet most prenatal vitamins fail to include vitamin K2.

DHA

There are several different forms of omega-3 fats, but DHA is the one that's most important during pregnancy. DHA is incorporated into the rapidly developing brain and eyes of the fetus in utero where it assists with the formation of neurons (brain cells) and protects the brain from inflammation and damage.[103] It remains crucially important during the first two years of infancy. If you plan to breastfeed, it's especially important to ensure your body has enough DHA, as your intake directly affects the amount in your milk.[104]

Many women are aware of the role of DHA in brain development, but few know how to get enough in their diet. You may have been told that you can get omega-3 fats from plant sources, such as flax seeds or chia seeds, but although these are healthy for other reasons, they are *not* going to boost your baby's brain development. That's because plant-sourced omega-3s come in a form called "ALA" and the type our brain and eyes need is "DHA." Your body lacks the ability to convert enough ALA to DHA to meet your baby's needs as the conversion rate is, at best, only 3.8%. Plus, if your diet is high in omega-6s (which happen to be concentrated in seeds, nuts, and vegetable oils common on a vegetarian diet), this conversion rate drops to 1.9%.[105] Vegetarian diets have significantly higher omega-6 to omega-3 ratios compared to diets that include animal foods. When I ran a comprehensive nutrition analysis on the sample prenatal vegan meal plan from the *Academy of Nutrition and Dietetics* and compared it to the meal plans in this book, the omega-6 to omega-3 ratio was over 10:1 in the vegan meal plan compared to 3:1 in mine.[106] The vegan meal plan contained 2.5x more omega-6 fats in total and had an unfavorable balance of fatty acids. Studies have shown that infants of women who consume a diet with a high omega-6 to omega-3 ratio are twice as likely to experience developmental delays by 6 months of age.[107] Mouse studies echo these findings, noting that an imbalanced ratio of these fats "impairs formation of the neocortical neuronal layer" in the offspring of these mice and leads to more anxious behavior.[108] This reaffirms the notion that there's a key window in development, particularly brain development, where inadequate nutrition can have lifelong consequences.

One study I want to highlight looked specifically at essential fatty acids in vegans (note: the average time a subject had been on a vegan diet was 7 years) compared to omnivores, including a set of mothers and their exclusively breastfed infants.[109] This study was before the era of vegan-derived DHA and before the popularity of fish oil supplements, so all mothers were unsupplemented. The results were striking. On average, DHA levels were 65% lower in plasma, 67% lower in red blood cells, and 61% lower in breast milk from vegans compared to omnivores. Following a similar trend, DHA levels in the red blood cells of infants were 69% lower in infants of vegan mothers compared to infants of omnivores (all exclusively breastfed). These results are not a one-off. A 2009 review of the research on vegetarian diets and DHA status found that the "proportions of DHA in plasma, blood cells, breast milk, and tissues are substantially lower in vegans and vegetarians compared with omnivores."[110] This raises major concerns when it comes to brain development of these infants. It also has implications for *your* brain health as a mother. Low intake of DHA during pregnancy, as a result of a vegetarian diet (or even a diet low in seafood), increases the odds of suffering from maternal anxiety.[111] In addition, women with a higher omega-6 to omega-3 ratio in their diet (9:1 or higher) are 2.5x more likely to suffer from postpartum depression.[112] Recall that the "well-planned" prenatal vegan meal plan from the *Academy of Nutrition and Dietetics* had an omega-6 to omega-3 ratio of 10:1.

The science is clear with DHA. You can eat all the walnuts, flaxseeds, and chia seeds you want, but you still won't get anywhere close to meeting your baby's DHA needs and you'll likely become depleted yourself. You must consume DHA *directly* to get enough. For those who do not eat fish or seafood, pasture-raised eggs and/or an algae-based DHA supplement (the only plant source of DHA) would be necessary. Also, in order to keep the omega-6 to omega-3 ratio at favorable levels, vegetable oils simply cannot be the primary source of fat in the diet.

Iron and Zinc

Lastly, certain minerals can be challenging to obtain on a vegetarian diet due to differences in absorption. Zinc and iron are the most notable examples. When it comes to iron, there are different forms available in foods. Heme iron is available in animal foods and is absorbed at about 25% efficiency (though some studies report 40% efficiency). Non-heme iron is the form found in plant foods and is absorbed poorly, generally ranging from 2-13%.[113] Iron absorption from whole grain cereals, for example, is extremely low at only 0.3 to 1.8%.[114] This is due to the presence of fiber, phytic acid, and other anti-nutrients that interfere with the absorption of minerals from whole grains and legumes.[115] For this reason, the RDA for iron is set 1.8x higher for vegetarians. Vegetarian women, on average, have lower iron stores and are more likely to be anemic.[116] Even among non-vegetarians, it's estimated that only 20% of women have adequate iron stores for pregnancy.[117] Inadequate iron intake during pregnancy is a risk factor for numerous pregnancy complications, including preeclampsia, hypothyroidism, and preterm birth. It may also impair fetal brain development, stunt growth, and increase your baby's lifetime risk of obesity, diabetes, and high blood pressure.[118]

Vegetarian diets also tend to be low in zinc. Over half of the zinc in an average American diet is obtained from animal foods (25% from beef alone). Animal protein not only tends to contain high amounts of zinc, but also significantly enhances zinc absorption. Much like iron, plant foods that are high in zinc, such as legumes, whole grains, nuts, and seeds, are also high in *inhibitors* of zinc absorption, including phytic acid. To account for the difference in absorption, zinc needs for vegetarians are set 50% higher than for non-vegetarians, but studies note that even this may not be enough to ensure adequate zinc status.[119] In one study, inadequate zinc status was found in 47% of vegans compared to only 11% of omnivores, despite the two groups consuming similar concentrations of zinc in their diets.[120] The authors attributed phytic acid and other inhibitors of zinc absorption to this difference. Zinc deficiency in pregnancy is dangerous as it's linked to higher odds of miscarriage, preterm delivery, stillbirth, placental inflammation, neural tube defects, and low birthweight.[121] Some research suggests that lack of zinc during pregnancy could have carryover effects for generation after generation. As one study points out: "It is clear that suboptimal zinc nutriture during pregnancy and early postnatal life (e.g., critical periods of development) can adversely affect the long-term health of the offspring and may predispose them to increased risk of chronic disease, which may persist for multiple generations."[122] The fact that zinc deficiency *now* could affect not only your baby, but your grandchildren as well, is worth taking to heart.

In summary, even minerals that are technically provided on a vegetarian or vegan diet may be poorly absorbed, which means that vegetarians are more likely to be deficient. A study from the *American Journal of Clinical Nutrition* sums it up well: "The iron and zinc from vegetarian diets are generally less bioavailable than from non-vegetarian diets because of reduced meat intake as well as the tendency to consume more phytic acid and other plant-based inhibitors of iron and zinc absorption."[123] That said, the richest sources of iron on a vegetarian diet are legumes, pumpkin seeds, cooked leafy green vegetables, and spirulina algae. For zinc, vegetarian sources include whole grains, nuts, seeds, and legumes. For optimal absorption, soak, sprout, or ferment grains, legumes, nuts, and seeds before consuming, as this decreases the content of phytic acid (and therefore enhances mineral absorption in your body).[124] Also, consuming these foods alongside acidic or high-vitamin C ingredients (like vinegar or lemon juice) and separate from high-calcium foods (like dairy) or high-tannin foods (like coffee and tea) can further enhance absorption of both iron and zinc.

Other Considerations

While my primary concern with vegetarian diets during pregnancy is inadequate micronutrient intake, as outlined above, there are other potential problems. Protein quality is one important issue, since non-animal sources of protein are "incomplete," meaning they lack all essential amino acids. As seasoned vegetarians know, this can be remedied by eating complementary proteins together, such as beans with rice or by having animal protein with any other plant protein (such as eggs or cheese paired with lentils). Plant proteins are also more difficult to digest, thanks to the presence of anti-nutrients, like phytates, tannins, lectins, and trypsin inhibitors.[125] Even if you try to eat extra plant-based proteins to make up for it, you need to consider glycine, which is universally lacking in vegetarian diets. In order to consume enough total protein, most vegetarians end up eating a fairly high-carbohydrate diet since all whole food plant proteins also naturally contain carbohydrates. It's no surprise that vegetarian women eat more carbohydrates, on average, than non-vegetarians.[126] In a study of eating patterns of omnivores compared to vegetarians among over 13,000 participants in the United States, average carbohydrate intake was 60% of calories while protein intake was <12% for vegetarians.[127] For lacto-ovo vegetarians, prioritizing eggs and low-carb dairy products (such as cheese and Greek yogurt), and favoring nuts, seeds, and legumes over grains can help shift the balance. Lastly, the common use of meat alternatives often introduces high amounts of processed soy into the diet, which is undesirable during pregnancy for reasons outlined in-depth in Chapter 4. Plant proteins do offer some nutritional benefits, like folate and fiber, but the research suggests they should not be your *sole* source of protein while pregnant.

Tips to Optimize a Vegetarian Diet

For some women, a vegetarian diet is non-negotiable. In this case, there are several important considerations when trying to optimize your nutrient intake. Let me be clear that I cannot ethically endorse a fully *vegan* diet during pregnancy, however with very careful planning and supplementation, a *vegetarian* diet that includes eggs and dairy (lacto-ovo vegetarian) *may* be able to meet the high micronutrient needs of pregnancy. If you choose to eat a vegetarian diet—or semi-vegetarian diet—while pregnant, please carefully consider implementing the following:

- Eat a minimum of 3 eggs per day (from pasture-raised hens). This will get you much closer to meeting your nutrient needs, providing 70% vitamin B12 (of current RDA), 35% vitamin A, 75% choline, and 40% DHA. If you do not regularly consume eggs, take a choline supplement, as this is rarely included in prenatal vitamins.

- Take an algae-based DHA supplement. This is particularly important if you do not eat eggs regularly, as this is the only significant source of DHA in a vegetarian diet. Additionally, some women make an exception while pregnant and breastfeeding to include some seafood, such as sardines, oysters, or salmon.
- Regularly include seaweed in your diet, as this provides iron and numerous trace minerals, including iodine. Spirulina algae would also be a wise supplement to provide glycine, iron, and trace minerals.
- Consider eating oysters several times a week. Though not a traditional vegetarian food, if you eat a plant-based diet purely for animal rights reasons, you may feel comfortable eating oysters since they do not have a central nervous system and therefore reportedly do not feel pain.[128] Oysters are one of the richest sources of vitamin B12 and also provide iron, zinc, selenium, iodine and DHA.
- Soak whole grains and beans/legumes in water for 7 hours (or overnight)—or—sprout them before cooking. This reduces the levels of phytic acid and tannins, which normally interfere with absorption of minerals, including iron, zinc, calcium, magnesium, and copper. Also, choosing bread made with sprouted grains or that has undergone traditional sourdough fermentation greatly enhances mineral absorption. For example, whole wheat sourdough bread has about half the phytic acid of regular whole wheat bread. In rat studies, consumption of whole wheat sourdough bread resulted in significantly higher absorption of iron, zinc, and magnesium.[129] You may also want to consume vitamin C or acidic foods alongside grains and legumes to enhance mineral absorption, especially iron.[130]
- Regularly eat full-fat dairy products from grass-fed/pasture-raised animals, especially fermented dairy products (yogurt, cheese, kefir). These will supply preformed vitamin A, vitamin K2, calcium, iodine, protein, probiotics, and numerous other nutrients. Try to eat dairy products separate from high-iron foods (like black beans and spinach), as calcium and iron compete for absorption.
- Ensure you take a high quality prenatal vitamin everyday. Be especially certain it contains vitamin B12, iron (in a highly absorbable form), and zinc. If your prenatal vitamin does not contain iron, take a separate iron supplement. See Chapter 6 for more information on what to look for in a prenatal vitamin and iron supplement.
- Consider where you can obtain glycine. As already noted, plant foods alone may not be sufficient. Some of my clients who had previously followed a vegetarian diet make an exception while pregnant for the well-being of their baby and choose to include some high-glycine animal foods. Bone broth, collagen or gelatin powder, and even fish (especially if eaten with the skin) may be more acceptable to those who otherwise abstain from meat. The best vegetarian sources

would be sesame seeds and spirulina algae, but the quantity needed to provide adequate glycine is rather impractical.

As you can see, this gets complicated. Some of my recommendations are to make specific exceptions to a vegetarian diet and/or rely more heavily on supplements, so you can optimize your nutrient intake. While this will work for some, not all women are well-suited to this way of eating, no matter how many supplements they take. For example, if you are among the 60% of women with a mutation in the MTHFR gene, I strongly encourage you to rethink a vegetarian diet. This common genetic variation increases the needs for certain nutrients involved in methylation. This includes, but is not limited to, choline, folate, vitamin B12, and glycine. Aside from folate, plant foods alone cannot supply these nutrients in sufficient quantities.

Summary

As you can see, real food is absolutely packed with health benefits beyond what you'll find in a prenatal vitamin. The synergistic effect of nutrients found in whole foods cannot be underestimated. From the fat-soluble vitamins to the interplay between choline and DHA, Mother Nature has your back. Of course, as I point out in this chapter, quite a few of these nutrient-dense foods that support a healthy pregnancy are the very foods you've been told to limit for unsubstantiated reasons. Don't be surprised if your healthcare provider or nutritionist doesn't know this information, but feel free to share it with them. If you find yourself questioning what to do or balancing conflicting opinions, return to this chapter and re-read the research on these foods. If you've been avoiding these foods or have been following a vegetarian diet, I hope this section helps explain the nutritional trade-offs and potential complications that may result from these dietary choices.

Of course, this chapter highlights just a few of the most critical foods that support a healthy pregnancy. So, it goes without saying, there are numerous foods beyond this list that you should include in your diet. The meal plans included in Chapter 5 will show you how I suggest incorporating these nutrient-dense foods, along with many other complementary foods, into your diet. There may also be some supplements to consider taking, which I'll cover in Chapter 6. But first, read the next chapter to learn what foods to avoid or limit during pregnancy, bearing in mind that my definitions are likely different than what you've read elsewhere.

Chapter 4:

Foods That *Don't* Build a Healthy Baby

"A large body of evidence supports the concept that human pregnancy outcome is significantly influenced by the nutritional status of the mother. The consumption of "poor diets" has been associated with an increased risk for pregnancy complications, including gross structural birth defects, prematurity, low birth weight, and an increased risk for neurobehavioral and immunological abnormalities after birth."
- Dr. Janet Uriu-Adams, University of California, Davis

Just as there are nutrient-dense foods that promote optimal development of your baby, there are foods that do the opposite. Foods that are contaminated with bacteria or viruses that can cause illness or contain known toxins are the most commonly discussed. When you look up "foods to avoid" in pregnancy, most of the ones you'll read about make the cut because of their propensity to cause food poisoning. Unfortunately, many of these foods are sources of the vital nutrients your baby needs to grow optimally. In some cases, strictly avoiding these "off limit foods" may do more harm than good.

On the other hand, there are other foods that are "safe" from a food poisoning perspective, but may not offer optimal nutrition for you and baby or may increase your chances of certain pregnancy complications. This second set of foods are often not mentioned—or not emphasized—in prenatal nutrition education, yet are just as important to be aware of. This chapter will review all of the above with special attention to the more controversial topics.

Common Sense About "Foods to Avoid" Lists

If you've been reading up on prenatal nutrition, you've probably seen the lengthy lists of foods to avoid. Soft cheeses, raw milk, certain fish (especially raw fish), undercooked meat, eggs with runny yolks, and deli meat are among the most popular to make the *Do Not Eat* lists.

In some ways, this is prudent advice. During pregnancy, your immune system makes some incredible adaptations to allow your baby to grow, and as a result, your body becomes slightly more susceptible to infections. Food poisoning—or foodborne illness, as researchers call it—can cause serious pregnancy complications. For example, infection with a type of bacteria called *Listeria* can potentially result in miscarriage or even stillbirth.[1]

This has led to the adoption of fairly strict prenatal nutrition guidelines around foods to avoid. But, do these guidelines have strong evidence to back them up or are we taking precautions to the extreme?

Eating on the "Safe Side" vs. Risking Nutrient Deficiencies

Unfortunately, strictly avoiding all foods that *could* cause foodborne illness can make it more difficult to meet your prenatal nutrition requirements. In fact, one study of nearly 7,500 women in Australia found that women who "consciously limit their consumption of potential *Listeria*-containing foods are likely to have suboptimal nutrient intake from foods," specifically fiber, folate, iron, vitamin E and calcium.[2] The study's authors concluded that "it appears reasonable to suggest that to balance the opposing risks, pregnant women should aim for moderate consumption of potential *Listeria*-containing foods as opposed to a low consumption or total exclusion, which comes at the expense of important nutrients for pregnancy."

While it's true that pregnant women are more susceptible to *Listeria*, it's extremely rare to become infected. In an analysis on *Listeria* risk among pregnant women using data from the U.S. Food and Drug Administration (FDA), the researchers estimated 1 case of listeria infection per 83,000 servings of deli meat or 5 million servings of soft cheese consumed by pregnant women.[3] By all accounts, that's a pretty minimal risk.

A separate analysis by Canadian researchers concluded: "If food is properly handled and stored, the risk of being infected with *Listeria* appears to be low. Therefore, pregnant women need not avoid soft-ripened cheeses or deli meats, so long as they are consumed in moderation and obtained from

Real Food for Pregnancy

reputable stores."[4] They go on to explain, "Despite the increased relative risk for pregnant women contracting *Listeria,* the absolute risk is extremely low, and avoiding deli meats altogether does appear to be rather punitive." I'd have to agree. All of these strict food rules can seem a bit like punishment.

Aside from missing out on the sheer pleasure of eating really tasty soft cheese or forbidden salami, you could be swapping out nutritious foods for less-healthy replacements. For example, it's not rare for me to have a pregnant client describe her choice to ditch eggs in the morning in favor of cereal, simply because she was warned that she *might* get sick from eating eggs with runny yolks. Though that one swap may seem minor, it could limit her intake of protein, choline, DHA, iodine, and a variety of other nutrients. In this case, she'd be replacing all the goodness of eggs with refined carbohydrates (and likely added sugars), which offer zero benefits and potential risks. Little does she know, the odds that an egg contains *Salmonella* are estimated to be between 1 in 12,000 to 1 in 30,000.[5] In other words, very rare. The odds are 7-fold lower if she eats eggs from an organic farm or from chickens raised on pasture.[6]

Another good example of biased information is the prenatal recommendation on fish. I outlined the risks and benefits of fish intake and mercury in the previous chapter; however, most women are not given enough information on fish to make an informed decision. One focus group on pregnant women in the United States found that, "Many women knew that fish might contain mercury, a neurotoxin, and had received advice to limit fish intake. Fewer women knew that fish contains DHA or what the function of DHA is. None of the women had received advice to eat fish, and most had not received information about which fish types contain more DHA or less mercury."[7] I'd also wager they never received information on selenium and its role in preventing mercury toxicity.

Sadly, the risks of mercury tend to make headlines more than the nutritional benefits of fish and seafood—and as a result, we have a lot more pregnant women missing out on the DHA, iodine, zinc, iron, vitamin B6, vitamin B12, glycine, and other nutrients that are abundant in many *safe-to-eat* types of fish. Essentially, this lack of information—or blatant misinformation—means that many women "would rather avoid fish than possibly harm themselves or their infants."[8] Not surprisingly, the benefits vs. risk equation is opposite in Japan. One Japanese physician, who had one pregnancy in Japan and her other two in the United States, wrote about her experience: "In Japan, it is commonly accepted that the benefits of fish oils override the risks of mercury intake from fish consumption."[9]

Aside from mercury, women are often warned to avoid eating raw fish or sushi due to risks of food poisoning, however that recommendation remains controversial. In Japan, consumption of raw fish is not only common during pregnancy, but *encouraged* for optimal fetal development. It is also condoned by the British National Health Service on their website: "It's usually safe to eat sushi and other dishes made with raw fish when you're pregnant."[10] A Canadian medical journal explains the rationale: "Seafood marketed for human consumption undergoes screening for microbial contamination, thus increasing the safety of commercially available products. Cooking is the most effective method for inactivation of parasites, although flash-freezing is also effective and is often used for sushi-grade fish. Pregnant women need not avoid raw fish if it is obtained from a reputable establishment, stored properly, and consumed soon after purchase."[11]

Even more interesting is that I noticed personally (and among many prenatal clients) that cravings for raw fish or sushi are sometimes heightened during pregnancy even when cooked fish was off-putting. This might be a sign your body is smarter than you think. It turns out that in some types of fish, including salmon, bioavailability of selenium is higher when it is eaten raw.[12] Given the role of selenium in preventing mercury toxicity, this could be your body's way of protecting you. Furthermore, some data has shown that omega-3 fats are more absorbable from raw fish than from cooked fish and that iodine levels are higher (iodine levels drop by up to 58% when fish is cooked).[13,14] Perhaps your body has your baby's brain development in mind. One important consideration, if you choose to eat raw fish, is to seek wild-caught instead of farmed fish in order to avoid exposure to antibiotic-resistant bacteria.[15]

The one exception I take to this is *raw* shellfish. Shellfish, such as oysters and clams, account for roughly 75% of seafood-associated outbreaks of foodborne illness.[16] In this case, my opinion is that the risks are not worth the benefits. Unless you're absolutely certain of the freshness and source, I'd ensure any shellfish you eat has been thoroughly cooked. Shellfish is incredibly nutrient-dense and I encourage you to eat *cooked* shellfish if you enjoy it.

Having worked in public policy myself, I can appreciate the rationale for blanket recommendations. However, you should be wary when taking them 100% literally, because in reality, there are no absolute safe or unsafe foods. Certain foods may be more likely to get contaminated, but paradoxically, are often not the foods associated with the majority of outbreaks.

In a U.S. Centers for Disease Control and Prevention (CDC) analysis of *Listeria* outbreaks from 2009-2011, cheese made from pasteurized milk (*not*

Real Food for Pregnancy

raw milk) was to blame for all but one of the outbreaks linked to dairy products.[17] The one outbreak tied to raw cheese was served at a wedding banquet, and catered events are notorious for improper food storage and handling. Of a total of 224 people infected with *Listeria* during those years, 147 became ill from eating raw cantaloupe. Another outbreak was traced back to raw, pre-cut celery. In 2016, the CDC investigated five outbreaks of *Salmonella*. One was due to eggs, but the remaining four were from plant foods, including alfalfa sprouts (two outbreaks), pistachios, and a vegan protein powder.[18]

I share these examples to drive home the point that no specific food is guaranteed safe and, likewise, no specific food is guaranteed dangerous. Pasteurized milk can still be contaminated during handling or storage. Nowadays, raw milk producers in the United States are under such strict scrutiny that many actually have bacterial counts far, far lower than commercial producers who can rely on pasteurization to kill bad bacteria. An analysis of raw milk from 21 artisan cheese producers in Vermont did not find a single sample positive for *Listeria, Salmonella,* or the dangerous strain of *E. coli* known as *O157:H7*.[19] They conclude: "Our results indicate that the majority of raw milk produced for small-scale artisan cheesemaking was of high microbiological quality with no detectable target pathogens despite the repeat sampling of farms." Perhaps that tasty raw milk cheddar is safer than you've been told.

Finally, allow me to play devil's advocate for a minute. Most of the conventional "foods to avoid" are of animal origin, however vegetables and fruits can be just as risky; they are not a guaranteed safe choice. If you're at an outdoor potluck in the summer heat with food sitting out for hours, you should be just as careful eating egg salad as you should with fruit salad or green salad. Plant foods, mostly fresh fruit and leafy vegetables, are the cause of 46% of food poisoning cases.[20] In fact, a 2013 analysis of outbreaks found that leafy green vegetables account for more food borne illnesses than any other food type and they are the second most frequent cause of hospitalizations due to food poisoning.[21] Yet, you never hear health officials warning pregnant moms to avoid eating salad. As one researcher puts it, "Fruit and vegetables are major components of a healthy diet, but eating fresh uncooked produce is not risk free."[22] This begs the question: Why should produce get a pass, while eggs with runny yolks, deli meat, and soft cheese get the scarlet letter?

After taking all of this into consideration, you can probably understand why I do not subscribe to conventional prenatal nutrition advice regarding foods to avoid. My stance may seem rogue, but there are a growing number of healthcare professionals who agree that stringent guidelines are no longer warranted, including these researchers who explain:

> *"Improved standards and surveillance have reduced the prevalence of contaminated foods at grocery stores. Therefore, it is no longer necessary for pregnant women to avoid foods like deli meats and soft cheeses (associated with Listeria); soft-cooked eggs (associated with Salmonella); or sushi and sashimi... As general guidelines to food safety, pregnant women should ensure that their food is obtained from reputable establishments; stored, handled, and cooked properly; and consumed in a timely manner."*[23]

When weighing the benefits and risks of eating certain foods, you must take into consideration the nutrients they contain as well as your chances of getting sick. The source and handling of *any* food can make an otherwise "safe" food a questionable choice. If, out of personal preference, you decide not to eat soft cheese, eggs with runny yolks, or deli meat, that's entirely OK. You can also opt for eggs with fully-cooked yolks and to eat deli meat that has been heated to steaming to lessen exposure to potential pathogens, while still benefiting from the nutrients in these foods. For those of you who choose otherwise, rest assured that the risks associated with eating such foods are likely minimal. Whatever your choice, take into consideration the following food safety precautions.

Food Safety Precautions

Even if you think you have an "iron gut," you can still get sick from eating improperly handled foods. Here are some tips to limit exposure to common foodborne pathogens:

- Trust your nose. If smells funny, don't eat it.
- Be smart about where you purchase perishable food. For example, an egg salad sandwich is probably not very fresh if purchased at a gas station compared to a nice deli.
- Avoid purchasing pre-cut vegetables or fruit, unless you plan to cook them before eating. Cut produce is far more likely to be contaminated with pathogens.[24]
- Cook at home more often. The majority of foodborne illnesses are linked to foods consumed at restaurants and ready-to-eat meals.[25]
- Defrost frozen meat in your refrigerator overnight (not on the counter). Do not store raw meat in your fridge for more than 2-3 days.
- Clean up before cooking and eating. Wash your hands and clean your counters, cutting boards, and anything that will come in contact with your food. Consider using a specific cutting board for meat only. You can use white vinegar to safely sanitize your kitchen.

- Be sure to wash your hands after handling raw meat (yes, before you grab the salt and pepper or touch your counters!).
- Separate raw and cooked foods to avoid cross-contamination. For example, if you are marinating raw meat, do not put fully-cooked meat back in the container it was marinated in (and do not consume the marinade, unless it is brought to a full boil first).
- Avoid raw shellfish.
- Refrigerate leftovers within 2 hours after cooking (sooner if your home is very warm).
- Consume refrigerated leftovers within 3-4 days (or freeze for long-term storage).
- If you doubt the freshness or source of any food, simply don't eat it.

Support Your Immune System

Aside from the above precautions, you can take additional steps to prevent foodborne illness by making your immune health a top priority in pregnancy. An estimated 80% of your immune system resides in your gut and what you eat directly affects your gut health. Here are a few ways you can boost your digestive and immune health:

- Eat fermented foods regularly to introduce probiotics into your diet, such as yogurt, kefir, sauerkraut, kimchi, kombucha, and naturally-fermented "pickled" vegetables. Ensure fermented vegetables are raw or unpasteurized (and from a reputable source); cooked or pasteurized products no longer contain live cultures.
- Eat foods rich in prebiotic fiber, which serves as food for the probiotics in your gut, such as vegetables (especially locally-grown cruciferous vegetables like cabbage, kale, and Brussels sprouts), fruit (especially berries and slightly under-ripe bananas), nuts, seeds (especially chia seeds), and legumes.[26]
- Include bone broth and slow-cooked meat in your diet regularly. The gelatin these foods contain helps maintain a healthy gut lining and thus improves your resilience to foodborne pathogens.
- Limit your intake of sugar and refined carbohydrates, as both are linked to suppressed immune function and imbalanced gut bacteria.[27]
- Know your farmer. Choose meat, poultry, dairy, and eggs from organic and pasture-raised sources to avoid exposure to antibiotic residues and pathogens. As previously mentioned, organic poultry farms have a 7-fold lower rate of *Salmonella* infection compared to commercial producers.[28] Cows raised by organic methods have significantly lower levels of antibiotic-resistant bacteria (which often

cause the most serious foodborne illnesses in humans) than those raised on conventional farms.[29] Small, artisan dairy farms following strict hygiene practices often have raw milk with bacterial counts lower than what's permitted in pasteurized dairy.[30] Once again, quality counts!

Foods to Limit or Avoid

The other category of foods to avoid are those that don't offer optimal nutrition for you and your baby, or may increase your chances of certain pregnancy complications. Some of these are commonly discussed, like alcohol and caffeine, while others are usually glossed over. At the end of the day, these foods/ingredients are simply not essential to your health, do not provide a rich source of nutrients to support your baby's development, and at a certain threshold of intake, could be harmful. The choice to limit or strictly avoid the following foods is up to you. I'll simply provide you with the research, so you can make an informed decision.

Alcohol

You're probably already aware that alcohol is best avoided during pregnancy. Alcohol readily crosses the placenta and can impact your baby's development. Fetal Alcohol Spectrum Disorders (FASDs), a collective term that includes a continuum of disorders seen in children exposed to alcohol in utero, is the main concern. FASDs shows up differently from one child to another, but the one common thread is intellectual or behavioral impairment. The most publicized and severe form of FASDs is Fetal Alcohol Syndrome, in which a child may have numerous developmental problems, including intellectual deficits, hearing problems, abnormal facial development, and stunted growth.[31]

There have been dozens of studies performed to better understand the risks of alcohol consumption in pregnancy, since it is still common in some parts of the world. One challenge in studying prenatal alcohol exposure is that researchers can't randomize studies and force some women to drink and others to abstain. That means studies rely on observing women who choose to drink and those who don't. Since most women have been told to abstain from alcohol, those who choose to drink may also not be heeding other advice, such as not smoking, not using drugs, or eating a healthy diet. For example, one frequently cited study concluded that having even 1 alcoholic drink per week while pregnant was associated with behavior problems in children.[32] But, when you examine the data a little closer, you might be surprised to learn that use of cocaine—*yes, cocaine*—was alarmingly high.

Real Food for Pregnancy

Nearly half (45%) of women who drank alcohol also used cocaine during their pregnancy compared to 18% cocaine use by non-drinkers (still a shocking number, if you ask me). Instead of naming this research paper *Prenatal Alcohol Exposure and Childhood Behavior at Age 6 to 7 years: Dose-response Effect*, a more accurate title would be something like *Illicit Drug Use in Pregnancy Linked to Childhood Behavior Problems.*

The other major challenge is defining what level of alcohol consumption is safe or unsafe and that's where things get a bit murky. In a review of 34 studies on prenatal alcohol exposure, binge drinking—more than 4 drinks on one occasion—was clearly detrimental to childhood cognition. That probably comes as no surprise. However, these researchers found that even mild to moderate alcohol consumption (up to 6 drinks per week) may impact children's behavior or cognition.[33] They conclude: "there is no known safe amount of alcohol to consume while pregnant."

Several studies have found conflicting results, concluding that low amounts of alcohol are *not* harmful. A study of 3,000 women in Australia examined the effects of drinking on behavior problems in children from ages 2 to 14. The women were split into 5 groups based on the level of alcohol they consumed during pregnancy: no alcohol, occasional drinking (1 drink/week), light drinking (2-6 drinks/week), moderate drinking (7-10 drinks/week) and heavy drinking (11 drinks/week). In this study, light to moderate prenatal alcohol consumption was not associated with behavioral problems. In fact, when you look at the original data, you can see that light drinkers apparently have children with *lower* rates of behavioral problems compared to those who abstained entirely.[34]

In another large, well-designed study of roughly 5,000 mothers and their children, researchers looked at prenatal drinking behaviors and a child's IQ at age 14. In this study, the women were stratified into 4 groups: no drinking, less than ½ glass per day, ½ to 1 glass per day, and more than 1 glass per day. This study found no evidence that alcohol consumption at an average of less than 1 glass per day had any significant impact on IQ scores, attention, or cognitive abilities.[35]

In an analysis of over 10,000 women (and their children), researchers found that speech and language skills in children were no different if their mothers either abstained or drank small amounts of alcohol during pregnancy. They defined small amounts of alcohol as less than 10 g per day.[36] For reference, a typical 12 oz beer (4-6% alcohol by volume) can contain anywhere from 11-17 g of alcohol and a typical 5 oz glass of wine (12% alcohol by volume) contains 14 g of alcohol. Nonetheless, these researchers caution that, "Healthcare providers should continue to advise abstinence from alcohol during pregnancy until further evidence on the effect of low-moderate gestational alcohol use becomes available... International guidelines have not reached consensus on safe alcohol recommendations for pregnant women."[37]

My conclusions about alcohol

When it comes to alcohol, the evidence is mixed. The general trend from the research is that very low amounts of alcohol are less likely to cause problems than large amounts, but there's also not a consensus that points to an amount that's guaranteed harmless. In my opinion, there also aren't enough nutritional benefits to justify regular alcohol consumption during pregnancy. It's likely that "the dose makes the poison," but the challenge remains defining what dose that is and if that dose is the same woman-to-woman. What one woman considers a small amount of alcohol can be quite a lot to another. Similarly, everyone's tolerance to alcohol varies. I certainly wouldn't sweat having a few sips of wine on occasion, but I wouldn't go so far to suggest you have several glasses to yourself every night, especially if you get "tipsy" easily. Again, that choice is ultimately yours to make. You are the only one who knows your alcohol tolerance.

Some of the reported harms of alcohol on fetal development, especially among heavy drinkers, may be due to the depletion of nutrients because the body must direct them towards detoxification of alcohol rather than fetal needs. These include B-vitamins (such as folate), vitamin A, glycine, selenium, zinc, and choline. This theory is supported by animal data showing alcohol-induced depletion of zinc in pregnant rats.[38] There's also human data to suggest that choline and its metabolites, which are essential to liver function, may be depleted with prenatal alcohol consumption.[39] This is important because these nutrients play a role in brain development and methylation. Thus, it's possible that requirements for certain nutrients may be higher for women who drink during pregnancy—and especially in those with low nutrient reserves or a poor diet—but this has yet to be studied.

At the end of the day, I'd want all available nutrients to go to my baby and not be directed towards detoxifying alcohol.

Note: The one exception I take is fermented beverages that have naturally very low amounts of alcohol and offer the benefits of probiotics, such as kombucha, a type of fermented tea. Kombucha is typically <0.5% alcohol by volume, so an 8 oz serving will provide less than 1 g of alcohol. Even overripe fruit can have alcohol concentrations higher than kombucha (ranging from 0.6-8.1% alcohol by volume).[40]

Real Food for Pregnancy

Caffeine

To have coffee or not to have coffee? That is the question. Luckily, it's a little more nuanced than that. The safety of caffeine in pregnancy is, not surprisingly, controversial. What we know is that caffeine crosses the placenta and that a baby's caffeine levels are similar to mom's. Also, the rate at which your body eliminates caffeine from your bloodstream decreases over the course of pregnancy.[41] Furthermore, higher maternal levels of caffeine can reduce placental blood flow, potentially limiting nutrient transfer to the baby.[42] Research from 20-30 years ago showed that a high intake of caffeine was associated with an increased risk of miscarriage and restricted fetal growth. This resulted in the precaution that pregnant women should not exceed intakes of 200 mg of caffeine per day.[43]

To put that into perspective, 8 oz of coffee has about 100 mg of caffeine, depending on brewing methods. The stronger you like your coffee, the more caffeine it contains. Also, remember that most of us consider 12 oz to be a proper "cup o' Joe." Other sources of caffeine are tea and chocolate—8 oz of black tea has roughly 30 mg (green, white, and oolong tea also contain caffeine, but in lower amounts); an ounce of dark chocolate has 20-30 mg.

Given that coffee consumption is so common, many researchers have continued to explore the effects of caffeine on pregnancy to try to confirm or refute the 200 mg precautionary limit. Unfortunately, these studies have found mixed results. A major review of data from 53 studies aimed at identifying a more evidence-based, safe level of caffeine in pregnancy came up empty-handed.[44] They found that while higher levels of caffeine were linked to higher odds of miscarriage, stillbirth, and low birth weight, there was no clear threshold at which caffeine was either safe or harmful. They concluded there was not enough evidence to change official recommendations on caffeine, noting: "A number of questions still remain to be answered. These include confirming causality, such as identifying whether caffeine is the causal agent, one of its metabolites, or whether the associations are completely explained by publication bias or caffeine being a marker of healthy pregnancy." It's also worth mentioning that for some women, soda—*not coffee*—is the major source of caffeine in the diet.[45] In this case, the refined sugar and additives in soda would confound any findings on caffeine.

Per usual in prenatal research, we may never have direct evidence because it's unethical to subject pregnant women to potential harm from consuming a lot of caffeine. At this time, it's wise to stay on the safe side and keep caffeine intake at or below 200 mg per day. That means up to 16 oz of coffee per day is probably A-ok. If you're not a coffee-drinker, you're probably in the clear, as it would be hard to consume excessive amounts of caffeine from tea or chocolate alone.

Note: If you drink coffee, consider the quality. Conventional coffee production involves the application of numerous pesticides. Buy coffee that is USDA certified organic or Rainforest Alliance approved to avoid pesticide residues. For more on pesticides, see Chapter 10.

Refined Carbohydrates

Carbohydrates that have been "refined" are those that have been processed heavily, most often to remove fiber and/or be turned into flour or starch. For example, whole wheat can be refined into white flour and whole corn can be refined into corn starch. Refined carbohydrates digest and absorb rapidly, causing a major spike in blood sugar. In other words, these foods have a high glycemic index. They also tend to have low nutrient-density, meaning they are primarily composed of carbohydrates while being low in vitamins, minerals, and antioxidants. These "filler foods" leave less room for more nutrient-dense foods in your diet.

Foods High in Refined Carbohydrates:

- Refined grain products, including anything made from white flour or "enriched" flour (bread, bagels, pizza, pasta, noodles, crackers, pretzels, chips, etc.)
- Breakfast cereal (yes, even those made from whole grains with no added sugar)
- "Puffed" grains (popcorn, rice cakes, etc.)
- "Instant" products, namely instant rice (or quick-cooking rice), instant noodles (like ramen), instant potatoes, and instant oatmeal (or quick oats)
- White rice

In general, the more refined carbohydrates you eat, the less nutritious your diet is overall. A study into the micronutrient content of prenatal diets found that intake of refined carbohydrates was the number one predictor of a nutrient-deficient diet. The authors of this study noted that "Changes in micronutrient intake were largely predicted by changes in carbohydrate quality. Specifically, higher starch intake predicted a less favorable micronutrient profile."[46] This is crucial to note because the average American consumes far more refined carbohydrates than they realize. In fact, 85% of grains consumed in the U.S. are in the form of refined grains.[47]

Real Food for Pregnancy

What about whole grains?

Aside from the refined carbohydrates listed above, it's important to recognize that even certain whole foods can provide a lot more carbohydrates and a lot fewer nutrients than you might expect. For example, many women think whole grains are a necessity in a prenatal diet, noting that they need to eat them to get enough fiber. However, even a "good" whole grain bread might have 2-5 g of fiber per slice, but 15-20 g total carbohydrates. Another example is brown rice, which offers only 3.5 g of fiber per cup, but a whopping 45 g of total carbohydrates. At the end of the day, these foods are mostly carbohydrates and not very "dense" in fiber.

It's worth noting you can get 5 g of fiber in just 2 tablespoons of coconut flour, ⅓ of an avocado, 1 tablespoon of chia seeds, or ¾ cup raspberries. Like non-starchy vegetables, these foods naturally come with much lower levels of total carbohydrates than grains and significantly more micronutrients. In other words, there are plenty of non-grain sources of fiber. The meal plans in this book, which contain limited quantities of grains, have 35-45 g of fiber per day, which is well above the recommended minimum intake of 28 g during pregnancy. For more examples of high-fiber, low-carb foods, see the section about constipation in Chapter 7.

Another rationale used to promote heavy intake of whole grains is their B-vitamin and mineral content. But if you compare nutrient levels in grains to that of other whole foods, like seafood, meat, and vegetables, it becomes clear that grains are far less nutritious than we've been led to believe. Compared to the above foods, whole grains have particularly low nutrient-density for the 13 vitamins and minerals most commonly lacking in American diets.[48] **Replace your typical serving of grains with a serving of vegetables and/or a larger portion of meat or fish and you're practically guaranteed to consume more B-vitamins, iron, magnesium, zinc, and calcium.**

When it comes to your blood sugar, whole grains are marginally better than refined grains, however they *still* raise your blood sugar significantly. In one study that compared white bread to whole wheat sourdough (made from freshly ground whole wheat flour that was "soured" through traditional fermentation; in other words, this was good sourdough), blood sugar responses did not follow the predicted trend. Rather surprisingly, some participants showed *higher* blood sugar levels from the *whole wheat sourdough* bread.[49] I'd still personally recommend the traditional whole wheat sourdough or a sprouted grain bread, since the fermentation process aids in digestion and nutrient absorption, as well as for the higher micronutrient levels (compared to white bread), however just because it's "natural" or "less processed" doesn't mean you get a free pass to eat unlimited amounts.

Lastly, an increasing number of people have health problems related to consumption of gluten, a protein found in certain grains, most notably wheat, rye, and barley.[50] Conventional medicine is slow to accept the existence of gluten-related disorders outside of classic celiac disease, however I frequently see non-celiac gluten sensitivity in my nutrition practice. If you've personally seen improvements in your health from eating a gluten-free diet, there's no need to reintroduce gluten-containing grains during pregnancy to make your diet more "nutritionally complete" or "well rounded." A gluten-free diet can absolutely meet your nutrient needs and may actually be more nutrient-dense if you opt to replace gluten-containing grains with whole foods (instead of replacing gluten with gluten-free flour and processed foods made with these refined carbohydrates).[51]

Most of us are accustomed to including grains in our diet—and that's ok—as long as they are eaten in relatively small quantities and they don't displace other more nutrient-dense foods, like vegetables, meat, fish, poultry, dairy, nuts, seeds, and legumes. For this reason, you'll see whole grains included in the meal plans in this book, just in small portions. I do this to give you some context, as it's surprisingly easy to overeat grains (and carbohydrates as a whole). One slice of sprouted grain bread with your eggs in the morning is far different than having a large bowl of oatmeal for breakfast, a sandwich for lunch, crackers as a snack, and whole wheat pasta for dinner all in the same day. If you follow a grain-free, gluten-free, paleo-inspired diet, or for any reason feel better 100% grain-free, you can easily replace the grains in the meal plans with other foods, as outlined in Chapter 5.

Sugar

It might be obvious to you already, but foods that contain high amounts of sugar (added *or* naturally occurring) are not the best choice during pregnancy. Excessive intake of sugar ups your chances of gaining too much weight during pregnancy and of your baby growing too large.[52] Eating too much sugar can also increase your chances of developing gestational diabetes.[53] A mom's sugar intake in pregnancy can predispose her children to asthma or eczema.[54] Plus, sugar tends to displace healthier foods, can be addictive, and may actually set up your child's brain to prefer sweet foods later in life.[55] Studies in mice have found that a high-sugar prenatal diet results in impaired brain development in the offspring and a predisposition for ADHD-like behavior, including low attention span and impulsive behavior.[56] Essentially, there are no studies that suggest sugar is *beneficial* in any way to pregnancy outcomes.

As you may already know, sugar is a hidden ingredient in many different food products. Food manufacturers know that ingredients are listed in descending order (major ingredient is first on the list), so they often include several different types of sugar in one product to make it appear lower in sugar overall. Don't be fooled. Check labels for sugar, in all of its possible names (see the below list). You can also look at the total grams of sugar to get a sense of how healthful the item is—*or isn't*. For reference, every 4 grams of sugar listed on a nutrition label is equivalent to one teaspoon of sugar. Added and naturally-occurring sugars are not separated out on nutrition labels, which is sometimes annoying and sometimes revealing when it comes to the sugar content of foods. Dried fruit, for example, is extremely concentrated in sugar. A mere ¼ cup of raisins has 25 g of sugar—that's more than 6 teaspoons!

Foods High in Sugar:

- Sugar: white sugar, brown sugar, raw sugar, evaporated cane juice, molasses, honey, agave nectar, syrups (like corn syrup, maple syrup, or brown rice syrup), date sugar, coconut sugar, maltodextrin, sucr*ose*, dextr*ose*, fruct*ose*, malt*ose*, etc. (if an ingredient ends in "-ose," it's a type of sugar).
- Sweets/Desserts: candy, ice cream, frozen yogurt, sorbet, cake, pastries, doughnuts, cookies, pie, popsicles, jam/jelly, etc.
- Sweet drinks: soda, punch, lemonade, fruit juice (even 100%, fresh-squeezed juice), sweet tea, flavored milk, aguas frescas, etc.
- Foods naturally high in sugar: dried fruit (dried cranberries, raisins, dates, etc.), fruit smoothies, juices, etc.
- Sauces made with a lot of sugar: ketchup, BBQ sauce, teriyaki sauce, honey mustard, etc.

Please know, I've never met a woman who abstained *entirely* from sugar while pregnant, myself included. There's the perfect world, then there's reality. So, when you *do* have a little sweet treat, remember to keep your portions small, eat them mindfully (savoring every bite), and perhaps consider eating a little less of other carbohydrate-rich foods with that meal, so your body doesn't get overwhelmed with a huge blood sugar spike. For example, if you want ice cream after dinner, you might opt for a lower-carbohydrate dinner and have an extra side of non-starchy vegetables instead of potatoes.

Also, be aware that less-processed sources of sugar, such as dried fruit, honey, and maple syrup, are still very concentrated in sugar. I prefer those to refined sweeteners like white sugar or corn syrup, thanks to their complex flavors and trace amounts of other nutrients, but they are *still sugar* and should be a minimal part of your overall diet. You'll get a sense for how I incorporate natural sweeteners in modest amounts in the desserts featured in the Recipe Appendix.

Artificial Sweeteners

Artificial sweeteners are a controversial topic; however, I believe that eating food as close to what our ancestors ate is almost always safest. Artificial sweeteners rely on chemicals that trick your body into tasting sweet. Research shows that the more your taste buds are *exposed* to sweet foods (from real or artificial sweeteners), the more your taste buds *prefer* sweet foods.

According to one scientist, "Artificial sweeteners, precisely because they are sweet, encourage sugar craving and sugar dependence. Repeated exposure trains flavor preference. A strong correlation exists between a person's customary intake of a flavor and his preferred intensity for that flavor."[57]

Simply put, the less we expose ourselves to sweet tastes, from naturally sweet foods or artificial sweeteners, the less our taste buds will crave them.

The other problem with artificial sweeteners is their effect on your blood sugar. For many years it was believed that artificial sweeteners do not *and cannot* raise blood sugar levels, but newer research flipped this thinking upside down when it was revealed that people who consumed the most artificial sweeteners were more likely to have blood sugar problems. It appears that artificial sweeteners interact with the microbes in your gut (probiotics), which leads to elevations in blood sugar. In one study, people saw a 2 to 4-fold increase in blood sugar after consuming artificial sweeteners (aspartame, sucralose, and saccharin were tested in this particular study).[58]

Artificial sweeteners don't just change the good bacteria in your gut, they can actually kill them. This is particularly true of Splenda (sucralose), which after only 12 weeks of use has been shown to significantly decrease populations of good bacteria in the gut (specifically, total anaerobes, bifidobacteria, lactobacilli, bacteroides, clostridia, and total aerobic bacteria were all decreased).[59] This happened with daily doses only *one fifth* of the "safe" level (called the Acceptable Daily Intake) set by the FDA.

There is so little we understand about how our microbiome—the populations of good bacteria in the body—affects our health, but it's a growing area of research, especially in the world of prenatal health. Since you pass on your microbes to your baby, it's best to do everything you can to support the natural and healthy populations of bacteria in your body. Probiotics may have far reaching beneficial effects on the immune system, blood sugar regulation, hormone balance, detoxification, and digestive health. For more on this topic, see the probiotic section in Chapter 6.

In addition to interfering with blood sugar balance and the gut microbiome, artificial sweeteners may impact thyroid hormones as well. Sucralose, in particular, has been shown to depress thyroid function, which could have a carryover effect on fetal brain development.[60] See Chapter 9 for more on thyroid health and Chapter 10 for additional chemicals that interfere with thyroid function.

Another problem with artificial sweeteners is that they may impact your child's propensity for obesity later in life. A 2017 study found that children of women who consumed artificial sweeteners on a daily basis during pregnancy were 1.6x more likely to be born large (macrosomia) and 1.9x more likely to be overweight or obese at age 7 compared to those who consumed none.[61] In addition, this study showed that drinking artificially-sweetened drinks during pregnancy in place of sugar-sweetened drinks (i.e. diet soda instead of regular soda) was linked to an increased risk of childhood obesity at 7 years, which was opposite of what the researchers expected. This echoes the findings from studies in adults in which artificial sweeteners, despite having zero calories and zero sugar, do not help with weight loss and may actually be linked to weight gain.

The authors of the above study sum it up well: "The high-intensity artificial sweeteners compared with glucose or sucrose may exacerbate glucose intolerance at a greater magnitude via alterations of gut microbiota, increase intestinal glucose absorption through apical glucose transporter 2 and promote excessive intake and weight gain via dysregulation of sweet taste and caloric reward."[62]

I suggest avoiding artificial sweeteners and simply getting used to things tasting less sweet. When you need an occasional treat, eat a small amount of the real thing or opt for one of the safe alternatives (see below).

Artificial Sweeteners to Avoid:

- Aspartame
- Sucralose
- Saccharin
- Acesulfame potassium
- Neotame

Safe Alternatives to Artificial Sweeteners

First of all, let me reiterate that when it comes to anything sweet, it's best to keep it to a minimum. That's easier said than done if you've had a sweet tooth for a while. If that's you and you want a sugar alternative, you can try either stevia or sugar alcohols.

Stevia-derived sweeteners (called steviosides) are extracted from the South American plant, stevia, and are generally considered safe during pregnancy. Unlike artificial sweeteners, which can raise blood sugar levels, stevia does not have that effect and may actually help reduce blood sugar levels.[63] Depending on the product, some can have a bitter aftertaste, so you might need to shop around to find one you like.

Sugar alcohols are another option. Despite the name, they don't contain the type of alcohol that makes you drunk. Sugar alcohols have a fraction of the calories, but the familiar granular texture and pleasant flavor of table sugar (with no strange aftertaste that some people notice with stevia). Keep in mind that some sugar alcohols can cause digestive discomfort, such as gas and diarrhea, so don't go overboard! The two sugar alcohols that are least likely to mess up your digestion are xylitol and erythritol. Erythritol tends to be the preferred choice amongst low-carb bakers and those with a sensitive gut.

Vegetable Oils

As I have explained in previous chapters, it's important that you eat enough fat during pregnancy. But, the type of fat you consume matters. Vegetable oils are those that are extracted from seed crops, like canola (rapeseed), soy, corn, safflower, and cottonseed. A better name for them would be "processed seed oils," but the way they are marketed in the grocery store is "vegetable oils." Prior to the last century, humans didn't have the ability to extract a significant quantity of vegetable oils from seed crops, meaning we didn't eat much of them. It takes intensive modern farming and sophisticated machinery to extract, refine, and deodorize vegetable oils, plus a slew of chemical solvents and acids to get the job done.

Although many health professionals praise vegetable oils for being healthy because they are low in saturated fat, this couldn't be more misguided. Despite the majority of people replacing animal fats with vegetable oils over the last 50 years, obesity, heart disease, diabetes, and numerous other chronic, inflammatory diseases are on the rise.[64]

Unsaturated fats, like those found in vegetable oils, are highly susceptible to damage and go rancid easily when they are exposed to air, are stored in clear plastic containers, or are heated by cooking. This creates highly toxic compounds called free radicals and reactive oxygen species, which are known contributors to pregnancy complications, including miscarriage, preterm labor, preeclampsia, and fetal growth restriction.[65]

Vegetables oils are high in a specific type of unsaturated fat called omega-6. These fats are considered pro-inflammatory, especially when consumed in large quantities compared to omega-3 fats, something that's almost guaranteed if you consume vegetable oils regularly.

The ideal ratio of omega-6 to omega-3 fats in the diet is somewhere from 1:1 to 4:1, yet unfortunately, recent estimates put this ratio closer to 10:1 among pregnant women (in some individuals, it's up to 30:1).[66,67] That's not reassuring given that "A high omega-6/omega-3 ratio, as is found in today's Western diets, promotes the pathogenesis of many diseases, including cardiovascular disease, cancer, osteoporosis, and inflammatory and autoimmune diseases."[68] This imbalance in essential fats is also problematic in pregnancy. One study found that consuming excess omega-6 fats (and not enough omega-3s) led to a surge in proinflammatory compounds called eicosanoids, which are associated with preterm labor.[69]

Brain development of your baby may also be influenced by the types of fats you eat. When psychomotor development of babies was measured at 9 months of age, it was found that mothers who consumed the most omega-6 fats had infants with delayed fine and gross motor skills.[70] This is not surprising, given that omega-6 fats compete with omega-3s within the body and may therefore prevent enough brain-boosting DHA from getting to the baby. Ultimately, this increases the odds of developmental delays in infants.[71]

Your child's metabolism may also be affected in the long run. In one study, children of mothers who ate the most omega-6 fats during pregnancy were more likely to be overweight and have excess body fat.[72] Obesity researchers warn that this effect may persist for generations, noting that "perinatal exposure to a high omega-6 diet results in a progressive accumulation of body fat across generations."[73] That means consuming too many vegetable oils now could affect not only your baby, but your future grandchildren.

The best way to limit your intake of omega-6 fats is to avoid the use of processed vegetable oils. Check the ingredient labels of snack foods, mayonnaise, salad dressings, and sauces. Avoid products made with soy, canola, cottonseed, safflower, peanut, or corn oils. Dine out less and cook more at home, as virtually all restaurants cook with cheap vegetable oils.

Commercial fried foods are the worst culprits, such as fries, onion rings, doughnuts, and potato chips, since they have been exposed to high heat (more heat exposure means higher levels of inflammatory free radicals).

When it comes to cooking, opt for saturated fats (like animal fats or coconut oil), which are naturally resistant to oxidation and breakdown. For things like salad dressing, consider making your own with extra-virgin olive oil, avocado oil, macadamia nut oil (or others listed in Chapter 2). These oils are naturally low in omega-6 fats and high in healthy monounsaturated fat.

Trans Fats

Trans fats are created when food companies take liquid vegetable oil and convert it into a solid when making shortening and margarine. They are the result of a process called "partial hydrogenation" and they show up in processed and fried foods because they extend the shelf life and last for a long time (so fast food joints don't have to replace the frying oil as often and Twinkies never go bad).

Unfortunately, these "partially hydrogenated oils" are quite harmful to your health. Not only are they linked to diabetes and cardiovascular disease outside of pregnancy, but they are known to contribute to adverse pregnancy outcomes. Since man-made trans fats are foreign to the human body, they can interfere with a variety of normal functions. The most worrying finding is that trans fats interfere with nutrient transport across the placenta. For example, trans fats disrupt normal essential fatty acid metabolism, meaning your baby may not get enough of the omega-3 fats needed for optimal brain and vision development.[74] Trans fats worsen insulin resistance, meaning your body has more trouble bringing your blood sugar down, and this effect may be passed on to your baby and increase their risk of diabetes later in life.[75] Even at relatively low levels of intake, trans fats are associated with lower birth weight, lower placental weight, and with a higher risk of preeclampsia.[76] They have been linked to fetal loss by interfering with normal placental function.[77] Lastly, a high intake of trans fats is a risk factor for preterm birth.[78]

Be vigilant about your intake of man-made trans fats. They have no benefits; only risks. Avoid foods made with "partially hydrogenated oils" such as shortening, margarine, fried foods, fast food, doughnuts, cakes, store-bought frosting, cookies, and pastries. You'll need to read the ingredients to ensure there are no hidden partially hydrogenated oils, because a labeling loophole allows food companies to include less than half a gram of trans fats *per serving* in products and still list (and advertise) "zero grams trans fats" or "trans fat free" on the packaging.

During pregnancy, when so many of us feel like we should be able to indulge, trans fats are the last thing you want indulge in! Use healthy saturated fats in place of trans fats, such as lard, butter, tallow, and coconut oil. After all, trans fats were created to replace these fats in the first place.

Note: I specify *man-made* trans fats in this section because there are actually several beneficial, naturally-occurring trans fats present in ruminant animals (such as cows and sheep). Trans fats from ruminants are the only source of *healthy* trans fats in the diet, so I want to be sure these are not mistakenly lumped together with man-made hydrogenated oils. The best known *healthy* trans fat is called conjugated linoleic acid (CLA), which has beneficial effects on metabolism, heart health, and cancer prevention.[79] In other words, naturally-occurring and man-made trans fats are polar opposites when it comes to your health. Food sources of CLA include beef, dairy products, lamb, and many types of game meat (grass-fed or grazing animals have higher levels of CLA).[80]

Soy

Despite what you've read about soy, it's not the health food you think it is, and it's especially problematic at a time when your nutrition matters most: before and during pregnancy. By now, you can appreciate how crucial certain nutrients are to a successful pregnancy. Unfortunately, there are several ways that soy works against you.

For one, soy inhibits mineral absorption. Soy is high in phytic acid, a substance that prevents absorption of essential minerals including calcium, magnesium, copper, iron, and zinc.[81] As you know, minerals play many important functions in your body, including building the skeleton and teeth of your baby (such as calcium), maintaining normal blood sugar levels (magnesium is crucial for this), and helping your baby's brain develop properly (like iron and zinc).

Soy, however, must undergo extensive fermentation for phytic acid to break down.[82] Traditionally fermented soy products, like miso, natto, soy sauce, and tempeh, are some of the few soy foods that are fermented long enough to significantly reduce phytic acid. The majority of soy consumed nowadays, however, is processed by modern methods that do not reduce phytic acid levels, such as soy flour and soy protein isolates (which you find in protein shakes, bars, veggie burgers, meat substitutes, low carb tortillas/breads, and many other foods).

Aside from the effects on mineral absorption, soy also interferes with protein digestion. That's because soy contains large amounts of naturally-occurring compounds called "anti-nutrients." Many of these anti-nutrients interfere with the normal action of digestive enzymes in the body, which can affect your ability to digest food and absorb the nutrients found within them.

One such anti-nutrient in soy is an "enzyme inhibitor" for the key protein-digesting enzyme called trypsin. Much like phytic acid, trypsin inhibitors in soy are particularly resistant to breakdown, even after extensive processing.[83] Intake of anything that interferes with the digestion and absorption of protein is likely not a good idea during pregnancy when needs for protein are increased. Sadly, many health professionals who simply focus on grams of protein will often recommend soy as preferred food for pregnant women, unaware that trypsin inhibitors even exist. This is especially common if they follow conventional dogma and promote a diet low in animal protein.

Goitrogens are another class of anti-nutrients present in high amounts in soy. Goitrogens are substances that interfere with the absorption of iodine, a mineral that's required for the production of thyroid hormones.

Your thyroid gland is under a lot of stress during pregnancy. Production of thyroid hormone increases by about 50% starting in the first trimester and remains elevated until delivery. Your baby is unable to produce its own thyroid hormones until the second trimester, meaning he or she is entirely dependent on yours up until that point.[84] Because of the key role of iodine and thyroid hormone in brain development, a lack of either in early pregnancy can result in lower IQ scores or, in a worst case scenario, permanent intellectual disability in your child.[85] It's hard to believe it, but "iodine deficiency remains the leading cause of preventable mental retardation worldwide."[86] Yes, it's *that* important.

Dietary iodine requirements are higher during pregnancy, yet many women fail to meet these targets. In the United States, where iodine deficiency is not considered a major public health problem, 57% of pregnant women don't consume enough.[87] Even mild prenatal iodine deficiency has been linked to hyperactivity and attention deficit disorders in children.[88] Limiting consumption of goitrogens from food, such as soy, is one way you can ensure you absorb enough iodine, maintain normal thyroid function, and ultimately support optimal brain development in your baby.

The importance of healthy thyroid function in pregnancy and your baby's brain development is virtually undisputed in the research. As explained in a 2016 study published in *The Lancet,* "Thyroid hormone is crucial for intrauterine neurodevelopment because it regulates migration, proliferation, and differentiation of fetal neuronal cells that form grey matter later in life, as well as synaptogenesis and myelination."[89]

The hormonal effects of soy are not limited to the thyroid gland. Soy contains high levels of phytoestrogens, or "plant estrogens," which mimic the effects of estrogen in the body, and can affect a number of hormones. There's a growing body of evidence from rodent studies showing that exposure to soy phytoestrogens in pregnancy can interfere with normal fertility, reproductive organ development in the fetus, and ability to carry pregnancies to term.[90] The anti-fertility effects seem to hold true for humans as well. A study of nearly 12,000 women found that those with the highest soy intakes reported the most difficulty conceiving.[91]

Another issue with soy is contamination with pesticide residues. The majority of it is grown on large conventional farms that rely on glyphosate, a pesticide, for weed control or as a desiccant (to dry the plant to allow for quicker harvest). Among the food crops that the U.S. Department of Agriculture sets maximum allowable pesticide residue levels, soy has one of the highest.[92] This is no surprise given that most soy is genetically modified. Conservative estimates are that 94% of soy crops in the United States are GMO (genetically modified organisms). The majority of GMO soy is modified in a way to make the plant withstand high-doses of glyphosate, the active ingredient in the pesticide commercially marketed as Roundup. Essentially, farmers can spray these "Roundup-Ready" GMO soy plants with pesticides at doses that would kill normal soy plants without doing any harm. It's no coincidence that "Roundup-Ready" soy has high amounts of pesticide residues—among the highest contamination of any of our foods.[93] If you have reservations about eating genetically modified foods, it's worth noting that GMOs have not been tested for safety on pregnant women or their unborn babies.

The reason I'm so concerned about the pesticide glyphosate is due to recent research showing how toxic it is to developing babies and how it interferes with key enzymes involved in hormone metabolism. It is known to harm human placental cells and embryos even at very low doses.[94] It has also been linked to birth defects and other reproductive problems, including hormone and placental abnormalities.[95] In rat studies, maternal exposure to glyphosate causes endocrine problems, behavioral changes, and "disturbs the masculinization process" in male offspring.[96]

This may explain why agricultural workers have more pregnancy complications, on average, than other women. Exposure to glyphosate in the first trimester is linked to a higher risk of gestational diabetes.[97] But, high levels of exposure are not needed to cause damage.

Scientists that study pesticide toxicity note that "Glyphosate and its commercial herbicides severely affect embryonic and placental cells, producing mitochondrial damage, necrosis and programmed cell death with doses far below the used agricultural concentrations."[98] In one study on human placental cells, researchers observed toxicity within 18 hours of exposure at concentrations far lower than agricultural use. The toxicity was even more pronounced over time or in the presence of Roundup adjuvants (meaning the ingredients *other than* glyphosate found in commercial Roundup).[99]

In addition to pesticide residues, soy can become contaminated with another toxin: aluminum. The presence of aluminum in soy products is believed to be due to leaching from the aluminum tanks in which soybeans are acid washed/processed, or in certain instances, from the addition of mineral salts (often aluminum chloride). Most commercial tofu, for example, is pressed in aluminum boxes (in place of the traditional wooden boxes), which leaches aluminum into the final product.

Aluminum is a toxic metal with no known beneficial effects in the human body. It preferentially accumulates in the brain and has been linked to neurological problems.[100] Perhaps this is why the American Academy of Pediatrics once had warnings against the use of soy formula, specifically citing aluminum toxicity as one of its concerns. It's well-established that soy formulas "contain high concentrations of phytate, aluminum, and phytoestrogens (isoflavones), which might have untoward effects."[101]

Aluminum readily crosses the placenta and, at least in studies on mice, has shown toxicity to placental and uterine cells.[102] Another study, which monitored outcomes of mice that were exposed to aluminum via their mother's diet during pregnancy and through lactation, found "significant and dose-dependent disturbance in the levels of neurotransmitters" in offspring, including serotonin and dopamine. These pups also had deficits in sensory motor reflexes and movement behaviors, as well as weight gain. The researchers' conclusion says it best: "Aluminum exposure during pregnancy has potential neurotoxic hazards to the in utero developing fetus brain."[103]

In a review of the evidence mounting against aluminum exposure during pregnancy, researchers concluded "experimental data suggest that oral exposure during pregnancy can produce significant changes in the tissue distribution of multiple essential trace elements, with

possible consequences on fetal metabolism."[104] Perhaps more frightening is the recent finding that aluminum and glyphosate may be even more toxic, particularly to the brain, when exposed together.[105] That would make soy a double whammy in this regard.

Since we'll likely never have randomized, controlled *human* studies on prenatal diets that are intentionally high or low in soy (for obvious ethical reasons), you can be proactive by limiting your intake of the anti-nutrients, estrogen-mimicking compounds, glyphosate residues, and aluminum found in soy products.

If you choose to consume soy during pregnancy, opt for fermented soy products, like soy sauce, miso, natto, and tempeh made from organically grown soybeans and only include them in your diet occasionally. At the very least, this averts the issues associated with mineral absorption and pesticide residues.

Summary

As you can see, there's a lot to consider when deciding what foods to avoid or limit during pregnancy. When weighing the benefits and risks of eating certain foods, you have to ask yourself: "Would this help build a healthy baby?" For some items, the answer is obvious. Nutrient-devoid products, like soda and cake offer no benefits. At the same time, virtually every whole food that offers nutritional benefits, like fresh vegetables and fish, can pose a food safety risk if mishandled. My hope is that you walk away with a better understanding of what's at stake when you choose to eat—*or avoid*—any particular food and can choose wisely.

Chapter 5:

Meal Plans

"Without knowledge, action is useless and knowledge without action is futile."
- Abu Bakr

By now, you've probably started taking a critical look at what foods you're eating, and you also have some ideas about what needs to shift. Or maybe I've overwhelmed you with too much research (sorry!) and you're feeling a bit stuck. This section is meant to help you see how all of this information comes together in the real world. After all, unless you can translate what you've learned onto your plate at meal time, what's the point in learning all of this?

Let me start by saying the meal plans in this book are not a prescription. They are not the *only* way to eat. They are simply a starting point. An outline. An inspiration board. They are my way of showing you how to fit nutrient-dense foods into your diet, how to balance macronutrients, and how to ensure your baby is getting the nutrition for optimal development.

Everybody's food preferences are unique, and to some degree, everyone's nutrient needs are unique, so you'll want to tweak these meal plans to fit *your* life. Nonetheless, as you learned in previous chapters, some general guidelines hold true: you require some protein and fat at each meal, you benefit from unrefined carbohydrates rather than processed ones, and you'll feel your best when eating whole foods that naturally balance your blood sugar levels.

I used the principles of The Plate Method, described in Chapter 2, to design these meals and snacks. I opted for a moderately-low carbohydrate template, as this will meet most pregnant women's needs. However, if you're struggling with gaining weight too quickly, have high blood sugar, or have high blood pressure, you can modify these meal plans to be lower carb. On the other hand, if you're very physically active, have trouble gaining weight, or otherwise feel better eating more carbohydrates, by all means, modify these meal plans with larger portions of carbs to fit your needs. I highly encourage you to incorporate mindful eating techniques along with input from your healthcare providers to find the right balance for *you*.

I intentionally did not specify the portion sizes for every single item on these meal plans. I generally suggest a minimum portion for protein, as this is what I have observed most frequently lacking for my prenatal clients. I also specify carbohydrate portions, as these are often the foods that are overdone. This is a general template that I *expect* you to modify. If 4 oz of protein is not enough for you to feel satisfied at a meal, by all means, eat more!

Calorie and macronutrient needs vary widely and therefore there's not a single meal plan that will work for all women.

On that note, feel free to swap out any items that don't agree with you. If you'd rather have pasture-raised pork than grass-fed beef, go for it. If you prefer cooking with coconut oil instead of butter, go for it. If you want asparagus at a meal instead of bell peppers and onions, that's your call. If you feel your best eating grain-free or legume-free, swap in another carbohydrate source at meals. The important point is to make these plans work for you, while still getting a good balance of nutrients. If you eat either dairy-free or grain-free, I include an example day for each.

Each of the meal plans includes 3 meals, 3 snacks, and an optional dessert. As I covered in previous sections, not everyone feels best having snacks, so let your hunger levels make that decision. You're welcome to follow the snacks listed or opt for another from the list that's included after the meal plans section. While I don't specify beverages within the daily meal plans, there is a list of healthy, low-sugar beverages included at the end of this chapter.

Believe me, I don't expect you to follow any of the meal plans to a "T." Refer back to Chapter 2 when making food swaps to ensure you're replacing one item with another that's nutritionally equivalent. Make an effort to specifically include the foods mentioned in Chapter 3 while minimizing or avoiding the foods covered in Chapter 4. Taking these extra steps will help you get enough essential vitamins, minerals, and other nutrients for you and your developing baby.

I include recipes for many of the items featured here in the Recipes Appendix at the end of the book. This book is by no means intended to be a cookbook; however, I specifically chose recipes that incorporate some of the nutrient-dense foods outlined in Chapter 3 (like liver and bone broth).

A Little Encouragement

Embracing a new way of eating can be hard. I want to remind you that you're human. There will be days where you eat a more nutritious diet than others—and that's OK. A lot of people have a pass/fail mindset with food, where if they have one less-than-stellar food choice, the rest of the day is "ruined," so they may as well eat whatever they want until the next day. Let me reassure you that shifting the way you eat is not like flipping a switch. It takes months, and sometimes *years* to fully embrace a new way of eating. Here you are doing the amazing feat of growing a new human *and* you're making the effort to eat more real food. This is not easy, so take it one recipe and one meal at a time.

The skills and taste preferences you develop now can help you—and your family—maintain good health for the rest of your life. Use the remaining months of your pregnancy to get comfortable in the kitchen, experiment with new foods, and develop a taste for real food. Your whole family will benefit.

7 Days of Real Food Meal Plans

Day 1

BREAKFAST

2-3 eggs, (from pasture-raised chickens) scrambled with spinach
Top with sharp cheddar cheese and diced tomatoes
1 orange

LUNCH

3-4 oz grilled lemon pepper salmon (wild-caught)
Asparagus, sautéed in butter
Riced cauliflower topped with fresh chives and butter
1 cup strawberries

DINNER

3-4 oz grass-fed beef burger wrapped in romaine lettuce
Top with pepper jack cheese, grilled onions, avocado, ketchup, mustard
½ cup roasted sweet potato fries

SNACKS (per your hunger)

1 nectarine + small handful of hazelnuts
carrot & cucumber slices + 12 plantain chips + guacamole
Celery + organic peanut butter

DESSERT (optional)

1 oz dark chocolate (75% cocoa or more) + almonds

Real Food for Pregnancy

Day 2

BREAKFAST

1 cup plain Greek yogurt (full-fat, unsweetened)
Fresh blueberries + macadamia nuts
Stevia + vanilla extract (optional, to taste)

LUNCH

1 cup beanless beef chili
½ cup black beans (optional)
Topped with shredded jack cheese, sour cream, salsa,
green onions, fresh lime
½ avocado

DINNER

2 salmon cakes (made with wild-caught salmon)
Mixed greens salad topped with sliced radishes, chopped almonds,
lemon-garlic dressing
½ cup fresh pineapple

SNACKS (per your hunger)

Olives + cherry tomatoes + mozzarella cheese + olive oil + fresh basil
1 oz grass-fed beef liver pate + cucumber slices or rice crackers
Hard-boiled egg + 1 slice sprouted grain bread + butter

DESSERT (optional)

Homemade berry sorbet

Day 3

BREAKFAST

Crustless spinach quiche
1-2 pork breakfast sausages (pasture-raised)
½ banana

LUNCH

2 cups homemade chicken & vegetable soup
½ cup cooked lentils (mixed into soup)
Arugula salad + lemon-herb dressing
Parmesan cheese

DINNER

3-4 oz grass-fed beef meatloaf
Roasted Brussels sprouts
½ cup roasted red potatoes

SNACKS (per your hunger)

Sardines packed in olive oil + rice crackers
1 apple + almond butter + cinnamon
½ cup plain Greek yogurt (full-fat) + 1 Tbsp chia seeds
+ vanilla extract + stevia (optional)

DESSERT (optional)

Fresh raspberries + homemade whipped cream

Real Food for Pregnancy

Day 4

BREAKFAST

Grain-free granola
1 cup whole milk, unsweetened kefir, or unsweetened almond milk
½ cup raspberries

LUNCH

3 oz lamb chop
Greek salad: romaine lettuce, ½ cup garbanzo beans, feta cheese, kalamata olives, cucumber and tomatoes
Vinaigrette dressing

DINNER

4 oz low-carb shepherd's pie
Lemon roasted broccoli
½ cup roasted sweet potato fries

SNACKS (per your hunger)

Cashews or pumpkin seeds + fresh blackberries
1 deviled egg (or a hard-boiled egg)
½ cup sweet potato fries (leftover) + 1 oz cheddar cheese

DESSERT (optional)

2 coconut macaroons

Day 5

BREAKFAST

1 cup full-fat cottage cheese
½ cup fresh mango or other fruit
Small handful of pecans
Dash of cinnamon + drizzle of honey (or stevia to taste)

LUNCH

Twice baked spaghetti squash
3-4 grass-fed beef meatballs
Cooked broccoli
1 slice buttered whole grain garlic bread (optional)

DINNER

1 cup coconut chicken curry
Roasted curried cauliflower
Spinach, sautéed in butter
½ cup potatoes or rice (optional)

SNACKS (per your hunger)

Sliced bell peppers and celery + ¼ cup spinach dip
Beef or turkey jerky
Nutty "granola" bar

DESSERT (optional)

Tart cherry gummies

Day 6 (Grain-Free Example)

BREAKFAST

2-3 eggs cooked in butter
Sautéed kale + fresh tomatoes
½ cup cooked sweet potato

LUNCH

3-4 oz baked halibut or cod (wild-caught)
Salad of romaine lettuce + shredded cabbage
Top salad with: sliced almonds, ½ cup sugar snap peas
Asian-style salad dressing
1 fresh mandarin tangerine

DINNER

3 oz chicken liver (from pasture-raised chicken) sautéed in butter
Sautéed spinach and onions
1 cup roasted butternut squash

SNACKS (per your hunger)

Small handful of almonds + 1 peach or nectarine
1 oz cheddar cheese + ½ cup black beans
Beef or turkey jerky

DESSERT (optional)

1 maple pots de creme (baked custard)

Day 7 (Dairy-Free Example)

BREAKFAST

2-3 egg omelet with veggies
Veggie filling: your choice of sautéed onion, red bell pepper,
chard or spinach, mushrooms
2 slices thick-cut bacon

LUNCH

Romaine lettuce leaves stuffed with 3-4 oz roasted turkey breast (with skin)
Top with tangy coleslaw, shredded beets, sliced green onion
1 cup roasted butternut squash

DINNER

3-4 oz slow cooker carnitas
Serve over riced cauliflower, roasted bell peppers, and onions
Top with salsa and fresh lime juice
½ avocado

SNACKS (per your hunger)

Walnuts + ½ cup blackberries or other fruit
Celery + organic peanut or almond butter
1 cup bone broth + nori seaweed snacks

DESSERT (optional)

Strawberries dipped in 1 oz melted dark chocolate (75-85% cocoa)

Snacks

Whenever I'm dreaming up snack ideas, I want to ensure they taste good, satisfy your hunger, and won't cause a huge blood sugar spike. In food terms, that means a balanced snack *always* contain a source of protein and fat to keep you satisfied and it *might* include some extra carbohydrates. Eating *just* carbohydrates for a snack, such as crackers or a piece of fruit ("naked carbohydrates"), tends to cause a spike followed by a steep drop in blood sugar, making you even *more* hungry by the time you're ready for your next meal. So, instead of plain crackers, match them with some cheese. And instead of a lone apple, pair it with some peanut butter.

Not everyone needs a significant amount of carbohydrates at snacks, so I include both a list of low-carb snacks and moderate-carb snacks to choose from. The moderate-carb snacks have roughly 15 g of carbohydrates each and make a good choice if you feel best eating a higher carbohydrate diet. These also work well before or after exercise, since your muscles will be using up energy (blood sugar) quicker at that time.

Snacks can help you eat slightly less at meals (preventing a spike in blood sugar, heartburn, and indigestion), and also prevent you from getting too hungry between meals, which can often help keep junk food cravings at bay. As always, use mindful eating to decide when and how much to have at your snacks.

Low-Carb Snack Ideas: (barely raise the blood sugar, if at all)

- Nuts or seeds - any kind (almonds, cashews, walnuts, pecans, macadamia nuts, pine nuts, sunflower seeds, etc.)
- ½ cup plain Greek yogurt + ¼ cup berries (may use stevia to sweeten)
- Beef or turkey jerky (look for one without MSG)
- Cheese, such as cheddar, jack, mozzarella, gouda, or string cheese
- ¼ cup blueberries or strawberries with unsweetened whipped cream
- Guacamole + fresh celery and bell pepper
- Small salad with pine nuts, balsamic dressing, and goat cheese
- Hard-boiled egg + salt and pepper
- Deviled egg
- Roasted nori (seaweed snacks) + avocado
- Cherry tomatoes, mozzarella, fresh basil, olive oil + balsamic vinegar
- Olives and dill pickles
- Kale chips + nuts
- ½ avocado with salt, pepper, and lemon juice
- Grilled chicken breast with pesto and Parmesan cheese

- Sardines + cucumber and bell pepper slices
- Canned oysters with lemon juice
- Roasted curried cauliflower with coconut milk + cashews
- Celery sticks with peanut butter or almond butter
- 1 oz dark chocolate + nuts (75% cacao or more; the darker, the better!)
- Grass-fed beef patty with cheese served over a small green salad
- Sautéed kale with bacon
- ¼ cup raspberries + ricotta or cottage cheese (stevia to sweeten)
- Dry salami + mozzarella cheese + cherry tomatoes

Moderate-Carb Snack Ideas: (raise the blood sugar a little)

- ½ cup homemade sweet potato fries + grilled chicken
- Quesadilla - 1 small corn tortilla + cheese + avocado + salsa + full-fat sour cream
- Taco - 1 small corn tortilla + chicken, beef, fish, or shrimp + cabbage + salsa + full-fat sour cream
- ½ cup beans or lentils + cheese
- Whole grain crackers + cheese, peanut butter, salami, or liver pate
- Whole grain crackers + sardines or canned oysters
- Medium apple + small handful of almonds or string cheese
- ½ banana + peanut or almond butter
- ½ cup fresh pineapple + cottage cheese
- ½ cup flavored Greek yogurt
- 1 cup milk + small handful of almonds
- ½ cup hummus + feta cheese + celery/carrot sticks
- ½ peanut butter sandwich on sprouted whole grain bread
- ½ sandwich with turkey or cheese (+ mustard, lettuce, tomato…)
- Open faced burger - grass-fed beef patty on 1 slice of whole grain bread
- Smoothie: ¼ cup berries, ½ cup plain Greek yogurt, 1 cup unsweetened almond milk. Stevia or vanilla extract to taste (bonus points for adding 1 Tbsp chia seeds and collagen protein!)

Beverages

Let's face it, drinking *just* water can get old. With the higher fluid needs during pregnancy (100 oz a day, remember?), you need options, so here are some things to keep in mind when you're planning what to drink.

Many drinks are a hidden source of sugar. Take fruit juice, for example. An 8 oz glass of orange juice has around 30 g of sugar, even the freshly-squeezed,

Real Food for Pregnancy

raw, with-the-pulp, organic kind. That amount of sugar is equivalent to what you get in 8 oz of soda. Even though the source is natural and fresh juice comes with more nutrients than soda, your blood sugar will respond almost identically: with a rapid spike. Like juice, smoothies are also packed with hidden sugar—some have 70 or 80 g a pop! Read the nutrition facts label before you buy.

My suggestion with drinks is to avoid drinks with naturally-occurring or added sugars, so you have more room in your diet to *eat* your carbohydrates. *Eat your fruit; don't drink it.* If you choose to have a sweetened drink, consider it your dessert.

Below are some examples of healthy beverages. These are all low in carbohydrates/sugars, except where noted.

Healthy Beverages

- Infused water: a great way to add flavor without much sugar
  - cucumber + lime
  - grapefruit + blueberries
  - peach + basil
  - strawberries or blackberries
  - orange, lemon, lime
  - strawberry + kiwi
  - apple + cinnamon sticks
  - mint + lime
  - pear + fresh ginger slices
- Sparkling water (flavored is OK, but make sure it's unsweetened)
- Unsweetened black, green, oolong, or white tea*
- Coffee (up to 16 oz per day if drinking fully caffeinated coffee)*
- Mint, ginger, rooibos (red tea) or raspberry leaf tea**
- Hot chocolate (made with unsweetened almond/coconut milk, unsweetened cocoa powder, and stevia)
- Unsweetened almond or coconut milk
- Coconut water (contains some natural sugar, but is a great source of electrolytes)
- Whole milk from pasture-raised animals (each 8 oz glass contains ~12 g carbs)
- Plain kefir (a type of fermented milk)
- Kombucha (a type of fermented tea; watch the sugar content, as it varies widely)
- Other fermented beverages, such as water kefir and kvass
- Green vegetable juice (such as celery, cucumber, spinach, kale, etc. Beware that carrot or beet juices are very high in sugar, as are fruits.)

- Bone broth (yes, it's savory, but it still counts towards your fluid intake!)

* Caffeinated drinks are best limited. Generally, it's suggested pregnant women consume no more than 200 mg of caffeine per day. 16 oz of coffee provides about 200 mg of caffeine. See Chapter 4 for a full explanation.

** Consult your healthcare provider about the use of red raspberry leaf. See Chapter 6 for more information.

Summary

Now that you have some ideas for meals, snacks, and beverages, it's time to create your perfect meal plan. Feel free to mix and match meals from different days. Let your feelings of hunger guide when and how much you eat and adjust your meal plan as needed. Remember to get creative in the kitchen! It's sometimes surprising how tasty real food can be.

Even when you slip up, or if nausea or food aversions have you eating less-than-perfectly, know that you can always return to these meal plans for inspiration and motivation. It's been said that the most effective diet is the one you don't even know you're on, meaning that enjoying your food is probably the only way to consistently stick to a certain way of eating.

Chapter 6:

Supplements

"The power of nutrition to influence health from one generation to the next is a fundamental concept that has transformed our understanding of health and disease. The health legacy of an individual is predetermined by a series of factors that occur long before birth and during the earliest days of life."
- Dr. Irma Silva-Zolezzi, Nestlé Research Center

By now you know I'm an advocate of getting your nutrients from food first before resorting to supplements. However, some nutrients are difficult to obtain in adequate amounts from food alone, especially if you're a picky eater or are facing food aversions.

Although I presented a lot of research on nutrients in Chapter 3, there's certainly more to say. This chapter will dive deeper into the nutrients you should keep on your radar when choosing prenatal supplements. You do not need to take every single supplement listed here to have a healthy pregnancy, but should you choose to take supplements, I want you to know what to look for and why these particular supplements may be beneficial. I will also point out food sources of key nutrients for those who prefer not to take supplements.

Prenatal Vitamins

It seems just about every healthcare provider recommends a prenatal vitamin, and for good reason. During pregnancy, many nutrient needs increase and some women are not able to meet these needs with diet alone. Researchers have found that intakes of vitamin D, vitamin E, iron, zinc, magnesium, and folate are often lower than recommended amounts in pregnant women.[1] Even women who eat a pretty nutrient-dense diet may fall short at some points during pregnancy. But not all prenatal vitamins are created equal, so here are a few things to keep in mind.

Most prenatal vitamins will list the the "Percent Daily Value" on the supplements facts label, and while it may be reassuring to scan the list and see "100% daily value" for each nutrient, it might be giving you a false sense of security. Some prenatal vitamins are less comprehensive than they seem, either lacking certain vitamins entirely or not including adequate amounts. It's important to keep in mind that most recommended dietary allowances (RDAs) for nutrients were set using data from adult men and adjusted via complex estimates to meet the needs of pregnancy. Also, they are set at a level to prevent severe deficiency, but not necessarily at a level for optimal nutrition.

As one study describes: "Nutrient requirements during pregnancy are usually calculated by adding an increment to the value for nonpregnant and nonlactating women that covers the cost of fetal growth and development and the associated changes in maternal tissue metabolism. This factorial approach, however, may not necessarily be correct because it does not take into account metabolic changes in absorption or excretion."[2]

Researchers have looked into the adequacy of current RDAs for pregnancy and, at least for some vitamins, actual needs may be higher than these estimates. For example, one study found that optimal vitamin B12 intake for pregnancy may be triple the current RDA.[3] Another study looked into vitamin B6 status during pregnancy, and among women meeting or exceeding the RDA, fully 58% had suboptimal blood levels at delivery, suggesting that the RDA is set too low.[4] Vitamin D needs are also significantly higher than the current RDA, likely by a factor of 10, as I describe later in this chapter. Given the above examples and the lack of solid data on numerous other nutrients, I think it's helpful to view prenatal vitamins as more of an insurance policy, meant to supplement, but *not replace* a nutrient-dense, real food diet.

Another consideration with a prenatal vitamin is that some nutrients occur in food in a different form than what's found in most supplements. Often the synthetic forms of nutrients used in supplements are not as well utilized by your body. Many supplement companies formulate their products with cost in mind, opting for the least expensive forms of vitamins rather than the most bioavailable. Look for a prenatal vitamin that contains what's called "activated" B vitamins, which are easier for your body to metabolize. It may cost more, but it's worth it.

Examples of "activated" B vitamins:

- Folate (L-methylfolate, also called 5-methyltetrahydrofolate)
- Vitamin B6 (pyridoxal-5"-phosphate)
- Vitamin B12 (methylcobalamin and/or adenosylcobalamin)

The correct form of folate is especially important (as opposed to synthetic "folic acid"), because researchers estimate that up to 60% of people have a reduced ability to use folic acid due to their genetics (a gene variant in the MTHFR enzyme) and therefore require the active form, L-methylfolate.[5] Inadequate folate intake, or supplementing with folic acid when you genetically cannot utilize it, increases the risk of neural tube defects. Luckily, food contains bioavailable forms of folate, not synthetic folic acid, so aside from what you get in a high quality prenatal vitamin, you can obtain folate by eating green leafy vegetables, legumes, liver, avocados, eggs, nuts and seeds.

In addition to choosing a prenatal with activated B vitamins, scan the label to be sure it's a comprehensive formula. Most often, I notice commercially available prenatal vitamins are lacking in iodine, vitamin B12, choline, magnesium, selenium, vitamin D, and vitamin K2. Some of these nutrients, like choline and minerals are "bulky," and therefore manufacturers leave them out or put in minimal amounts to keep the total number of pills down. Some formulas also completely leave out preformed vitamin A (retinol), opting for the less potent beta carotene. Retinol supplementation in high doses (over 10,000 IU per day) is contraindicated in pregnancy, but I have yet to see a prenatal vitamin with excessive amounts. You'll recall from Chapter 3 that a large percentage of pregnant women don't consume enough vitamin A from their diets, especially women who don't eat liver, and that beta carotene is not a reliable source of vitamin A. In other words, your prenatal vitamin should contain *at least a portion* of its vitamin A in the active form (it's often listed as retinyl palmitate on supplement labels).

Lastly, consider *how* you take your prenatal vitamin. Take it alongside a meal or snack rather than on an empty stomach, as this improves absorption and minimizes side effects, like nausea. Most of the quality prenatal vitamins require several capsules for a full daily dosage (usually the one-a-day formulas have absolute minimum quantities of vitamins and/or leave out certain nutrients). Your body can only absorb so many nutrients at one time, so to get the most out of your prenatal vitamin, you might consider splitting your dosage throughout the day. For example, if the prenatal vitamin you choose calls for 3 capsules per day, you might take 1 with each meal or 2 with breakfast and 1 with lunch. Some women find that taking a prenatal close to bedtime interferes with sleep (B vitamins can boost your energy levels); if that's you, take it earlier in the day.

If I can summarize my thoughts on prenatal vitamins in one sentence, it's this: **A prenatal vitamin is an insurance policy, but don't assume that you can get "everything" you need in a pill.**

Clearly, there's a lot to consider when choosing a high-quality prenatal vitamin. With hundreds on the market, sorting through all the options can get confusing. Because manufacturers change formulations from time to time, I decided to publish a list of recommendations on my website instead of within the book. This way, you can rest assured that my list is up-to-date.

Get my recommendations on prenatal vitamins at
www.realfoodforpregnancy.com/pnv/.

Vitamin D

While a prenatal vitamin and real food diet will cover a lot of your vitamin needs, it might not contain enough vitamin D to prevent deficiency. Vitamin D is unique in that it's the only vitamin that you make from the sun. It turns out that your diet is *not* the primary source of this nutrient, and in fact, sun exposure accounts for 90% of vitamin D in the body in those who do not supplement.[6]

However, there are a wide variety of factors that influence your ability to produce enough vitamin D from the sun. This may explain why rates of deficiency vary considerably across the globe. Nonetheless, studies estimate the prevalence of vitamin D deficiency in pregnant women worldwide ranges between 20-85%, with rates of deficiency reaching 98% in some areas.[7,8]

If you have naturally darker skin, you're are at a 6-fold higher risk for deficiency, in part due to higher levels of the pigment melanin in the skin that inhibits vitamin D production from sun exposure.[3] So keep in mind that the darker your skin tone, the more sun exposure you'll need to meet your body's demand for vitamin D. Other factors that contribute to vitamin D deficiency are avoidance of sun during midday (when your ability to make vitamin D is highest), inability to produce vitamin D from the sun in the winter in regions far from the equator (>33 degrees North or South), use of sunscreen, and wearing protective clothing.

The Institute for Medicine sets the RDA for vitamin D at 600 IU/day; however, several studies have found this level of intake to be insufficient to maintain normal vitamin D levels throughout pregnancy.[9,10] Vitamin D deficiency during pregnancy puts you at higher risk for preeclampsia, having a low birth weight infant, and gestational diabetes (according to two major meta analyses).[11,12]

Aside from preventing pregnancy complications, adequate maternal vitamin D is of crucial importance to your baby. In infants with rickets (a disorder that leads to soft, weak bones), 81% of mothers had severe vitamin D deficiency while pregnant (<10 ng/ml).[13] Even more concerning is the long-term impact on the health of a child born to a mother with vitamin D deficiency. A 2006 study from *The Lancet* found that bone development remained hindered at age 9 in children of mothers who were vitamin D deficient during their pregnancies.[14] Maternal vitamin D deficiency may also be associated with childhood risk of asthma, language impairment, schizophrenia, type 1 diabetes, and multiple sclerosis.[15,16,17,18,19,20]

The question then remains: How much vitamin D do you need and how can you get enough?

A well-designed study from 2011 helped to answer this question. This was a double-blind, placebo-controlled, randomized controlled trial on vitamin D supplementation in 450 women that tested three levels of supplementation: 400 IU, 2,000 IU, and 4,000 IU per day. Their blood levels of vitamin D were measured throughout pregnancy and at their baby's birth.

In short, the study found that supplementing with vitamin D at higher doses was not only safe, but significantly more effective at raising blood levels of vitamin D in both mother and baby.[21] Only 50% percent of women receiving 400 IU/day had sufficient serum vitamin D levels when they gave birth, compared to 70.8% and 82.0% in the 2,000 IU and 4,000 IU groups, respectively. A similar pattern was seen in infant vitamin D sufficiency with 39.7%, 58.2% and 78.6% achieving normal vitamin D levels at birth in the 400 IU, 2,000IU, and 4,000 IU groups, respectively.

Despite supplementing with levels well above the RDA, no side effects were noted and not a single participant experienced excessive blood levels of vitamin D. Also, women receiving higher doses of vitamin D supplements had significantly lower rates of pregnancy complications, including gestational diabetes. In light of the staggering rates of deficiency and the safety of supplementing with vitamin D, I believe all pregnant women should be screened for vitamin D deficiency.

Unfortunately, the American Congress of Obstetricians and Gynecologists, an organization that heavily influences prenatal care guidelines, isn't on board with universal screening. They suggest pregnant women should be screened for vitamin D deficiency *only* if they are ethnic minorities, live in cold climates, reside in northern latitudes, wear sunscreen or protective clothing, or are vegetarian.[22] However, knowing that at least two-thirds of the United States is above the 33 degree North parallel (denoted roughly by drawing a line from Long Beach, CA to Atlanta, GA), we can recognize that most American women are living at a latitude where they are unable to produce enough (or any) vitamin D from sun exposure during the winter. In other words, the proactive answer is to test *every* woman.

If your provider has not already checked your vitamin D levels, request this simple lab test at your next visit. It's called "25-hydroxy vitamin D." Optimal blood levels are discussed in Chapter 9. Keep in mind that most prenatal vitamins only contain 400 to 600 IU of vitamin D, which is nowhere near enough to keep your vitamin D at normal levels without regular midday sun exposure. I recommend a supplement of 4,000 IU per day for maintenance and possibly higher amounts if you are deficient. Some researchers suggest that the RDA for vitamin D should be closer to 7,000 or 8,000 IU per day (more than 10x the current RDA), but again, your dosage can be fine-tuned by having your blood levels of vitamin D measured by your doctor.[23,24]

When shopping for vitamin D supplements, there are two forms commonly available: vitamin D3 (cholecalciferol) and vitamin D2 (ergocalciferol). Vitamin D3 is more effective at raising and maintaining vitamin D levels in the body, and is chemically identical to the form of vitamin D that your body produces from sun exposure.[25] In short, always opt for vitamin D3. Since vitamin D is a fat-soluble nutrient, you can ensure you absorb it well by taking your supplement alongside a meal or snack that contains fat (such as any of the meals or snacks found in Chapter 5).

Lastly, there are several nutrients required for vitamin D metabolism, namely vitamin A, vitamin K2, zinc, and magnesium.[26] These nutrients should be provided in your prenatal vitamin and in your diet. Be sure to read the section on magnesium in this chapter and refer to Chapter 3 for food sources of the other nutrients.

Omega-3 Fats and Fish Oil

As mentioned in previous chapters, the specific omega-3 fatty acid called DHA is essential to obtain through your diet or supplements during pregnancy. DHA is incorporated into your baby's rapidly developing brain and eyes in utero, where it assists with the formation of neurons (brain cells) and protects the brain from inflammation and damage.[27] During the last 3 months of pregnancy, your baby accumulates an average of 67 mg of DHA *every day*.[28] It continues to be important to your baby's brain development until at least 2 years of age.

At minimum, aim to consume 300 mg of DHA per day to provide enough for yourself and your baby, though studies have shown benefits with higher doses. In one study, women were supplemented with 2,200 mg of DHA per day, or a placebo (olive oil), for the last 20 weeks of pregnancy. At 2 ½ years

Real Food for Pregnancy

of age, infants of DHA-supplemented mothers scored significantly better on hand-eye coordination tests.[29] Another study showed better problem-solving skills in kids at age 4 when their mothers supplemented with ~1,200 mg of DHA during pregnancy.[30]

It is absolutely possible to meet your DHA needs from diet alone if you consume 2-3 servings of cold water, fatty fish each week, such as salmon, herring, sardines, trout, fish eggs (roe), or mussels. Eggs from pasture-raised chickens (or those fed flaxseeds, marketed as "omega-3 eggs") and meat, organs, and dairy obtained from grass-fed, pasture-raised animals are other (although less concentrated) sources of DHA. To put it into perspective, 3 oz of sardines or wild Alaskan sockeye salmon contains upwards of 1,400 mg of DHA, while 3 oz of grass-fed beef contains 100 mg. One pasture-raised egg contains about 100 mg. Fish eggs, one of the most concentrated sources of DHA, can have up to 1,900 mg per oz. Algae is the only plant source of DHA, but concentration of DHA varies considerably from species to species (in other words, an algae-based DHA supplement is a good option, but *eating* algae is not reliable).

If you dislike the above food sources or simply do not eat them regularly, you'll definitely want to consider a DHA supplement. A high quality fish oil, cod liver oil, krill oil, or algae oil can provide you with DHA. Ensure that your DHA supplement also contains EPA, another type of omega-3 fat that improves the transport of DHA across the placenta.[31] Fish and seafood naturally contains a blend of DHA and EPA, however some brands of fish oil separate the two fatty acids (another hat tip to the genius of real food). If you opt for cod liver oil, keep in mind that it also contains vitamins A and D (though levels vary considerably brand to brand), so you'll want to factor that into your other supplements and make sure you're not exceeding recommended intakes, particularly for vitamin A. You'll also want to choose a high-quality brand of fish oil that has been tested to be free of contaminants, like heavy metals and PCBs.

While I'm in full support of DHA supplementation, it's important to recognize that seafood provides nutrients other than DHA that makes it beneficial to consume during pregnancy, as outlined in Chapter 3. Of note, you may not consume enough iodine without eating seafood or seaweed directly. Given the importance of iodine for brain development and thyroid function, at the very least, ensure your prenatal vitamin contains the RDA for iodine if you dislike seafood.

Note About Flaxseed Oil

Some prenatal nutrition educational materials have incorrect information about omega-3 fats and fail to separate the difference between omega-3 fats and DHA, however these terms are not interchangeable. As discussed in the section on vegetarian diets in Chapter 3, not all omega-3 fats are a source of DHA and your body lacks the ability to convert plant-sourced omega-3 into DHA in sufficient quantities. In other words, flaxseed oil is *not a source of DHA*. The only plant-based source of DHA is algae-based DHA supplements. Repeat after me: flaxseed oil is *not* a replacement for fish oil.

Probiotics

Probiotics are the "good bacteria" that live within and on our bodies. Bacteria outnumber human cells 10:1, colonizing everything from your digestive system to your skin to your vagina. Think about that for a minute. We are made of more bacterial cells than we are human cells (fully 90%), so it behooves us to pay attention to them.

The bacteria in your body (also called your "microbiome") are always in a state of flux based on what you eat, how you sleep, your stress levels, and more. Most of these bacteria live in your gut, however probiotics impact a lot more than digestive health. For example, it's estimated that up to 80% of your immune system is actually located in your gut.

Maintaining a healthy microbiome is important for your overall health and can also influence your risk of pregnancy complications. An imbalance of healthy-to-unhealthy bacteria may increase your risk of preterm birth, preeclampsia, gestational diabetes, and excessive weight gain during pregnancy.[32] Consumption of foods rich in probiotics during pregnancy is linked to lower rates of preterm birth and preeclampsia, which researchers attribute to reduced inflammation in the placenta.[33] Probiotic supplements taken during pregnancy may also result in better blood sugar levels. In one study, probiotic supplements were shown to reduce the risk of gestational diabetes by up to 23%.[34] Among women who have gestational diabetes, probiotic supplements have been shown to lower the risk of having a large baby.[35]

Recent research has shown that the placenta, previously believed to be sterile, is rich with bacteria that are transferred to the developing baby throughout gestation.[36] Prior to this, it was believed an infant's first contact with bacteria was through the birth canal. That gives extra incentive to maintain a healthy microbiome throughout your pregnancy.

One important way to preserve your microbiome is to avoid unnecessary exposure to antibiotics. Antibiotics kill bacteria—both good and bad—which can have lasting consequences for your baby. One study found that maternal exposure to antibiotics during the second and third trimester increased a child's risk of obesity by 84%.[37] Prenatal antibiotic exposure has also been linked to higher rates of allergies, asthma, and eczema in infants.[38,39,40] In contrast, supporting the microbiome through probiotic supplementation in late pregnancy (and while breastfeeding) may protect against infant allergies, eczema, colic, spitting up, and more.[41,42]

One way to ensure your body has a healthy balance of bacteria is to regularly consume fermented foods, nature's original probiotic "supplement." Kefir, yogurt, aged cheese, raw sauerkraut, kimchi, lacto-fermented vegetables (like pickles), raw apple cider vinegar, fermented beverages (water kefir or kombucha), miso, and natto. For fermented vegetables, ensure they are unpasteurized (raw), otherwise the beneficial bacteria will no longer be alive. Don't assume that supplements are always more potent than food. For example, a tablespoon of sauerkraut juice contains a whopping 1.5 *trillion* CFU (which refers to the number of bacterial cells otherwise known as "colony forming units").[43] Kefir contains equally high concentrations of probiotics (more than yogurt).[44] This is actually quite a bit considering that most probiotic supplements measure potency by the millions or billions, *not trillions.*

It's also important to eat a wide variety of foods that contain *prebiotic* fibers, which serve as a food source to these bacteria and sustain their populations in your gut. This includes eating fiber-rich foods like vegetables, nuts, seeds, coconut, legumes, and high-fiber fruits (like berries). The meal plans in Chapter 5 contain an ideal amount of fiber at 35-45 grams per day. Foods that contain a specific type of prebiotic called resistant starch are also beneficial.[45] This includes slightly unripe bananas (those that are still a bit green), legumes, cashews, and potatoes that have been cooked and cooled (like you'd have in potato salad). Limiting added sugars and refined carbohydrates also fosters the growth of healthy bacteria rather than harmful ones. This not only supports healthy digestion, but helps prevent bacterial vaginosis and yeast infections.[46]

Should you choose to supplement with probiotics, find a product that contains at least 30 billion CFUs of bacteria per serving. That might sound like a lot, but keep in mind you have over 100 *trillion* bacterial cells in your body, so when you see a product boasting "1 billion CFU per serving," it's like a drop in the bucket. Good quality probiotic supplements will list the individual strains and the quantities of each strain on the label. Look for one that contains both *Lactobacilllus* and *Bifidus* strains.

You might also consider a probiotic supplement with strains of bacteria specific to the vagina, to prevent unwanted strains of bacteria from growing (unwanted strains include Group B *streptococcus* (GBS) and the bacteria associated with bacterial vaginosis).[47] Ultimately, the goal is that your vagina is home to beneficial bacteria so that your baby is "seeded" with healthy bacteria during birth. Two strains that fit the bill are *Lactobacillus rhamnosus*, GR-1® and *Lactobacillus reuteri*, RC-14® which have over 25 years of clinical data supporting their use and efficacy.[48] These two strains were used in a well-designed, randomized trial of 99 pregnant women who tested positive for GBS at 35-37 weeks. Half of the women received probiotic treatment (containing 10 billion CFU of each strain), while the other half received a placebo. A repeat screen for GBS was completed at the time of admission to the hospital for delivery to see if the bacteria was still present. Among the women who received probiotics, *43% tested negative* for GBS compared to only 18% in the placebo group.[49] In other words, probiotics have the potential to favorably shift the microbial balance in the vagina.

Calcium

I rarely recommend calcium supplements, but because this is a common question, I'll address it here. Unlike many other nutrients, calcium needs do not increase during pregnancy. Also, most women obtain enough calcium from food alone. An analysis on calcium intake in Americans (eating a standard American diet—i.e. not healthy foods) found that women aged 19-30 years consume an average of 838 mg of calcium from their diets. This number is even higher in women over 30.[50] The recommended intake for pregnancy is 1000 mg, so you certainly do not need an additional high-dose calcium supplement to reach your needs. In addition, calcium absorption in the intestines doubles during pregnancy, making the calcium from your food easier for your body to assimilate.[51] I find that most women have no trouble meeting their calcium needs from food alone provided that they consume a nutrient-dense, real food diet (as outlined in this book). My meal plans have an average of 1,200-1,500 mg of calcium per day; no fortified foods or supplements needed.

What I see more often than low calcium intake is inadequate consumption of complementary nutrients, such as vitamin D, vitamin K2, and magnesium. These nutrients are required for your body to optimally process calcium and build strong bones.

However, some women may need to pay careful attention to their calcium intake, particularly those who do not consume dairy products. There are many non-dairy calcium sources including green leafy vegetables, bok choy, broccoli, almonds, sesame seeds, chia seeds, and sardines or salmon canned *with the bones.* If you avoid dairy, make an extra effort to include some of the above foods in your diet every day. Unless you are averse to all of these foods or have another medical issue that necessitates supplementation, skip the calcium supplement. If you have high blood pressure or are at risk for preeclampsia, some studies have found benefits from calcium (and magnesium) supplementation. See Chapter 7 for details.

If you choose to take a calcium supplement, at the direction of your healthcare provider, be aware that calcium and iron compete for absorption. This can be a problem for the many women who enter pregnancy with low iron status. The best way around this is to take your calcium at a separate time from an iron supplement and/or iron-rich foods.

Magnesium

Unlike calcium, magnesium deficiency is quite common. In fact, according to recent estimates, 48% of Americans consume inadequate magnesium from food.[52] Magnesium deficiency is even more common during pregnancy, and research has found that magnesium depletion, especially in the presence of calcium excess, can predispose women to vascular complications of pregnancy (such as preeclampsia). Women with gestational diabetes are also commonly deficient in magnesium.[53]

Though most women don't have obvious symptoms of magnesium deficiency, muscle cramps are a good sign you're not getting enough, and research has shown that supplementing with magnesium reduces pregnancy-induced leg cramps.[54] Magnesium supplements may also reduce the risk of high blood pressure in pregnancy.[55] One side effect of magnesium deficiency is nausea, and anecdotally some women have noticed less morning sickness when supplementing with magnesium or when eating more magnesium-rich foods.

Your best food sources of magnesium are seaweed, green leafy vegetables, pumpkin seeds, Brazil nuts, sunflower seeds, sesame seeds, almonds, cashews, chia seeds, avocados, unsweetened cocoa powder (or dark chocolate), bone broth, and green herbs including chives, cilantro, parsley, mint, dill, sage, and basil. However, the widespread use of aggressive farming practices, such as heavy pesticide application, has depleted the soil of magnesium on many commercial farms.[56] As a result, food grown in these soils is often magnesium-deficient. Organic and biodynamic farms typically have higher magnesium in the soil, which is then taken up by the crops, so when possible, source your food from small farms where attention is placed on soil fertility.[57]

If you take magnesium as a supplement (orally), be aware that a common side effect is diarrhea. The form of magnesium you take matters, with magnesium glycinate being one of the best absorbed forms and the least likely to cause GI side effects. If you can benefit from faster transit time (i.e. you're constipated), magnesium citrate is a good choice. To minimize any potential digestive effects, I recommend starting magnesium supplements at a low dose, such as 100 mg, and gradually increasing to up to 300 mg per day. Consult your healthcare provider if you take higher doses.

You can also absorb a significant amount of magnesium through your skin by taking Epsom salt baths or foot soaks (Epsom salt is magnesium sulfate).[58] If you opt for a full bath, just be careful with the water temperature and avoid overheating, since hyperthermia is a risk factor for certain birth defects.[59] Topical magnesium sprays are another option (often called "magnesium oil"), which are simply a mixture of water and magnesium chloride.

Iron

During pregnancy, iron needs are 1.5x higher than usual due to a massive increase in red blood cell production, as well as increased iron needs to support the growth of your baby and placenta.[60] The recommended intake of iron is 27 mg per day in pregnancy, compared to 18 mg in non-pregnant women. Iron plays a key role in fetal development, which is why it's fairly routine to check iron status during pregnancy. Iron deficiency increases your risk of premature birth and having a low birthweight infant.[61] It can also impair your thyroid function, which can lead to neurodevelopmental delays for your baby.[62]

This information often results in women taking iron supplements in an effort to be proactive, however iron supplements can be a double-edged sword. Many iron supplements are poorly absorbed or have unwanted side effects like constipation, nausea, and heartburn.[63] In a study of nearly 500 pregnant women who took iron supplements, 45% reported side effects and of those who stopped taking iron, 89% did so because the side effects were "unbearable."[64]

I recommend you get as much iron through your diet as possible, particularly from animal foods, which is well-absorbed and without side effects. Iron from animal foods comes in a form called heme iron, which is absorbed 2-4x better than plant-sourced non-heme iron.[65] This is partly due to the form of iron and also because plant foods contain compounds that inhibit iron absorption, such as phytic acid, oxalates, and certain polyphenols. This explains why the RDA for iron is 1.8x higher for vegetarians. The best source of iron, by far, is liver

Real Food for Pregnancy

and organ meats. Red meat, game meat, oysters, sardines, dark meat poultry (like chicken legs and thighs) are also reliable sources.

Foods rich in heme iron (per 3 oz portion; in order of most to least):

- Chicken liver - 9.9 mg
- Oysters - 5.7 mg
- Beef liver - 5.6 mg
- Beef heart - 5.4 mg
- Venison - 3.8 mg
- Ground bison - 2.7 mg
- Sardines - 2.4 mg
- Ground beef - 2.3 mg
- Clams - 2.3 mg
- Lamb - 1.7 mg
- Ground turkey - 1.7 mg
- Chicken thighs - 1.2 mg
- Chicken breast - 0.9 mg
- Wild salmon - 0.5 mg

There are several ways you can enhance iron absorption from your diet. First, consume iron-rich foods along with a source of vitamin C or other acidic ingredients, such as marinating meat in a vinegar-based marinade, adding ground meat to tomato sauce, or eating citrus alongside an iron-rich meal. Second, avoid eating iron-rich foods with calcium-rich foods, calcium supplements or antacids, as these minerals can compete for absorption. Third, consider cooking in cast iron pans, which can "fortify" your food. In one study, non-acidic foods, like eggs and potatoes, averaged a 5-fold increase in iron content after cooking in cast iron, and tomato sauce (acidic) had a 29-fold increase in iron content.[66] Cast iron pans are a favorite in my kitchen for this very reason.

Your doctor will monitor your iron status during pregnancy and let you know if you're falling short. In my experience, the majority of women following my dietary advice do not require an iron supplement to maintain sufficient iron levels throughout pregnancy. If they do, it's typically in the third trimester. If you need to supplement—or your diet is not sufficient to meet your needs—opt for a well-absorbed form of iron, like iron bisglycinate. Steer clear of ferrous fumarate or ferrous sulfate, which (unfortunately) are the most commonly prescribed forms of iron, but have twice the rate of side effects and are less efficiently absorbed compared to iron bisglycinate.[67]

Alternatively, you can take dessicated liver (if you don't regularly consume liver) or spirulina, a type of algae, to obtain iron. Dessicated liver supplements have a long history of use, and although modern studies on its efficacy are lacking, older research found that it was more effective than iron supplements for treating pregnancy-related anemia.[68] Spirulina algae is also a good choice. In a study that supplemented pregnant women with either spirulina (1500 mg per day) or iron (90 mg ferrous sulfate), significantly lower rates of anemia were found in the spirulina group.[69] In addition to being more effective at raising hemoglobin levels, spirulina was better tolerated and did not cause constipation. Additional benefits of spirulina are covered in Chapter 10.

Gelatin and Collagen

As outlined in Chapter 3, gelatin and collagen are the major dietary source of the amino acid glycine, which is "conditionally essential" during pregnancy, meaning you need to get it from your diet.[70] Gelatin and collagen are abundant in the connective tissues, bones, and skin of animal foods. If you regularly consume bone broth, slow-cooked meat, poultry with the skin, cracklings or pork rinds, and meat on the bone, you'll likely get enough gelatin and collagen in your diet.

If you're not able to do so, you can obtain glycine by supplementing with pure collagen or gelatin powder. Either can be mixed into foods, like hot beverages, soups, or smoothies. The only difference is that gelatin will cause a liquid to solidify once it cools down (like Jello), while collagen will not. Nutritionally, however, they are the same. An easy way to incorporate it is by adding a tablespoon of collagen powder to your morning tea or coffee, stirring it into yogurt, or mixing it into a bowl of soup. If you like gelatin desserts, try using unsweetened gelatin powder mixed with 100% fruit juice to make your own (see Tart Cherry Gummies in the Recipe Appendix). As with all animal foods, the source is important. Seek gelatin and collagen from grass-fed or pasture-raised animals.

Chia Seeds

Although chia seeds are a real food, I chose to include them in this section because they are often used like a supplement. Chia seeds offer several nutritional perks. They are rich in minerals including calcium, magnesium, iron, and potassium, and are loaded with fiber (while they also contain omega-3 fats, they cannot provide you with DHA, as explained earlier in this chapter).

Chia seeds are unique in that they have an ideal balance of soluble to insoluble fiber, meaning they can help regulate bowel movements whether you tend towards constipation or diarrhea. These fibers also serve as prebiotics, which help maintain healthy bacteria levels in the intestines. You'll notice that when chia seeds come in contact with water they release a clear gel around the seed. This gel holds onto water during intestinal transit, which is how it helps to normalize digestion and stool consistency. Chia "gel" also slows how quickly carbohydrates are digested and absorbed, thereby regulating blood sugar. Some women consume chia seeds before meals to reduce their post-meal blood sugar.

When taking chia seeds, start with a small amount, like 1 teaspoon, and work your way up to 1-2 tablespoons per day. They do not need to be ground into a powder to be digested, unlike flaxseeds, so you can use them whole. Of course, you can use ground chia seeds if you prefer. Just be sure to store them in the refrigerator or freezer in an airtight container, since they contain unsaturated fats that easily go rancid.

How to Use Chia Seeds:

- Chia Gel - mix 1 tablespoon with 8 oz of water, let sit for at least 5 minutes before drinking
- Chia Pudding - mix 1 tablespoon with 3 oz of unsweetened almond milk and other ingredients for extra flavor (such as maple syrup or stevia, cinnamon, cacao powder, or vanilla extract) and let sit for 5 minutes before consuming
- Add to protein shakes, smoothies, or any drink
- Mix into yogurt or applesauce

Herbs

Virtually every pregnant client of mine has questions about herbs. This topic is one I didn't plan to include in the book because, as a science junkie, I find it disheartening how poorly researched this topic is. As one reviewer explains, "About half of pregnant women try a wide range of herbal treatments, although the efficacy and safety of such remedies are poorly known."[71]

Historically, many cultures promote the use of specific herbs to help with common discomforts of pregnancy, however, high quality data is simply lacking on many of them. This shortage of data leads doctors to warn against the use of herbs, not because of evidence of harm, but from lack of safety data. There are, however, several herbs with a long history of use in pregnancy and scientific evidence to support their safety.

Red Raspberry Leaf

One example of such an herb is red raspberry leaf (not to be confused with raspberry-flavored tea or raspberries themselves). It is literally the leaves of the raspberry plant and although it has a pleasant flavor, it tastes nothing like raspberries. This herb is typically consumed as a tea, but can also be consumed as a powder, in capsules, or as a tincture. Many herbalists and midwives suggest supplementing with red raspberry leaf in the second or third trimester to help "strengthen, tone or prepare uterus, soften or prepare cervix, and induce or ease labour."[72] The beneficial effects of red raspberry leaf tea have been documented in mainstream medical literature since as early as 1941, in which it was noted that it can relax uterine muscle.[73] There are mixed opinions on first trimester use of the herb, though some prenatal vitamins contain small amounts.

Nutritionally, raspberry leaves are rich in minerals, vitamin C, and certain antioxidants, including rutin, which is known to reduce inflammation.[74] In studies on lab animals, "Some of the constituents, such as flavonoids, have repeatedly been shown to have a relaxing effect on smooth muscle."[75] Research hasn't conclusively shown it to help shorten or ease labor, but they also haven't found adverse effects of red raspberry leaf supplementation in pregnant women.[76] Personally, I find the flavor mild, and the potential (though anecdotal) benefits worth giving it a try. At the very least, you'll have an antioxidant and mineral-rich beverage to enjoy.

Ginger

Ginger is the most well-studied herb used during pregnancy, and has been proven effective in the treatment of nausea and vomiting.[77] Ginger has been used for centuries to reduce nausea and is the only herb that is almost universally considered safe in pregnancy by conventional standards.[78] You can try ginger tea, crystallized ginger (dried, sweetened ginger slices), or a ginger supplement in doses of up to 250 mg every 6 hours to treat nausea.[79] Note that ginger ale or ginger sodas usually don't have enough actual ginger to be effective. See Chapter 7 for more tips on managing nausea.

Chamomile

Often used as tea, chamomile may aid in relaxation and encourage restful sleep. Chamomile is one of the most commonly consumed herbs in pregnancy, yet safety data is lacking. Some research suggests that it may stimulate uterine contractions.[80] A recent study found that among women who were 40 weeks or further along in pregnancy, chamomile supplements (at high doses of 3,000 mg/day) were effective at initiating labor. "Labor started in 92.5% of the chamomile group and 62.5% of the placebo group one week from the start of taking capsules."[81] It's worth noting that an occasional cup of chamomile tea likely isn't strong enough to stimulate contractions, but nonetheless, caution should be taken when consuming large quantities during pregnancy or if there are any signs of preterm labor. I wouldn't encourage you to drink gallons of the stuff, but as researchers note, "there have not been any credible reports of toxicity caused by this common beverage tea."[82] Taken postpartum, chamomile may act as a galactogogue (increases milk supply), improve sleep quality, and help reduce postpartum depression.[83,84]

Other Herbs and General Considerations

Additional herbs that appear to be safe in pregnancy include echinacea (for short-term immune support, like colds and flus), cranberry (for urinary tract infections), St. John's wort (for depression), and ashwagandha (for overall stress and adrenal support).[85,86,87] Across the globe, a variety of other herbs have been traditionally used during pregnancy, which varies region to region. The data is sparse and inconsistent on the safety of herbs as a whole, which makes it difficult for me to fully endorse or warn against their use (beyond those specifically addressed in this section). Based on how clinical studies are performed and the ethical dilemma of testing pregnant women, we'll likely never have clear "Yes, this is always safe" answers when it comes to herbs. Herbalism, when practiced correctly, is highly individualized both in combinations of herbs and dosing. What's effective for one person might be harmful, or not have any effect, for another. Many people assume that herbs are natural and therefore always safe, but that's not always the case. Certain herbs can cause birth defects or other developmental problems.[88]

Use of culinary herbs is likely not a problem, so by all means, don't skip the oregano or parsley in your favorite recipe. Where you want to be cautious is with supplemental herbs, especially those taken consistently for long periods of time and/or in high doses. Formulations that are concentrated, such as herbal extracts or essential oils, deserve extra caution. This is especially true for early pregnancy use (first trimester), when the embryo is most susceptible to damage. For example, a study on mouse embryos exposed to 5 common essential oils (sage, oregano, thyme, cinnamon, and clove) found that all except thyme had negative effects on embryonic development.[89] How that translates to human pregnancy is unknown.

Another consideration, if you choose to take herbal supplements, is the quality. Since dietary supplements are not heavily regulated, there is a risk of contamination with other substances, such as pharmaceutical drugs (unlabelled) or heavy metals.[90] Use of adulterated or mislabeled herbs have been linked to adverse pregnancy outcomes.[91] So, not only do you want to be careful with the specific herbs you are taking, but you want to ensure you obtain herbs from a reputable source. My motto is: when in doubt, leave it out. I recommend seeking the advice of a trusted health professional or trained herbalist (with knowledge of pregnancy) before choosing to supplement with herbs.

Other Supplements

As previously mentioned, this list of supplements is not exhaustive; it covers the basics. Depending on your personal health concerns, you may consider additional supplements. For example, a sublingual vitamin B12 supplement may be helpful if you have health problems (like low stomach acid) that prevents adequate absorption of this nutrient or if you know you are deficient. Choline supplements (such as choline bitartrate or sunflower lecithin) may be helpful if your diet does not always contain sufficient amounts (see Chapter 3). If you are nauseous, you might consider vitamin B6—alone or in addition to ginger (see Chapter 7). Chlorella or spirulina, both of which are types of algae, may have some protective effects on toxin exposure (see Chapter 10). Selenium, if your prenatal vitamin does not contain it, may be helpful if you have thyroid problems or heavy metal exposure (see Chapters 9 and 10). This list could go on and on, but these types of questions are best discussed with a knowledgeable healthcare provider with an extensive background in prenatal nutrition.

Summary

Clearly, supplements are not a black and white topic. There are many considerations when choosing to supplement, including the nutrient intake from your diet and specific health concerns (like your genetics or pregnancy complications). My hope is that this chapter has given you an overview of the most common supplements and what to look for on the labels. When deciding which supplements to take, and what dosages are right for you, it's helpful to consult with your healthcare provider.

Remember, if you need help choosing a prenatal vitamin, I share my recommendations here: **www.realfoodforpregnancy.com/pnv/**.

Chapter 7:

Pregnancy Expectations & Common Complaints

"Pregnancy creates profound anatomical, physiological, and biochemical changes to support growth and development of the fetus. Changes begin soon after fertilization and continue throughout gestation. Most of these remarkable adaptations occur in response to physiologic stimuli provided by the fetus, as well as significant hormonal alterations. Although physiologic alterations are a part of gestational evolution, they often can be misinterpreted as disease or compromise."
- Col. Keiko Torgersen, Nurse Corps, U.S. Air Force

Pregnancy is full of ups and downs. Some days you feel energized and ready to take on the world and others you feel, well, not so great. Although every woman's experience of pregnancy is unique, you'll likely have a lot of questions about the new and ever-changing symptoms that arise.

Maybe you'll ask: Am I gaining too much weight? Is heartburn normal? Will the nausea and food aversions ever end? Can I do anything to keep my blood pressure and blood sugar in check? Why is my digestion weird?

For the symptoms that are nutrition-related (at least on some level), I want to dig a little deeper into the reasons why these symptoms may arise and what you can do to manage them. I've noticed that a lot of pregnant women are bombarded with "just you wait" comments about how horrible they will feel in the coming weeks (I certainly was when I was pregnant). It left me rather anxious about what annoyances the next stage would bring. In an effort to not be *that* person, I decided to structure this chapter by topic rather than the stage in pregnancy when it most often occurs. That way you can look up your concern and move right along without worrying about the heartburn and constipation that supposedly "every" woman deals with in the third trimester ('cause you might get lucky and bypass them entirely).

In truth, there's a huge range of symptoms you may or *may not* experience and there's no set time for you to experience them. I remember when I first started working clinically in prenatal nutrition at a high-risk obstetric practice (meaning a high percentage of our clients had complications during pregnancy) and had to field questions about all sorts of symptoms. The funny thing about being a nutritionist is that you're automatically less intimidating than a doctor, so women really opened up to me about all sorts of symptoms. Of course, not being a doctor myself, I'd often consult with the doc to understand what was normal. After all, I needed to know whether offering reassurance and coping strategies was best or if they really needed medical attention. After several years in this position, I realized the vast majority of symptoms that I heard about were totally normal, often fleeting, managed with simple strategies, and overall nothing to be concerned about.

Please know I'm not encouraging you to ignore symptoms or keep information from your healthcare provider, rather I want to ease the panic when you see the scale going up or when you struggle with food aversions. Trust your instincts and absolutely seek medical attention if your symptoms are unusual or severe.

Fast forward to my own pregnancy, and I was able to experience first-hand the ups and downs of growing a baby, with the only expectation that there is no "normal." I had hoped my body, after more than a decade of eating nutrient-dense foods, would handle the stresses of pregnancy with ease. And, for the most part, that was true. But when a wave of nausea would hit or heartburn would act up, I was reassured that it's all temporary and remembered to ride the waves rather than swim against the current.

In this chapter, I'll delve into some of the more common pregnancy expectations and complaints to offer my perspective, evidence-based research, and simple solutions to help make your pregnancy as smooth and as comfortable as possible.

Nausea and Vomiting

Nausea and vomiting in pregnancy are often referred to as morning sickness, but this is such a misnomer. For a lot of pregnant women, *any-time-of-day* sickness is a better description. Your nausea may last for a few weeks, a few months, and—I'm sorry to say—it may even stick around for your whole pregnancy. Most often, nausea is a fleeting symptom that occurs in the first few months, then gradually eases up. In approximately 60% of women, nausea and vomiting will resolve by the end of the first trimester (13 weeks) and if it doesn't, know that only 9% of women experience it past 20 weeks.[1]

Real Food for Pregnancy

It's so tough when you want to do everything to nourish your baby, and yet your body is rejecting food. Hang in there.

In order to figure out your best way to manage it, the first step is to observe what triggers your nausea. Is it strong odors? Time of day? Certain foods? Movement? Getting out of bed too quickly? Allowing yourself to get too hungry? Overeating? Undereating? Imbalanced meals? Eating too fast? Drinking too much fluid at mealtimes?

Most women benefit from smaller, more frequent snacks in place of large meals when nausea is at its worst. This helps prevent you from getting too hungry/full or from your blood sugar dropping, both common nausea triggers. When you're nauseated or anticipate throwing up, it can be hard to want to eat. Carbohydrates tend to be the easiest-to-digest foods, meaning they often digest *before* you throw up, so at least you can get *some calories* in. I know it's contrary to my suggestions in earlier chapters, but if you're having trouble stomaching *any* food, opt for things like fruit, cooked sweet potatoes, a smoothie, or rice. (See the section on food aversions and cravings below for a possible physiological basis for carb cravings in the first trimester.) Just be aware that sharp blood sugar fluctuations are another nausea trigger, so once you can tolerate a small amount of carbohydrates, try to follow it with a small portion of protein or fat-containing foods to stabilize your blood sugar, such as nuts, cheese, avocado, Greek yogurt, scrambled eggs, or beef jerky. Yes, you may be eating more carbohydrates for the time being and that's OK. Just try to opt for the least-processed carbohydrates whenever possible and read those ingredient labels to keep pesky additives out. It's far too easy to get hooked on sugary cereals and candy. Do your best to "keep it real" with carbs.

Protein shakes are a great option during this time, though again, check the ingredients on protein powders. I prefer unsweetened versions, such as grass-fed whey protein or organic rice protein (or a combo formula that combines rice with other plant proteins—aside from soy protein, of course) blended up with yogurt, kefir, coconut milk, or almond milk for liquid and ½ to 1 cup of fruit for flavor. For extra "staying power," again if your current nausea situation allows, a tablespoon of nut butter or coconut oil, or even half of an avocado, can add healthy fats. You may also be able to "hide" things like greens and collagen powder in it to give you a nutritional boost. Some of my clients have even opened the capsules of their prenatal vitamin into their shake, as this was the only way they could get it down in the first trimester. Grab your blender and experiment.

Some women wake up nauseous first thing in the morning (perhaps where the term "morning sickness" originated) and find it helpful to keep a snack at their bedside. Saltine crackers are a classic, but I personally found that the steep blood sugar spike I got from them only worsened my nausea. Roasted, salted cashews were my bedside snack of choice. I'd nosh on a few before even sitting up in bed and that seemed to do the trick (most mornings, anyways). It can also help to ease out of bed slowly if you notice that quick movements worsen your nausea.

Protein at breakfast is especially helpful for maintaining blood sugar balance throughout the day, which can help alleviate nausea the rest of the day. Even if you can only get down a sip of a protein shake, or 2 bites of egg, or a few almonds, it can still help in the long run.

If you find that having an overly full stomach is a nausea trigger, try eating slowly and mindfully. Ideally, stop eating when you're comfortably satisfied, but not stuffed. For more on mindful eating, see Chapter 2. Also, avoid drinking large quantities of water or other beverages with meals and instead try to sip on them throughout the day.

Some women find that sour or salty foods help mitigate their nausea, which perhaps explains why pickles are a common pregnancy food craving. In India and Mexico, sweet/sour foods (such as tamarind) are traditionally recommended to ease nausea. Other options to try include lemon water, tangy popsicles (homemade versions with citrus juice work well), avocado with salt and lemon juice, and unsweetened dried cherries (a good balance of sweet and tart, like nature's sour candy). Or try my recipe for Tart Cherry Gummies in the Recipe Appendix, which is a healthier alternative to sweet and sour gummy candy.

If you find certain odors are a trigger, you may want to have others cook your meals for you or simply avoid places with strong smells (like seafood restaurants or the perfume section of a department store). I remember feeling nauseated while cooking certain foods, but if my husband cooked and I was nowhere near the kitchen, I had no problem eating a full meal. Cold foods are often better tolerated, probably since they don't smell as much as hot, cooked foods. You may find that chilled beverages, popsicles, frozen berries, or yogurt help get you through tough days. As you can gather, none of this is a perfect science and you have to be a bit of a detective to test out what will work for you. This is not the time to beat yourself up about not eating perfectly or having imbalanced meals. Just celebrate when you can keep something down!

Although unpleasant odors are a nausea trigger, some smells may actually help reduce nausea. Aromatherapy with pure lavender and peppermint essential oils is both safe during pregnancy and effective at alleviating nausea. One study tested the effects of diffusing a combination of both essential oils (4 drops lavender + 1 drop peppermint) on a group of about 100 pregnant women and found that it significantly eased nausea symptoms in most women.[2]

Beyond the above tweaks, certain supplements can be effective for managing nausea. One of the most common is vitamin B6, usually given in doses of 10-25 mg every 8 hours.[3] I've found the active form of vitamin B6, pyridoxal-5'-phosphate, to be more effective for my clients (as opposed to the type found in most supplements, called pyridoxine). In addition, you can try munching on vitamin B6-rich foods, like avocados, bananas, pistachios, and sunflower seeds. Meat, fish, and poultry are also good sources of vitamin B6, but are often not that appealing when you're nauseous (if you can eat them, go for it!). Ginger has been used for centuries to reduce nausea and is clinically shown to be both safe and effective in pregnancy.[4] Several forms of ginger are good options: ginger tea, crystallized ginger (dried, sweetened ginger slices), and a ginger supplements (often sold in capsules). If you opt for supplemental ginger, it's considered safe to take doses of up to 250 mg every 6 hours.[5] Ginger ale or ginger sodas usually don't have enough actual ginger to be effective. Some women find that magnesium lessens their morning sickness, though this has yet to be clinically studied. You can take a magnesium supplement (see Chapter 6), use a topical magnesium spray, or do a relaxing bath or foot bath with Epsom salts to boost your levels.

Acupressure or acupuncture is effective for some women. The most commonly used pressure point is located on the wrist, called P6 or Nei Guan.[6] P6 is located 3-fingers-distance below the crease of your wrist on your inner arm. One company even manufactures a little wristband (Sea-Band) designed to put pressure on this exact spot. Given that there are no side effects, it's worth a shot!

If and when you throw up, be sure to replenish lost fluids and electrolytes with homemade bone broth, diluted juice, coconut water, and anything salty (or try my recipe for a homemade electrolyte replenishment drink, below). Potassium-rich foods are helpful at this time, such as avocados, bananas, potatoes, sweet potatoes, winter squash, and oranges. Magnesium-rich foods, as outlined in Chapter 6, are also beneficial. If you are unable to keep *anything* down (food or fluids), call your medical provider, as dehydration while pregnant can be dangerous. A very small percentage of women have a severe form of nausea called hyperemesis gravidarum, in which case medication and other interventions may be warranted. If your vomiting is severe, don't wait to talk to your doctor or seek emergency medical services.

Lily's Electrolyte Replenishment Drink:

- 1 quart coconut water (unsweetened)
- ¼ teaspoon sea salt (such as Himalayan pink salt)
- ½ cup fruit juice (such as 100% pineapple, orange, or apple juice)
- Juice of 1 lemon
- 10 drops trace mineral concentrate (optional)

Sip on the electrolyte replenishment drink throughout the day and especially after vomiting. Store leftovers in the refrigerator.

To summarize, although there's no "cure" for nausea in pregnancy, there are many little things you can try to ease your symptoms:

- Eat small, frequent meals/snacks (never get too hungry or too full).
- Balance your blood sugar—aim to include some protein and fat when you eat, even if the portion is small (protein at breakfast is especially helpful).
- Try a protein shake.
- Eat slowly and mindfully.
- Try salty, sour, or cold foods.
- Avoid drinking too much liquid at meal times.
- Keep a snack at your bedside and move slowly first thing in the morning.
- Avoid strong odors—let someone else cook for you!
- Diffuse essential oils (4 drops lavender oil + 1 drop peppermint oil).
- Consider supplementing with ginger, vitamin B6, and/or magnesium.
- Try acupressure or acupuncture.
- If you throw up, replenish fluids and electrolytes.

Lastly, reassure yourself that this is temporary and the human body is an incredible machine. Human beings would not have been able to survive famines without a complex system to make up for a temporary lack of nutrition. When my nausea was at its worst, I remember feeling nervous that I couldn't eat all the nutrient-dense foods that I knew were so important for my baby's development. But, I had to trust that my body could handle the demands and draw from my nutrient reserves for the short term. They did, the nausea eventually went away, and I had a very healthy baby despite an imperfect diet in my first trimester. (Full disclosure: salt & vinegar chips were a lifesaver on bad days. Ideal? No. Better than starving? Yes.) If you're

Real Food for Pregnancy

struggling with nausea, take heart that you *will* get through this and you *will* be able to return to a more balanced diet when it passes.

Researchers are still trying to figure out why nausea and vomiting are so common in pregnancy. Theories include hormonal triggers (likely placental hormones), B vitamin deficiencies, your body's attempt to protect you from eating spoiled or unsafe food (like rotten meat or poisonous wild plants), and even thyroid health. Currently, the most compelling theory is that metabolites of your thyroid hormones are to blame and that morning sickness is simply a sign that your thyroid is healthy. Essentially, your body is shunting iodine and thyroid hormone to your baby to promote optimal development.[7] In fact, *lack of nausea* may be an indication that you should have your thyroid hormones tested. As annoying as it is, perhaps it's reassuring to know that experiencing nausea is linked to positive pregnancy outcomes.[8] *(If you don't have nausea, don't panic. Plenty of women have healthy babies and miraculously escape nausea. Enjoy it!)*

Food Aversions and Cravings

Pickles and ice cream are what most people imagine when they think of pregnancy cravings. Up to 90% of women experience cravings during pregnancy, with most occurring during the first and second trimesters.[9] Food aversions tend to go hand in hand with nausea. It's not a matter of "I don't want to eat that" or "I'm in the mood for something else." It's more of a "If I smell, taste, see, or even *think* of that food, I'm gonna hurl." No one really knows why pregnancy causes certain cravings or food aversions, but plenty of theories are out there, ranging from metabolic and hormonal changes to nutritional deficits, to even cultural and psychosocial factors.

For most health-conscious moms, cravings and aversions come with a lot of self judgement and guilt. "I really *want* to like eggs right now, but all my body wants is crackers!" I, too, had a lot of those thoughts when food aversions were at their height. For myself and my clients, putting some context behind *why* food aversions or cravings might be happening helps you accept the current state of affairs and stay positive. In this section, I'll address both cravings and aversions, possible causes, and some strategies to manage them.

For the most part, cravings and aversions are nothing to fear and not a sign that anything is wrong. With the exception of cravings for non-food items (termed "pica"), pregnancy cravings may not always be a bad thing and, within reason, I'm a proponent of following your body's lead.

For one, the metabolic shifts that are going on in your body unbeknownst to you could be a driving force for both cravings and aversions. In the first trimester, many women crave carbohydrates, even if they were following a low-carb diet before conceiving. This may be your body's attempt to build up maternal fat stores that it can draw from in later pregnancy and postpartum (for breastfeeding). In early pregnancy, your pancreas undergoes dramatic changes to prepare for the impending insulin resistance that accompanies the second half of pregnancy. The number of insulin-producing beta cells increases as does the production of insulin.[10] In fact, insulin production may triple during pregnancy.[11] For a short time, typically before 11 weeks, insulin resistance hits an all time low and your blood sugar levels fall. It's reasonable to view carbohydrate cravings during this phase as a physiological response to lower blood sugar; in other words, it's an adaptation to this stage of pregnancy. As long as you're mindful about eating a variety and balance of foods (or moving that direction after protein aversions or nausea subsides) and prioritizing unprocessed carbohydrates, you have nothing to worry about. That means choosing things like whole fruit instead of fruit-flavored candy and whole grain crackers in lieu of sugary cereal. In my experience, most women can gradually ease back to eating a lower-carb diet in the second trimester.

Some cravings can be a sign of nutritional deficits. The most extreme examples are cravings for non-food items (pica), like laundry starch and dirt. Pica is more prevalent in those deficient in certain minerals, namely iron, zinc, and calcium. Cravings for ice, in particular, can be a sign of iron deficiency.[12] If you're having odd cravings, let your healthcare provider know and consider getting screened for anemia and other nutrient deficiencies.

Non-food cravings aside, there is merit to the theory that some cravings are driven by nutritional needs. For example, cravings for raw fish or sushi may be a sign your body needs more iodine or omega-3 fats. Iodine needs double during pregnancy and along with omega-3 fats, are needed for your baby's brain development. Some data shows that omega-3 fats are more absorbable from raw fish than cooked fish.[13] Iodine levels decline by up to 58% when fish is cooked.[14] Plus, the selenium in fish that helps prevent mercury toxicity is also better absorbed when fish is uncooked.[15] This "odd" craving may be your body's way of ensuring you provide the building blocks for baby's rapidly growing brain while protecting you from mercury. (See Chapter 4 for food safety precautions.)

Another commonly craved group of foods are dairy products, which is even reported by women who were previously dairy-free prior to conception. Many women with lactose intolerance report that it "disappears" during pregnancy. You might expect that calcium needs are the driving force behind this craving, but I suspect that iodine is a more likely culprit. In populations where seafood and seaweed consumption are relatively low (like the United

States), dairy products are a major source of iodine.[16] If you normally feel well avoiding dairy, but find yourself with an unexplained urge to have yogurt or cottage cheese for breakfast, this might be the reason for it.

Salt cravings are another way that your body may be looking out for you. As explained in Chapter 2 (and in more detail in this chapter in the section on high blood pressure), your body's requirements for salt go up during pregnancy.[17] This is not a craving to be ignored.

There are other examples of food aversions or cravings being protective beyond meeting nutritional needs. For example, the first trimester is when most food aversions appear (alongside nausea) and this coincides with the time when your baby is most vulnerable to outside toxins.[18] Many of the food aversions reported in the first trimester are to vegetables, particularly the bitter-tasting varieties. Virtually all plant foods contain what's called "secondary compounds," which serve as defense mechanisms from fungi, insects, and other pests. Many double as antioxidants and are beneficial in small quantities, but can be harmful if over-consumed. As one study points out, "it has been speculated that an increase in taste and olfactory sensitivity may serve to discourage consumption of potentially toxic foods in pregnancy, and could also be responsible for changing food preferences and patterns of consumption."[19] That being said, most vegetables available today are a far cry from the vegetation our ancestors would have eaten and contain much lower amounts of potentially toxic compounds than wild plants, so if you're *not* averse to vegetables, know it's absolutely beneficial to keep eating them.[20]

Meat, fish, and eggs are another category of food aversions common in the first half of pregnancy. Some research speculates that prior to modern hygiene and safe food storage (like refrigeration), these foods were a common source of pathogens and infections, which could pose a danger to a mother and her baby.[21,22] In other words, meat aversions are practically etched into our DNA from thousands of years ago. Nowadays, this may work against us, since avoiding meat often means eating more processed foods that provide few micronutrients, but excessive amounts of sugar and calories. If you're not careful, these once protective food aversions can lead you to overeat empty calories or undereat nutrient-dense foods, resulting in other health problems, like excessive weight gain and gestational diabetes. Currently, roughly half of all pregnant women in the United States exceed their recommended weight gain goals and many cite "pregnancy cravings" as a driver of weight gain.[23]

Some food aversions or cravings may be, in part, related to hormonally-driven shifts in sensitivity to smells. In one study, 65% of women reported changes in odor perception during pregnancy.[24] Given that your perception of smell affects taste, it makes sense that certain foods are less palatable during pregnancy. For example, many pregnant women quit drinking coffee due to an aversion to its taste or smell, which researchers think is related to a higher sensitivity to bitter flavors in pregnancy (and may be protective against excessive caffeine intake).[25] Changes in taste perception often coincide with cravings in the first trimester, though researchers aren't entirely sure why.[26] Many of my clients have a preference for cold foods in the first trimester, like smoothies and popsicles, which may be because they don't smell as strong.

Certain foods may be responsible for food cravings in and of themselves. Research has repeatedly shown that high-glycemic foods (like sugar) trigger changes in your brain's neurotransmitters that mimic drug addiction. One study performed on rats who were regularly offered sugar for several weeks, followed by a week where no sugar was offered, found that "the effects of sugar addiction, withdrawal and relapse are similar to those of drugs of abuse."[27] Another study concluded: "Sugar is noteworthy as a substance that releases opioids and dopamine and thus might be expected to have addictive potential."[28] If you're finding yourself craving high-sugar and high-glycemic foods, like candy, cereal, baked goods, and bread (especially beyond the first trimester nausea phase), it's possible that pregnancy isn't the only driving force, but rather your body is simply habituated to crave the "highs" you experience when you eat them.

It's tricky to break the cycle, but it can be done. Research has shown that a nutrient-dense diet results in fewer cravings and better regulation of hunger cues.[29] Women given low-glycemic versus high-glycemic foods report significantly lower hunger levels and greater satiety.[30] And even a modest increase in carbohydrates at a meal contributes to an "earlier rise and fall in postprandial glucose concentrations and an earlier return of appetite."[31] In other words, the real food, lower-carb approach described in this book can help you minimize sugar cravings and frequent hunger pangs. Stabilizing your blood sugar levels by eating enough protein, fat, and high-fiber vegetables, while minimizing your intake of processed carbohydrates, is the golden ticket. Eating enough protein and fat at breakfast seems to be particularly important, as this sets the stage for your blood sugar regulation for the rest of the day and is shown to reduce overeating at lunch and dinner (hence why the meal plans in this book reflect that advice).[32]

As I mentioned in the nausea section, carbohydrate cravings are quite common, especially in the first trimester. I find that they only become problematic if cravings drive overconsumption of *highly processed* carbohydrates and result in nutritional imbalances, elevated blood sugar, or excess weight gain. Once your nausea and aversions lessen, do your best to shift the balance from a carb-heavy diet to a more balanced approach (as outlined in Chapter 2). It won't be an overnight shift, so be gentle with yourself during the transition and follow your body's lead, knowing that carbohydrate needs are entirely individual.

The above theories offer a physiologic rationale for cravings or food aversions, but some researchers point the finger at cultural or psychological factors. In many western countries, food cravings are a hallmark of pregnancy. I find it both shocking and reassuring to learn that the word "craving" doesn't have a suitable translation in many other languages nor is it an expected side effect of pregnancy in some cultures.[33] I remember being repeatedly asked what my cravings were while pregnant to the point that I'd often just choose a random food to end the annoying inquiries (I had more aversions than overt "cravings"). My thought at the time was, Perhaps if I wasn't craving a food at the time, I wasn't "normal." Or perhaps our view of what's normal is warped.

In our media-driven world, where thinness and dietary restraint is idealized, some research has found that pregnancy is a "socially acceptable time for women to indulge," especially as women view their bodies in a more functional way and are encouraged to "eat for two."[34] Psychologically, pregnancy might make you feel like you don't have to worry about your weight for once in your life, making it easier to claim a "pregnancy craving." Other research has found that "pregnancy acts as a time for women to legitimize seemingly excessive food intake, disregarding any previous attitudes and intentions to eat less."[35] That quote is slightly offensive and sexist, but it does make you pause. My takeaway is that it's worth it to get curious about your food cravings and eating behaviors, so you don't accidentally fall into one of these traps.

As you can see, there are dozens of possible reasons for any craving, food aversion, or absence of either. Hopefully, this section has put it into context—at least somewhat. If you're finding yourself struggling, know that most cravings or food aversions are temporary. Aside from cravings for food that's dangerous (meaning toxic or non-food items), allowing yourself to avoid foods that you don't want to eat and indulge in the ones that you do—within reason, of course—is probably harmless. I highly encourage you to incorporate mindful eating and to approach your cravings and aversions with curiosity, especially if you feel that they are negatively impacting your day-to-day life or your health. Mindful eating has been specifically shown to reduce binge eating and emotional eating.[36] Mindfulness practices allow you to approach eating without judgement or guilt. There will be times when you don't eat as healthy as usual and that's ok. Understanding and accepting where you're at on any given day makes it easier to naturally shift back to a real food-focused diet.

Many of my clients have found that a combination of hunger awareness (mindful eating) and better blood sugar balance (through a real food diet) are helpful for navigating food aversions and minimizing cravings.

To summarize, consider the reasons for cravings and food aversions; they may:

- Help you consume enough beneficial nutrients (or may be a sign of a nutrient deficiency).
- Protect you from toxins or food poisoning.
- Be one way to get through the nausea phase (carbohydrate cravings).
- Help you avoid strong odors.
- Be a sign of an imbalanced diet (too high in sugar, refined carbs, or processed food).
- Prevent you from having low blood sugar.
- Be the result of cultural expectations to have pregnancy cravings.
- Offer a reminder to eat mindfully and honor your hunger/fullness cues.

Heartburn

Heartburn and reflux are annoyances that can happen at any time in pregnancy, but most often rear their fiery heads in the second and third trimesters. Many women describe it as a burning sensation behind the breastbone, in the upper chest, or the throat. Pregnancy predisposes you to heartburn and reflux for several reasons that are out of your control: your baby pushing up on your stomach (which increases intra-abdominal pressure), increased levels of progesterone (which relaxes the lower esophageal sphincter), and slower intestinal motility.[37] Your stomach is also naturally more acidic due to placental production of gastrin, a hormone that tells the stomach to pump out hydrochloric acid. It's no wonder that 50-80% of women complain of heartburn at some point in their pregnancies.[38]

As tempting as it is to just pop an antacid, try to avoid them. You have acid in your stomach for several important reasons: to kill harmful bacteria, viruses and fungi, to help you absorb minerals (like iron and calcium), to digest protein, and to absorb vitamin B12. By decreasing the acid in your stomach, you run the risk of food poisoning, digestive problems and nutrient deficiencies. Plus, some heartburn is a result of too little acid, not too much. This is why diluted apple cider vinegar is a common home remedy for heartburn.

Also, over-the-counter antacids may also expose you to harmful levels of aluminum, a known neurotoxin. As one researcher puts it, "Over-the-counter antacids are the most important source for human aluminium exposure from a quantitative point of view. However, aluminium can act as a powerful neurological toxicant and provoke embryonic and fetal toxic effects in animals and humans after gestational exposure."[39] For more on the risks of aluminum in pregnancy, see Chapter 10.

Luckily, lifestyle changes are often effective for managing heartburn. Distension of your stomach caused by eating too much food or drinking too much liquid at mealtimes is a known heartburn trigger.[40] So, opt for small meals and snacks rather than big portions and aim to sip on liquids throughout the day rather than drink large amounts during meals. In addition, think of the composition of your meals. High blood sugar causes your lower esophageal sphincter to relax, which means that stomach acid can more easily enter your esophagus.[41] The more carbohydrates you eat, the higher your blood sugar, and the more likely you are to experience heartburn. This provides yet another reason to watch your intake of carbohydrates, especially refined carbohydrates and simple sugars. A lower-carbohydrate diet has been found to be clinically effective for managing heartburn and reflux.[42] If your heartburn flares up specifically at night, try eating an earlier, smaller dinner and consider elevating the head of your bed.

Some heartburn is the result of food sensitivities or eating irritating foods.[43] The most common culprits I've observed in practice are sugary foods, spicy foods, caffeine (coffee or tea), chocolate, acidic foods (like citrus or tomatoes), dairy, and gluten. That said, reactions to foods are highly individual, so if you suspect certain foods trigger your heartburn, keep a detailed food diary to help narrow down the list.

If the above options aren't enough, you can try acupressure or acupuncture. The same acupressure point that's used to help manage nausea, Nei Guan or P6, mentioned earlier in this chapter, is effective for heartburn in some individuals.[44]

Lastly, consider your posture. As your pregnancy progresses and there's less and less room in your torso, slouchy posture becomes especially problematic. If you sit with your shoulders hunched and your belly compressed, guess what? There's *even less* room for your internal organs to find space around your baby, and your poor stomach doesn't have anywhere to go. Make an effort to sit up straight with your weight directly over your sitz bones (rather than tucking your hips under you) and imagine a string is attached to the crown of your head pulling you up ever so slightly. It might sound silly, but simple posture adjustments can go a long way toward alleviating heartburn.

To summarize, try the following if you're experiencing heartburn:

- If possible, don't use antacids (and consider the possibility of acid levels being *too low*).
- Avoid eating too much at meals (practice mindful eating).
- Drink most of your liquids *between* meals.
- Try a splash of apple cider vinegar diluted in a small amount of water before meals.
- Lower your intake of carbohydrates, especially sugar and refined carbs.
- For nighttime heartburn, eat an earlier, smaller dinner and elevate the head of your bed.
- Keep a food diary to help identify your trigger foods.
- Try acupressure or acupuncture.
- Practice good posture.

For many of my clients, simple lifestyle shifts are enough to keep heartburn at bay. Sometimes though, your baby is just taking up too much room in your torso and it's not possible to escape the annoyance of heartburn entirely. For heartburn that started during pregnancy, at least you have a timeline for when it'll go away.

Constipation and Hemorrhoids

If you're having trouble going to the bathroom, you're not alone. It's estimated that anywhere from 10-40% of women will experience constipation in pregnancy.[45] Potential causes of constipation include elevated hormone levels, your uterus physically obstructing your colon, decreased activity levels, lower levels of motilin (a gastric hormone that controls intestinal motility), enhanced water and electrolyte absorption in the colon, and the use of iron or calcium supplements.[46]

Constipation often results in hemorrhoids, which are swollen veins in the lowest part of your rectum and anus that can cause pain or bleeding while having a bowel movement. Researchers have the following to say about hemorrhoids: "their development or aggravation during pregnancy is no doubt related to increased pressure in rectal veins caused by restriction of venous return by the enlarged uterus as well as by constipation related to pregnancy."[47] As you can see, many of the culprits for both constipation and hemorrhoids are out of your control, but that doesn't mean you're out of options. The following advice applies to both complaints.

I'm sure you've heard it before, but getting the right amount of fiber and fluids is important. When increasing your intake of fiber, you'll want to do so gradually and right alongside an increase in fluids, otherwise you can make your constipation worse. Fiber comes in two forms in food: soluble and insoluble. Ideally, you'll want to consume a good balance of the two. Many fiber supplements are based on soluble fiber (the kind that dissolves in water), but soluble fiber alone is not very effective at improving constipation. Instead, opt for whole food sources of fiber that naturally contain a good balance of soluble and insoluble fiber, such as lentils, beans, berries, non-starchy vegetables, shredded coconut or coconut flour, almonds, and avocados. Vegetables are particularly helpful for constipation and often increasing your vegetable intake to 1-2 cups per meal will do the trick all on its own.

Chia seeds and flax seeds are other whole food options, though most people treat them as fiber supplements. In working with hundreds of pregnant women one-on-one, I personally prefer chia seeds, since I've observed that flax seeds can make constipation worse in some individuals. Unlike flax seeds, chia seeds do not need to be ground into a powder before consuming. For every tablespoon of chia seeds, you'll want to consume at least an additional 8 oz of water. For more on chia seeds, see Chapter 6.

Although many people think of grains as a good fiber source, they aren't your best option. Whole grains have a relatively small amount of fiber compared to the quantity of carbohydrates, which I call the fiber-to-carbohydrate ratio. For example, 1 cup of brown rice has 45 grams of carbohydrates, but only 3.5 grams of fiber, while lentils have a similar amount of carbohydrates, but a whopping 16 grams of fiber. While pregnant, aim for 28 g of fiber at minimum per day (the meal plans in this book contain 35-45 g). If you try to get all of your fiber from whole grains, you'll end up eating a very high-carbohydrate and less nutrient-dense diet. Instead, consider the following fiber-rich foods.

Examples of high-fiber foods (with a high fiber-to-carbohydrate ratio):

- ½ avocado: 7g fiber (8g total carbohydrates)
- ½ cup lentils: 8g fiber (20g total carbohydrates)
- 1 cup blackberries: 8g fiber (14g total carbohydrates)
- 1 cup raspberries: 7g fiber (12g total carbohydrates)
- 2 Tbsp coconut flour: 5g fiber (8g total carbohydrates)
- 1 Tbsp chia seeds: 5g fiber (5.5g total carbohydrates)
- 1 cup cauliflower: 5g fiber (6g total carbohydrates)
- 1 cup cooked cabbage: 4g fiber (9g total carbohydrates)
- 12 spears asparagus: 3g fiber (3.5g total carbohydrates)

- ¼ cup almonds: 4g fiber (8g total carbohydrates)
- 2 Tbsp cocoa powder, unsweetened: 4g fiber (6g total carbohydrates)

Beyond fiber and fluids, consider your intake of fats. Eating enough fat is key to having regular, easy-to-pass bowel movements for several reasons. First, dietary fats and oils help to lubricate, for lack of a better word, your intestines and keep bowel movements from becoming too dry and hard. Second, fat stimulates the release of bile from the gall bladder, which naturally stimulates peristalsis (movement of your intestines) and facilitates "propulsive contractions" of your colon.[48] In other words, *fat helps you poop*. If you're following my nutrition advice, you'll likely get enough fat in your diet, but a lot of women have spent decades hearing that "fat is bad" and subconsciously continue to restrict their intake even when they move towards incorporating more real food into their diet.

If you're holding back on cooking with fat, if you're skimming fat from your soups, or if you're using the least possible amount of oil when dressing your salad—*and you're constipated*—it's clearly time to get comfortable eating more fat. Liberally incorporate more fat into your diet, such as adding more butter to your vegetables, using heavy cream in your coffee or tea, eating more avocado, eating the crispy skin from your chicken wings, *not* draining the pan of fat after cooking meat, and *not* blotting your bacon of every last drop of grease. You can also try adding 1 tablespoon of coconut oil to your breakfast, which many find effective at triggering a morning bowel movement.

Aside from dietary shifts, there may be some changes in posture or movement that can help. Exercise naturally helps stimulate the bowels. Simply going for a daily walk may be enough, but specific exercises that involve gentle twists (like you might do in yoga or Pilates) help give your intestines a gentle massage and may help things move along. Notice that I emphasize the word *gentle* when referring to twisting movements. Twisting stretches performed in a controlled, mindful manner are safe, but twists with sudden starts or stops are best avoided during pregnancy to avoid joint injuries. See Chapter 8 for more on prenatal exercise.

Another consideration is the position you take to go to the bathroom. Traditional cultures did not sit on toilets; rather, they squatted to poop. This position puts your colon and pelvic floor muscles in the proper alignment to have an easy bowel movement without straining. Or as the researchers put it, the "sensation of satisfactory bowel emptying in sitting defecation posture necessitates excessive expulsive effort compared to the squatting posture."[49] Squatting to poop may also help prevent or alleviate hemorrhoids.[50] To mimic a squat while still being able to use your toilet, there are a number of foot stools on the market, like the Squatty Potty®, that you can have at the

Real Food for Pregnancy

foot of your toilet and still be in an ideal position. It's also helpful to try not to push too much when having a bowel movement to avoid straining. When you have the urge to poop, head to the bathroom as soon as possible and wait until your body starts moving your bowel movement down *before* you actively push. By the way, this is excellent preparation for labor, as it helps you learn to relax your pelvic floor muscles and encourages blood flow to the area, both of which lower your chances of having perineal tears.

Lastly, take a look at your supplement regimen. Some supplements can make constipation worse while others alleviate it. Magnesium supplements are commonly used and although I'm a proponent of magnesium glycinate for its superior absorption, it's unlikely to help with constipation. In the case of constipation, you actually want a magnesium supplement that's *less* efficiently absorbed, such as magnesium citrate. The goal is that the magnesium will remain in your intestines and draw water into the bowel to soften your stools (this is called an osmotic laxative). Some other forms of magnesium are *very* poorly absorbed and rather harsh on the digestion, often causing cramps and diarrhea (this includes magnesium oxide and magnesium sulfate). Steer clear of these unless you're under medical supervision.

Probiotics are often helpful for improving constipation. Having the right balance of bacteria in your gut helps you digest your food and keeps it moving through at the right pace. Regularly consuming fermented foods, as discussed in previous chapters, is helpful, as is taking a probiotic supplement. One study showed a daily probiotic containing a combination of *Lactobacillus* and *Bifidus* strains was effective at treating constipation in pregnancy, and also had the unexpected benefit of reducing acid reflux.[51]

Some supplements, however, worsen constipation. Use of iron supplements is significantly linked to constipation during pregnancy. This is one reason I strongly suggest getting most of your iron from food, and if needed, opting for a well-absorbed form of iron that doesn't have this side effect.[52] See Chapter 6 for more information on iron supplements. Calcium supplements, especially when taken without magnesium, can also cause constipation.[53] Even if you're not taking calcium directly, you might be unknowingly consuming it through antacids (like Tums®).

To summarize, try the following if you're experiencing constipation:

- Drink enough fluids (100 oz per day or more).
- Eat more fiber-rich foods (with a high fiber-to-carbohydrate ratio).
- Consider chia seeds.

- Eat more fat.
- Move more.
- Squat to poop.
- Consider taking magnesium citrate and a probiotic supplement.
- Avoid calcium and iron supplements, unless medically indicated.

Weight Gain

When it comes to weight gain during pregnancy, there's a huge range of what's normal and healthy. I shy away from talking numbers as much as possible, but sometimes having a little context is helpful. Research has shown that when you're given accurate information about weight gain goals during pregnancy, you're more likely to gain within that range.[54] Please keep this in mind as you go through this section and know that my intention is not to body-shame in any way; my intention is only to inform and help you have the healthiest pregnancy, no matter what your weight is. The last thing I want you to do is dwell on a number on the scale.

Gaining too little or too much weight throughout your pregnancy is linked to a number of problems, including your likelihood of having a small or large baby, your risk of developing gestational diabetes, preeclampsia, and for having complications at delivery.[55] Up until the past 50 years, the concern over weight gain in pregnancy was focused on maternal undernutrition and low birth weight, but current research suggests the opposite problem is now more prevalent.

In the United States, roughly half of all women gain more than the recommended amount of weight during pregnancy. From 1990 to 2003, there was a 20-25% increase in women gaining 40 pounds or more during their pregnancies in America.[56] This is becoming a major concern because studies have "consistently shown maternal overweight and obesity during pregnancy to be significant risk factors for higher birth weight and neonatal adiposity; and for childhood obesity and later life metabolic dysregulation."[57] So as much as I'd like to say that "weight is just a number," the research tells us that we shouldn't ignore it.

Why are women gaining more weight during pregnancy these days?

Research suggests that the increased consumption of high-glycemic carbohydrates may be to blame for the rise in excessive prenatal weight gain (as well as big babies) seen in Western countries. Dietary surveys in the United States from the 1970s compared to the last decade show a steady

Real Food for Pregnancy

increase in carbohydrate consumption coupled with lower fat and protein intake.[58] One study found that average prenatal weight gain among women eating a low-glycemic diet was 23 pounds compared to 41 pounds in women who ate more high-glycemic carbohydrates.[59] In addition, all measures of infant size and fat mass were significantly higher in the women eating a high-glycemic diet.

For many women who gain beyond the guidelines, some of these extra pounds stick around postpartum. One researcher puts it this way: "pregnancy may serve as an inciting factor that leads to increased body weight 15 to 20 years postpartum."[60] This means that your weight gain during pregnancy can impact your weight and risk of metabolic problems later in life.

How much weight should I gain?

There's not a one-size-fits-all recommendation for prenatal weight gain. A lot of what determines your "ideal" weight gain is your pre-pregnancy weight. You can use online calculators (such as http://www.bmi-calculator.net/) to determine your body mass index (BMI) and see if you fall into the underweight, normal weight, overweight, or obese category.

Although BMI is not a perfect measure (mainly because it has no way of differentiating lean tissue vs. fatty tissue), it's the most convenient way to estimate a weight gain goal. Clearly, if you are big-boned or have a lot of muscle mass, you'll want to use your best judgement when interpreting your BMI and weight gain goals; some muscular women will have a BMI in the "obese" category even if they have a healthy body fat percentage. I also think it's helpful to take into account your height. A woman who is 4'11" may want to err on the lower end of her BMI's weight gain range while a woman who is 5'11" may want to aim for the higher end.

The Institute of Medicine suggests the following weight gain ranges for pregnant women (use your *pre-pregnancy* weight to calculate your BMI):

- Underweight (BMI <18.5) 28-40 lbs
- Normal weight (BMI 18.5-25) 25-35 lbs
- Overweight (BMI 25-30) 15-25 lbs
- Obese (BMI >30) 11-20 lbs

Interestingly, prenatal weight gain goals are not universal across the globe. In parts of Western Europe, India, Africa, the Philippines, and Chile, weight gain targets are at the lower end of the Institute of Medicine ranges, with targets ranging from 18-33 lbs for normal weight women.[61] Clearly "normal" weight gain in pregnancy is a moving target.

The idea of gaining weight during pregnancy gives a lot of women anxiety, but it's nothing to be scared of. Your body is growing another human, it's growing a brand new organ (your placenta), your breast tissue is changing to prepare to produce milk, you have several *pounds* of extra fluids, and your body (naturally) accumulates some fat. Weight gain does not always follow a linear path. If you're having nausea or food aversions, there may be some points in your pregnancy when your weight gain is at a standstill or when you lose some weight. Then there may be times when you suddenly gain several pounds in a week (this is common in the latter half of pregnancy). The hormonal shifts going on in your body sometimes take the reins, even if you're not consciously eating larger portions. Don't worry. It usually evens out by the end.

That said, If you experience rapid weight gain (more than 4 pounds in a week), and especially if it's accompanied by swelling or water retention, contact your medical provider to rule out complications, such as preeclampsia or high blood sugar.

Many women expect to only gain weight in the second half of pregnancy and then feel surprised or worried if/when they feel puffy and bloated in the first trimester. Let me reassure you that this is normal. In the first half of pregnancy, your body is in an anabolic state, meaning it's trying to store energy (build up your fat stores) for later on. Your body is also working overtime to grow the placenta (which, on its own, can weigh several pounds). Although your baby is small at this stage and doesn't account for much of this weight gain or "puffiness," your body is doing other (very important) work to prepare a home for your baby. A weight gain of 3-7 lbs in the first trimester is pretty typical for an average-sized woman.

In the second half of pregnancy, your body switches to a catabolic state, where it attempts to shunt as many nutrients as it can to your rapidly growing baby.[62] This is when your body often makes use of your maternal fat stores to fuel your baby. Although your belly is probably huge, you might feel a bit leaner in other parts of your body. This too, is normal. (And if you're simply feeling huge *everywhere*, that's normal too!)

If your BMI puts you in the overweight or obese category at the time of conception, like 60% of moms in the United States, you may benefit from less weight gain or even no weight gain at all.[63] The Institute of Medicine ranges are a helpful guide, but some research suggests these goals could be fine-tuned. In a very large study of over 120,000 obese women, the most favorable pregnancy outcomes were found in women who gained *below* the Institute of Medicine ranges, specifically noting a lower risk of preeclampsia, C-section delivery, and chances of having a big baby. The researchers suggest that women with a BMI >35 gain 0-9 lbs and with a BMI >40 gain no weight or *lose* up to 9 lbs over the course of their pregnancies.[64] This may sound extreme or impossible, but in my practice, I've observed hundreds of healthy pregnancies where women at these BMI ranges barely gained weight or even finished their pregnancies weighing less. I attribute a lot of these results to women changing their eating habits to more nutrient-dense foods, incorporating mindful eating, and having the metabolic efficiency of pregnancy on their side. Since I have never promoted calorie counting or deprivation diets, it certainly was not because they were "starving" (believe me, when I observe weight loss, I want to make sure my clients are honoring their hunger cues and not purposefully undereating). Their bodies were simply re-distributing some of their stored energy to the baby.

Some of the research I point out in this section might sound frightening. You may be reassured to hear that some research has shown that an infant's risk of growing too large or accumulating too much fat during gestation is a reflection of poor diet quality, rather than pre-pregnancy weight or even total caloric intake.[65] In other words, we can't blame everything on weight.

No matter where your weight was preconception and where you are now, try to focus your attention on consuming high quality, nutrient-dense foods, eating mindfully, and moving your body in a way that feels good to you instead of obsessing over the scale or stressing about what you could have done in the past to be at a different weight. Remember that weight gain goals are not etched in stone. The outcomes of your pregnancy are not dictated by your weight alone; it's simply one of many factors to consider.

High Blood Pressure

High blood pressure affects up to 10% of all pregnancies.[66] Normally, blood pressure levels trend down in early pregnancy, then gradually increase to pre-pregnancy levels as you get closer to delivery.[67] If your blood pressure is elevated (typically defined as $\geq$ 140/90 mmHg), there's a higher risk of certain complications, notably having a low birthweight baby and going into preterm labor. In some cases, high blood pressure can can progress into preeclampsia.

Preeclampsia involves high protein levels in the urine and swelling (edema) in addition to high blood pressure. These symptoms are signs of dysfunction of the lining of your blood vessels and, in some cases, can lead to organ damage.[68] There's been extensive research into the origins of high blood pressure and preeclampsia and researchers still don't have perfectly clear answers on how to prevent or treat it. There is more than one cause of high blood pressure and it's helpful to work with an experienced medical provider to understand your unique case. My aim with this section is to give you some insight into the role that nutrition and lifestyle tweaks can play in regulating your blood pressure. Please understand that while some cases of high blood pressure and preeclampsia can be managed with lifestyle choices, this is not true for all cases. That said, the following is a summary of the evidence on managing high blood pressure naturally.

Many women are told to reduce their salt intake to lower their blood pressure. Unfortunately, this is outdated and unfounded advice. As I explained in Chapter 2, salt is vital to many functions in your body and is even more important in pregnancy. In spite of what you've heard, salt often does not have an impact on blood pressure. In fact, only about 25% of the population is salt-sensitive (meaning, only 25% of people will see their blood pressure drop on a low-salt diet or go up on a high-salt diet). Plus, 15% of the population will see their blood pressure *go up on a low-salt diet.*[69]

Pregnancy-induced high blood pressure seems especially non-responsive to salt restriction. Studies on pregnant women show that a low-salt diet neither prevents nor controls preeclampsia.[70] In fact, it can actually make it worse. Inadequate salt intake can lead to unwanted consequences, like dehydration, that only compounds the stress your body faces when you have preeclampsia. As one study concludes, "a low-salt diet is not only ineffective, but also accelerates volume depletion in preeclampsia."[71] A low-salt diet is also known to disrupt blood sugar balance.[72] Even more concerning is the fact that salt restriction can impede your baby's growth and may affect his or her risk for disease later in life. As one researcher explains, "Salt is one of the integral components for normal growth of fetuses. Salt restriction during pregnancy is connected to intrauterine growth restriction or death, low birth weight, organ underdevelopment and dysfunction in adulthood probably through gene-mediated mechanism."[73] It is also "well reported that during critical developmental periods, salt restriction might affect fetal hormonal, vascular, and renal systems to regulate fluid homeostasis in the fetus."[74] Even a Cochrane review—a highly respected source of evidence-based analyses—concluded that advice to lower salt intake in pregnancy should not be recommended.[75]

In simple language, a low salt diet is not a good idea while pregnant, and could be even worse for women who have preeclampsia. Given that preeclampsia is associated with growth restriction in babies, it makes you wonder how much of that is to blame on the diagnosis itself or the low-salt diet these women were prescribed.

Consuming more salt—*not less*—may actually improve your blood pressure. As early as 1958, in a study of over 2,000 women, researchers noted lower

Real Food for Pregnancy

levels of preeclampsia in women who consumed higher levels of salt.[76] In addition, they observed a reduction in blood pressure and edema (swelling) in women when additional salt was added to their diets. In light of this information, these researchers advised women with signs of preeclampsia to "measure out each morning four heaped teaspoonfuls of table salt and to see that by night they had taken all of it." This resulted in "spontaneous recovery" from preeclampsia (called toxemia in this era) for the majority of the women. They noted that "The extra dose of salt had to be taken up to the time of delivery; otherwise the symptoms of toxemia recurred," which suggests that salt was indeed playing a crucial role in treating their condition. Recent studies have replicated this finding, noting that higher salt intake during pregnancy lowers blood pressure and lessens the severity of preeclampsia.[77,78] In addition, a 2014 study concluded that "Extra salt in the diet seems to be essential for the health of a pregnant woman, her fetus, placental development, and appropriate function."[79]

If you happen to fall into the small percentage of people who are salt-sensitive (meaning your blood pressure goes up if you eat too much salt), know that research has shown that salt-sensitivity is frequently driven by other dietary factors. One of the key players in salt sensitivity is over-consumption of a type of sugar called fructose.[80] Before drastically reducing your salt intake, it would be wise to cut out sugary beverages and other concentrated sources of fructose (especially high-fructose corn syrup and fruit juice). In a study of nearly 33,000 pregnant women, those who ate the most added sugars (like sugar-sweetened drinks) were more likely to develop preeclampsia.[81] Another reason to limit fructose is that it's the number one driver of elevated triglycerides, a type of fat in your blood that's a marker of inflammation and is generally higher in women with preeclampsia.[82]

Fructose isn't the only type of sugar that causes problems, though. High blood pressure and high blood *sugar* tend to go hand in hand, so eating excessive amounts of sugar (or even carbohydrates, which break down into sugar in your body), is unwise. We know that insulin resistance in the first trimester, a hallmark of blood sugar imbalance, may actually predict preeclampsia later in pregnancy.[83] Also, women with gestational diabetes have a 1.5 fold higher risk for developing preeclampsia.[84] Luckily, your blood sugar is something that you can shift by changing your diet. Research has shown that a lower-carbohydrate diet tends to reduce the severity of high blood pressure.[85] There's no better time than the present to get proactive about your food choices and switch to a lower-carb, low-glycemic diet.

Aside from reducing your intake of sugar and processed carbohydrates, there are certain foods and nutrients you can emphasize to help normalize your blood pressure. For one, foods that help to lower inflammation often help lower blood pressure as well. Women with preeclampsia tend to have lower levels of healthful omega-3 fats and an excess of omega-6 fats.[86] If you're not already doing so, ditch the processed vegetable oils (a major source of omega-6s), and aim to include more foods rich in omega-3 fats, including salmon, sardines, eggs from pasture-raised chickens, and pasture-raised meat. Refer back to Chapter 2 for recommended healthy fats. You also want to be sure you're not consuming trans fats in your diet as they have been linked to vascular complications in pregnancy. Trans fat intake, even at relatively low levels, is associated with lower birth weight, lower placental weight, and with a higher risk of preeclampsia.[87] For more on trans fats, see Chapter 4.

Protein intake is especially important when it comes to maintaining normal blood pressure. Your entire cardiovascular system is under a tremendous amount of stress during pregnancy, as it has to cope with higher levels of fluids, hormonal shifts, and expanding blood vessels. Protein-rich foods supply the raw materials to help your body meet these demands, so it's no surprise that low protein intake is a risk factor for developing preeclampsia.[88] One amino acid, called glycine, can be especially helpful for regulating blood pressure. As you may recall from previous chapters, glycine needs increase dramatically during pregnancy. One of the functions of glycine is in the production of elastin, a structural protein that allows your blood vessels to expand and contract. Glycine is also protective against oxidative stress, a hallmark of preeclampsia, and glycine has been shown to reduce blood pressure and blood sugar in studies.[89] Women with preeclampsia excrete less glycine in their urine, suggesting increased demands for glycine and/or depleted maternal stores.[90] The best sources of glycine are the connective tissues, skin, and bones of animal foods, like you consume when you eat bone broth, slow-cooked meat (like pot roast and stews), chicken with the skin, pork cracklings (fried pork skin), and collagen or gelatin powder. Refer to Chapter 3 for additional information on the food sources of glycine.

Another nutrient that may protect against preeclampsia is choline. It appears that choline plays a role in placental function and may enhance the transfer of nutrients to your baby, a process that's disrupted in preeclampsia.[91] In rodent studies, supplementation with choline prevents preeclampsia and reduces placental inflammation.[92,93] Studies on human placental cells confirm these results, noting that "choline inadequacy may contribute to placental dysfunction and the development of disorders related to placental insufficiency."[94] Supplementing pregnant women with high amounts of choline in the second and third trimester (930 mg, which is roughly double the current recommended intake) has been shown to improve vascular function of the placenta and "mitigate some of the pathological antecedents of preeclampsia."[95] Theoretically, this makes a lot of sense. The placenta shares a lot of similar functions to the liver and choline is particularly

Real Food for Pregnancy

protective to liver function. Consumption of foods that provide high amounts of choline, namely egg yolks and liver, also supply a variety of micronutrients that are anti-inflammatory. If you're not already doing so, incorporate these two nutrient-dense foods into your diet. Refer back to Chapter 3 for more information on the benefits of these foods.

Other foods that help to lower blood pressure include fresh vegetables and fruits that are rich in both potassium and antioxidants, such as green leafy vegetables, tomatoes, Brussels sprouts, mushrooms, winter squash, avocados, oranges, and broccoli. Berries are especially high in antioxidants and studies suggest they may help lower your blood pressure.[96] You might be tempted to take an antioxidant supplement, however supplemental antioxidants (like vitamins C and E) have shown mixed results in research studies.[97] Instead, I recommend relying on real food as your source of antioxidants.

Sometimes there are good reasons to supplement, though. When it comes to high blood pressure, consider your intake of magnesium, calcium, and vitamin D. Numerous studies have linked vitamin D deficiency with preeclampsia, so be sure to have your vitamin D levels tested and supplement accordingly.[98] Early pregnancy vitamin D supplementation appears to be especially beneficial.[99] Women with preeclampsia tend to have lower intakes of calcium and magnesium, so it's not a bad idea to supplement with both.[100] In severe cases of preeclampsia, women are admitted to the hospital and receive an IV with magnesium sulfate. Interestingly, supplementing with magnesium starting in the second trimester reduces the risk of high blood pressure.[101] Though I'm not a proponent of routine calcium supplements in pregnancy, I make an exception in the case of preeclampsia. Some studies have found that supplementing with calcium, even in doses of just 500 mg per day, can help alleviate high blood pressure in pregnancy and may reduce related complications.[102] One study found that a combination supplement with calcium, magnesium, zinc, and vitamin D significantly reduced blood pressure in pregnant moms at risk for preeclampsia.[103] Given the role of complementary nutrients in calcium utilization, I would suggest a combined supplement (like the one just mentioned), rather than calcium alone. Iodine is another mineral that may influence the risk of preeclampsia, and some researchers suggest it may help with the treatment of preeclampsia.[104,105] See Chapter 6 for more information on supplements and Chapter 9 for information on getting your vitamin D levels tested.

Finally, there are other lifestyle factors—beyond food and supplements—that affect your blood pressure. Exercise is especially helpful to maintain lower blood pressure, and moderate exercise may help prevent preeclampsia.[106] One study showed that pregnant women who did not exercise were 3x more likely to develop high blood pressure compared to those who exercised 3 days per week for roughly an hour at a time.[107]

Stress and anxiety are known contributors to both high blood pressure and preeclampsia.[108] At the same time, as I'm sure you can relate, there's no shortage of worries while pregnant. You can, however, lower your stress levels with simple, everyday practices. Studies have shown that a mindfulness practice can effectively lower anxiety symptoms by half (or more).[109] Often a mindfulness practice is as simple as paying attention to your breathing patterns, consciously scanning the sensations in your body, or actively relaxing your muscles, one by one, as you go from head to toe. There's no right or wrong way to de-stress, just find a practice that works for you. See Chapter 11 for a deeper discussion of stress management and self care.

To summarize, the following may help if you're experiencing high blood pressure:

- Do not excessively restrict salt intake. Use high-quality unrefined sea salt to taste.
- Drink enough fluids.
- Limit added sugars, especially fructose.
- Eat a lower-carb, low-glycemic diet. Ditch the refined grains.
- Avoid vegetable oils and trans fats. Eat more omega-3 fats.
- Consume adequate amounts of protein, especially glycine-rich sources of protein.
- Ensure you consume enough choline.
- Eat more high-antioxidant fresh produce.
- Consider supplementing with magnesium, calcium, and vitamin D.
- Exercise regularly.
- Find ways to manage your stress and anxiety.

As you can see, high blood pressure during pregnancy can be related to many areas of your life, from food, to supplements, to exercise, and even stress management. While there are a lot of potential lifestyle tweaks to try, be aware that some high blood pressure requires the help of medication to manage it, and that's ok. It's helpful to work with an experienced medical provider who can determine the underlying cause of your high blood pressure and help you find the right balance of natural treatments and medical management.

High Blood Sugar

Gestational diabetes, or high blood sugar that either develops or is first recognized during pregnancy, is a complex topic and has been the focus of most of my professional work as a dietitian. Over the past few decades, research has made several things clear: blood sugar is naturally meant to run *lower* during pregnancy; many women unknowingly come into pregnancy with high blood sugar (prediabetes); and even mildly elevated blood sugar carries risks for mom and baby. I'll do my best to go through the most important points here, and if you want to learn more, I have an entire book on this topic, *Real Food for Gestational Diabetes*. If you find yourself with this diagnosis, you'll know where to go for additional guidance.

There are many metabolic changes going on inside your body that can affect your blood sugar, particularly in the second half of pregnancy. Placental hormones along with weight gain make your body more insulin resistant in an attempt to send as many nutrients to your rapidly growing baby as possible. Normally, this doesn't result in high blood sugar because your body has planned ahead and triggered your pancreas to increase the production of insulin (by up to 3x normal levels).[110] In fact, blood sugar tends to run about *20% lower* during pregnancy.[111] However, in the case of gestational diabetes, your body may not be able to keep up with insulin production, and/or your insulin resistance may be so high that your body cannot maintain normal blood sugar levels without significant changes to your diet, exercise, or supplement habits (and in some cases, requires the help of medication or insulin).

Nowadays, researchers have recognized that many cases of gestational diabetes are actually undiagnosed prediabetes or type 2 diabetes, meaning we can't just point the finger at placental hormones or gestational weight gain in every case. An elevated first trimester hemoglobin A1c, which is a reflection of several months of average blood sugar levels, accurately predicts gestational diabetes in 98.4% of cases.[112] In other words, for some women, blood sugar was elevated *before* they got pregnant. This, in part, explains why gestational diabetes is on the rise, right alongside population-wide increases in type 2 diabetes, and now affects up to 18% of pregnancies.[113] This makes it the most common pregnancy complication, by far.

Why does blood sugar matter?

To put it simply, your body is *obsessed* with keeping your blood sugar fairly low during pregnancy. High blood sugar is a known cause of birth defects and can impact your baby's growth, development, and metabolic health for life.[114] Your baby's blood sugar levels are a direct reflection of your own.

When they run high, your baby's pancreas must compensate by secreting high levels of insulin. One side effect of high insulin and blood sugar levels is higher percentage body fat. This explains why babies of moms with uncontrolled gestational diabetes risk being born too large, not because they are exuberantly healthy, but because they have accumulated excess body fat. They also run the risk of having low blood sugar (hypoglycemia) after birth. Once the umbilical cord is cut, the constant supply of sugar stops, yet the baby's body is still pumping out lots of insulin. The result can be life-threatening hypoglycemia.

Though these may seem like problems that only affect the time immediately during or after birth, we now know that these babies can have altered metabolism for life. Being exposed to elevated blood sugar can "turn on" the genes that predispose your infant to obesity, diabetes and heart disease in their lifetime. As mentioned in Chapter 1 of this book, this effect is called "fetal programming." Children of mothers with gestational diabetes face a 6-fold higher risk of blood sugar problems and obesity by the time they are teenagers.[115]

These statistics have a physiologic explanation. Fetal production of insulin—the response to high maternal blood sugar—can be measured by insulin levels in the amniotic fluid. High levels of insulin in amniotic fluid have been linked to obesity in children at adolescence.[116] I don't mean to scare you, but I think it's important to understand how and why blood sugar can impact your pregnancy and your baby. Before I go any further, please know that even moms who are given an "official" diagnosis of gestational diabetes can avoid these outcomes and have perfectly healthy pregnancies *if they maintain normal blood sugar levels*. Blood sugar levels are far more important than a label.

That said, every pregnant mother—with or without "official" gestational diabetes—owes it to herself and her baby to keep her blood sugar under control. Research is showing us that even mildly elevated blood sugar during pregnancy is linked to serious problems. For example, the landmark Hyperglycemia and Adverse Pregnancy Outcomes study (HAPO), which studied 23,316 women with gestational diabetes and their infants, found that mildly elevated fasting blood sugar levels (which are blood sugar readings taken first thing in the morning) were linked to high insulin levels in infants at birth and macrosomia, meaning the baby is larger than normal at birth. In that study, women with an average fasting blood sugar of 90 mg/dl or less had a large baby only 10% of the time, compared to 25-35% in women whose average fasting blood sugar was 100 mg/dl or higher.[117] That's a substantial difference for what most would think is a relatively minor 10-point elevation in blood sugar. A more recent study out of Stanford University found a significantly higher risk of congenital heart defects in babies born to women with mildly elevated blood sugar (even below the diagnostic criteria for gestational diabetes).[118]

The bottom line: your blood sugar levels in pregnancy matter. Clearly, the adverse "fetal programming" typically attributed to gestational diabetes may be occurring to mothers who experience only slightly elevated blood sugar. That's why I believe *every* pregnant woman should have her blood sugar in mind while pregnant and eat in a way that naturally supports healthy blood sugar regulation. This takes the strain off of an already overworked pancreas.

How can I maintain lower blood sugar?

The good news is that blood sugar is highly responsive to lifestyle changes. First and foremost, the most important step to lower your blood sugar is to understand that the only nutrient that significantly and directly raises your blood sugar is carbohydrates. With gestational diabetes, you'll need to watch your total intake of carbohydrates and pay close attention to the quality and quantity of carbohydrates you eat. This makes sense given that one way to describe gestational diabetes is "carbohydrate intolerance in pregnancy."

This advice may seem obvious, but unfortunately, the conventional nutrition advice for gestational diabetes ignores this basic truth and pushes a high carbohydrate diet (no less than 175 g per day). It's silly when you stop to think about it. If you're given the diagnosis of "carbohydrate intolerance," why would you be told to eat a bunch of carbohydrates? If you think about the way that gestational diabetes is most commonly screened for—with a glucose tolerance test that contains 50+ grams of glucose—why would anyone think you'd have normal blood sugar after eating 50+ grams of carbohydrates (which turn into glucose in your body) at almost every meal?

It's no wonder that roughly 40% of women with gestational diabetes will require insulin and/or medication to lower their blood sugar when they're consistently filling up their carbohydrate-intolerant bodies with lots of carbohydrates.[119] It's not their fault; it's what they've been instructed to do by well-meaning, but misinformed, clinicians. This is a major reason I developed my "real food approach" to manage gestational diabetes. Women were not "failing the diet," *the diet was failing them.* The safety and efficacy of a low-carb, nutrient-dense diet during pregnancy is clear: it supports better blood sugar regulation and ensures the optimal development of your baby.

One research study found that eating a lower-glycemic diet reduces the chances that a woman will require insulin by fully 50%.[120] A separate study found that a lower glycemic meal plan "acutely halves day-long maternal glucose levels and reduces glucose variability, providing further evidence to support the utility of a low glycemic diet in pregnancy."[121] In other words, your diet plays a huge role in your blood sugar levels, and cutting out the processed carbohydrates goes a long way in helping to manage your blood sugar.

With gestational diabetes, however, you'll likely have to do more than just cut out the processed carbohydrates; you'll need to be careful with carbohydrates from all sources. You'll want to use a glucose meter to test your blood sugar first thing in the morning (called fasting blood sugar) and 1-2 hours after each meal. This will help you identify when your blood sugar is high, so you can take action. (See Chapter 9 for target blood sugar levels during pregnancy, as they differ from non-pregnancy targets.)

For example, if your blood sugar is consistently high after meals, it's often a sign that you're eating too many carbohydrates. Even if those carbohydrates are from whole foods, like fruit or yogurt or sweet potatoes, they still raise your blood sugar and the portion size that's right for you might not work for another woman. Plus, the combination of foods that you eat at meals and snacks can affect how quickly and/or how high your blood sugar goes after eating. Often, eating smaller portions of carbohydrates alongside an adequate amount of protein and fat (and non-starchy vegetables) results in the best blood sugar levels. While there are some general principles that are helpful when starting out, know that blood sugar responses to foods can be highly individual, some of which can only be identified by using a blood sugar meter and testing yourself. Return back to Chapter 2 for more information about carbohydrates, food combining, and mindful eating, which are all extremely helpful for managing blood sugar levels.

While your diet is undeniably the most important factor in regulating your blood sugar, exercise is the runner up. Regular exercise can help lower your overall blood sugar (fasting and post-meals), it decreases insulin resistance, and it can reduce the need for medication.[122] In general, women who exercise tend to gain less weight in pregnancy, which also helps lower their insulin resistance.

How can I avoid gestational diabetes?

That's the million dollar question. Sometimes gestational diabetes is out of your control; sometimes there are things you can do modify these risks. If you've already been diagnosed, please do not dwell on "why" for too long. For example, if diabetes runs in your family, you suspect you had undiagnosed prediabetes, are an older mom, or started your pregnancy at a higher weight, statistics simply show that gestational diabetes (or more accurately, insulin resistance) is more common. You can't rewind the clock to lose weight preconception or change your family medical history, and the important thing is to focus on what *is* in your control: how you eat and care for your body *now*.

If you haven't been diagnosed and want to try to avoid it, there is some research showing that lifestyle factors can lessen the risk of gestational diabetes, at least for *some women*. For one, be sure you eat enough protein. That's because your pancreas, the organ that produces insulin, undergoes dramatic changes in early pregnancy as it prepares to pump out roughly triple the amount of insulin (this is to overcome the innate insulin resistance of late pregnancy *and* to keep your blood sugar in that nice 20%-lower-than-usual zone). In order to do this, the pancreas needs enough of certain amino acids, which suggests that inadequate protein consumption (particularly during the first trimester) is a risk factor for gestational diabetes.[123]

Next, you'll want to watch your intake of carbohydrates, especially refined carbohydrates. Women who drink juice or eat too much cereal, cookies, and pastries, have higher rates of gestational diabetes (interestingly, lower rates are found in women who regularly eat nuts).[124] Excessive fruit intake in pregnancy is also linked to higher odds for developing gestational diabetes, especially high-glycemic fruit.[125] This is logical, given that high-glycemic carbohydrates result in big spikes in blood sugar and may, for some women, exceed the insulin-secreting capacity of their pancreas.

High-glycemic carbohydrates are a double whammy because they not only drive the blood sugar up, but they are consistently linked to excess weight gain. Gaining too much weight drives up insulin resistance and then the cycle continues.

As one researcher describes, "Altering the type of carbohydrate eaten (high- v. low-glycemic sources) changes postprandial glucose and insulin responses in both pregnant and non-pregnant women, and a consistent change in the type of carbohydrate eaten during pregnancy influences both the rate of feto-placental growth and maternal weight gain. Eating primarily high-glycemic carbohydrate results in feto-placental overgrowth and excessive maternal weight gain, while intake of low-glycemic carbohydrate produces infants with birth weights between the 25th and the 50th percentile and normal maternal weight gain."[126]

Remember that how much you move your body is another powerful tool for regulating your blood sugar. Women who exercise regularly in pregnancy lower their chances of having gestational diabetes by up to 78%.[127] If that's not motivation to get moving, I don't know what is.

Nutrient deficiencies can also play a role in blood sugar metabolism. Deficiency in vitamin D has specifically been linked to insulin resistance and a higher chance of developing gestational diabetes.[128] Magnesium also plays a role in insulin resistance and women with low magnesium levels are more likely to develop gestational diabetes.[129] Supplementing with magnesium (250 mg/day) in women already diagnosed with gestational diabetes has been shown to significantly lower blood sugar levels and result in better infant outcomes.[130]

Nitty gritty research out of the way, know that simply following the nutrition advice in this book will help lessen your risk of gestational diabetes. Without going into all the details, there are numerous micronutrients that help with blood sugar regulation (beyond those mentioned above), so a more nutrient-dense diet that supplies these vitamins, minerals, and antioxidants is incredibly important.

If you suspect you have blood sugar issues or have been diagnosed with gestational diabetes, consult my other book, *Real Food for Gestational Diabetes*, which walks you step-by-step through coping with this diagnosis. It includes extensive discussions about fine-tuning a meal plan for optimal blood sugar control, what you need to know about blood sugar-lowering medications, and much more.

This section specifically focused on action steps to help with blood sugar management, but I'm sure you have questions about screening for gestational diabetes. Rest assured, I tackle this controversial and confusing topic in Chapter 9.

Summary

I hope this chapter has helped put some of the most common pregnancy complaints into context and given you food for thought. There's often so much fear, confusion, and misinformation about these topics, and when you're in the thick of it, sometimes it can feel like you have no control over what's happening. Understanding *why* you might be experiencing a symptom or pregnancy complaint often helps point to the solution. With that information, you're put back into the driver's seat and can choose to take a bumpy road a little slower or find another route altogether.

As you now know, many pregnancy complaints are, at least *somewhat*, in your control to manage. Often, you have the power to address them by making some changes in your lifestyle. Even when there are several possibilities, having a strategy or a checklist can make all the difference. So, before you rush ahead to the next section, jot some notes down and a make a commitment to yourself (and your baby) to act on your newfound insight.

Speaking of action, the next chapter is all about how moving your body can impact your pregnancy. What the evidence says about exercise during pregnancy may be different than what you've heard from friends. In my experience, pregnant women will usually do less (not more) exercise unless they are given accurate information, so I'm thrilled to spend some time covering everything you need to know about prenatal exercise.

Chapter 8:

Exercise

"Pregnancy is no longer a contraindication for physical activity, but is rather recognized as a window of opportunity for behavior modification. It is safe to continue or start most types of exercise…"
- Dr. Ylva Trolle Lagerros, Karolinska Institutet

We all know exercise is healthy, but somehow this becomes a controversial topic when you add pregnancy to the mix. Centuries ago, expecting moms engaged in a lot of the same activities while pregnant as they did preconception; nowadays, there's a lot of fear surrounding prenatal exercise. While there are some considerations and adjustments to make, particularly during the final months of pregnancy, exercise is generally a very good thing for both you and baby.

The American Congress of Obstetricians and Gynecologists (ACOG), which provides professional guidelines for prenatal medical providers across the United States, suggests that pregnant women "engage in 30 minutes or more of moderate exercise on most, if not all, days of the week" unless they have medical contraindications. Despite this recommendation, only half of physicians recommend physical activity to pregnant patients, even though there's no compelling evidence that exercise is harmful to pregnant women or their babies.[1]

This may partly explain why most women tend to reduce the duration and intensity of exercise over the course of their pregnancies.[2] A 2017 study found that only 15% of women meet the ACOG exercise goals.[3] My goal with this chapter is to give you accurate, evidence-based information on prenatal exercise as well as practical tips on how to modify your movements to be comfortable and safe in pregnancy.

You might be wondering what a nutritionist knows about exercise, but you should know that in addition to my nutrition background, I'm also a certified Pilates Instructor. I've taught Pilates to many women throughout their pregnancies and postpartum, and have worked under the direction of women's health physical therapists (those who deal with things like pelvic organ prolapse and abdominal separation), so I have quite a bit to share with you.

Overall Benefits of Exercise

Research has repeatedly shown beneficial effects of prenatal exercise on pregnancy outcomes. As one researcher puts it, "the scientific evidence is indisputable."[4] Women who remain active tend to gain less weight during pregnancy, have lower chances of developing gestational diabetes or preeclampsia, and recover faster from childbirth.[5,6]

In fact, a large study of over 21,000 women found that sedentary women had a 2.3x higher risk for developing gestational diabetes.[7] A different study found that inactive women were 3x more likely to develop high blood pressure, 1.5x more likely to exceed their weight gain goals, and 2.5x more likely to have a macrosomic baby when compared to women who exercised 3 days per week.[8] Exercise strengthens the pelvic floor and improves aerobic capacity, both of which may help you cope with labor.[9] Plus, women who exercise tend to be less likely to require C-sections.[10] If exercise were a drug, every pregnant mama would be taking it.

Beyond the physical benefits, exercise has mental and emotional effects as well, helping to relieve stress, anxiety, and depression.[4] Exercise makes it easier to stay in-tune with your body as it changes throughout the pregnancy. This mind-body awareness can help you choose exercises that help prevent lower back pain, reduce hunching in the shoulders, and reduce the chance of injury. Prenatal yoga has specifically been shown to help reduce anxiety, depression, stress, sleep disturbances, and lower back pain.[11]

In general, women who exercise during their pregnancies are more likely to return to regular exercise postpartum and have an easier time losing the weight they gained during pregnancy.

Benefits of Exercise for Your Baby

One of the biggest reasons women are afraid to exercise is that they're worried they might hurt the baby. However, most researchers agree that the benefits outweigh the risks when it comes to exercise during pregnancy. Fears around diverting blood flow from the baby, increasing the risk of miscarriage, or causing harm if the heart rate goes up have been shown to be nothing but old wives' tales.

Real Food for Pregnancy

Interestingly, we now know that while uterine blood flow *does* decrease slightly during exercise, oxygen delivery to the baby remains unchanged thanks to several complex metabolic shifts.[12] In other words, your body is smarter than you think. Also, research has found that regular exercise in pregnancy increases fetal heart rate variability, which may benefit brain and nervous system development.[13] Numerous research studies confirm that exercise improves brain development. One study notes that, "Compared to the newborns of mothers who were inactive during their pregnancy, the children of exercising pregnant women are born with more mature brains."[14] These benefits appear to extend beyond infancy, as children of active moms show better oral skills and academic performance later in childhood.[15]

Beyond the benefits to brain development, we see a decreased risk of obesity, type 2 diabetes, and metabolic syndrome in children of moms who exercised in pregnancy.[16] One researcher sums it up eloquently: "Evidence continues to grow in support of the notion that exercise during pregnancy is beneficial for fetal health and well-being, extending into childhood. Benefits for offspring are observable related to body weight and composition, cardiovascular health, and nervous system development. Exercise during pregnancy may elicit a prenatal programming effect, creating a healthy environment in utero during a critical time of organ development."[17]

If you're having trouble wrapping your mind around this, think of it this way: The increased circulation you experience during exercise brings new blood, nutrients, and oxygen to your baby. And remember, the only way your baby is getting nourishment and excreting waste is through *your* circulation, so keep that blood moving!

Starting an Exercise Program

The ideal exercise program for you will vary based on your individual abilities, preferences and fitness level before pregnancy. In general, aim for 30 minutes of exercise every day (or minimum of 150 min per week), including both strength/resistance exercise and aerobic exercise.[18]

If you're not used to exercising, start slow, such as adding a 10 minute walk after lunch. Once that becomes easy, you can gradually add more until you reach 30 minutes of physical activity in total over the course of the day, keeping in mind you can exercise for longer if it feels good. Some women choose to break up their activity into shorter stints. For some, a short walk several times a day is more realistic than doing a full workout. For others, they prefer a longer workout 3-4 days a week. It's up to you and how your body feels. It's worth it to think about the types of activity you actually like to do, because exercise is about making your pregnancy easier and healthier, not punishing yourself. I often prefer the word "movement" to "exercise" for that reason.

If you do not already exercise, be sure to check with your doctor or medical provider to rule out any specific contraindications or situations in which exercise should be avoided. You can also discuss any medical targets with them, like blood sugar levels if you have gestational diabetes.

Exercise Precautions for Pregnancy

There are some considerations pregnant women should take to make sure the exercise regimen they choose is safe and effective. Once you have your medical provider's approval, there are a few things to keep in mind.

First is to become aware that your body is going through amazing and necessary changes to accommodate your growing baby. Pregnancy causes an increase in blood volume, cardiac output and respiratory rate, which may make it feel like it's hard to catch your breath. In the third trimester, this is compounded by the fact that baby is larger and pressing up into your chest cavity, thus limiting your lung capacity (and therefore oxygen intake). Listen to your body and use the "talk test," described below, to assess your efforts and limits.

Talk Test

The talk test is a pretty simple method to assess your exertion. If you're having trouble breathing, can't catch your breath, or are unable to say a short sentence, you are exercising too hard. Slow down and catch your breath. An increase in heart rate and respiration is fine, just not to the point where you cannot get enough oxygen or start to feel faint. You're exercising at a good level if you have a noticeable increase in heart rate and are still able to carry on a light conversation. I realize this advice is vague; however, the "talk test" correlates better to exertion during pregnancy than any other measure.[19] As physiotherapist Marika Hart, says, "You should be able to talk, but not be able to sing."

Heart Rate

Many women want to check their heart rate to monitor their body during exercise. However, you may be surprised to learn that heart rate does not correlate with exertion during pregnancy nor is there a set guideline on what heart rate is ideal (or too high) during pregnancy.[4]

In general, the fear is that if you exercise too hard, your body will divert blood flow from the placenta to working muscles, which would result in heart rate changes in the fetus. This however, is not supported by research. Studies show that moderately strenuous exercise does not induce fetal distress or decrease fetal heart rate in healthy pregnant women.[20] That said, if you work out at a high intensity or are an elite athlete, working with a qualified health and fitness professional would be ideal. For the other 99% of us, rest assured that moderate aerobic activity throughout your pregnancy is nothing to fear.

Don't Over-Stretch

During pregnancy your body releases a hormone called relaxin, which, as the name suggests, helps *relax* your ligaments. Without relaxin, your pelvis would not be able to widen and allow you to birth your baby vaginally! It's actually a pretty neat system when you think about it.

The only downside is that some women can feel as if their joints are a little *too* loose. Joint instability and discomfort, especially in the pubic symphysis (pubic bone) and sacroiliac joints (very low back and hips) is fairly common.[21] This makes activities like jumping and twists or turns with sudden starts or stops potentially problematic. For some, deep lunges can put too much strain on the hips/sacrum and cause pain. Use caution with stretching and yoga, especially in the third trimester when you're carrying around the extra weight of your baby (and of course, your placenta, amniotic fluid, etc.). Know your limits and don't push it. It's easy to accidentally stretch too far and pull a muscle during pregnancy.

Also keep in mind that higher impact activities, including running, may become uncomfortable. Prenatal weight gain can increase forces on the knees and hips, especially during activities like running. If you were running regularly prior to conception, it's generally considered safe to continue during pregnancy, but *do* listen to your body. If it becomes uncomfortable, opt for lower impact activities like walking, swimming, moderate hiking or using an elliptical machine. Lower impact aerobics ease stress on those joints and also reduces pressure on your pelvic floor muscles (which can ultimately help prevent incontinence and pelvic organ prolapse). With any physical discomfort from exercise, it's wise to *not* "work through the pain."

Posture, Alignment, and Back Pain

Exercise is only beneficial and safe if you do it with good form. This is even more important during pregnancy, when your body has to cope with a shift in your center of gravity, and often, a lot more weight. As your belly grows, it pulls you forward. Many women tend to jut their hips forward and lean back or tuck their tailbone in an attempt to counterbalance the weight of their baby, but this may put your body out of alignment and aggravate back or hip pain.

Instead of allowing the weight of your baby to pull you forward, consciously try to get taller by imagining a string pulling you up from the crown of your head. With proper alignment, your head should be directly over your shoulders (ears aligned with shoulders), shoulders centered over your rib cage, rib cage centered over your hips, hips over your knees, knees over your ankles, and weight evenly distributed between the balls of your feet and your heels. It's a lot to think about!

If your breasts have grown or if you're not conscious of your posture, you may also experience upper back pain, as your shoulders begin to hunch forward and close in towards your chest. To offset this tendency, regularly stretch your chest muscles and strengthen the muscles of your upper back (between the shoulder blades). Imagine your collar bones lifting up, away from your belly, and gently widening towards the sides of your body. Hunching in the shoulders tends to get worse postpartum when you spend so much time feeding and holding your baby, so developing good posture now is really helpful in the long run.

Back pain is compounded when abdominal muscles are weak, since the abdominal muscles help you maintain alignment and "lift" in your spine. Exercises that involve core stabilization and/or an exercise ball have been shown effective to alleviate lower back pain and pelvic girdle pain that is so common in pregnancy.[22] Below I'll review some sample exercises to help you with this.

Proper Alignment

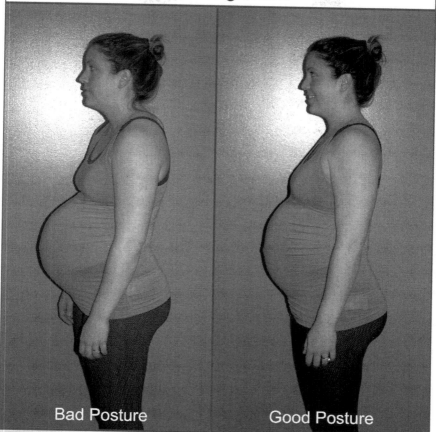

Bad Posture | Good Posture

The above photos are taken just minutes apart in a woman who is 40 weeks pregnant. In the example of "bad posture," notice the arching in her lower back and the tilt of her pelvis as she allows the weight of the baby to pull her forward. Also, note how her shoulders and upper back are hunched, causing her head to jut forward and strain her neck.

In the example of "good posture," she uses her abdominal and back muscles to lift and hold the baby close to her spine. This aligns her spine, reducing compression and pain in the lower back and neck. She has lengthened her spine, lifted her ribcage, and very literally created space for the baby in her torso. Also notice the length in her neck, the openness in her chest, and the position of her head directly over her shoulders.

Abdominal, Back, and Pelvic Floor Strength

The muscles of your core, which includes your abdominal, back, and pelvic floor muscles, are under a lot of pressure in pregnancy. As a Pilates teacher, I've repeatedly observed, firsthand, the beneficial effects of regular, properly performed core exercise on strength, stabilization, and flexibility during pregnancy. Pilates is an excellent option for expecting moms because it combines aerobic and strength exercise into one workout. It also works within the normal range of motion for joints, strengthens small stabilizing muscles, focuses on alignment, and is low-impact, thus reducing the risk of overstretching ligaments or injuring joints.

Pilates focuses attention on the abdominal, back, and pelvic floor muscles, which all tend to get weak during pregnancy. And yet, it is these muscles that are critical in maintaining healthy posture and vaginally birthing a baby.

Pelvic floor exercises, in particular, can help manage one pregnancy and postpartum annoyance that no one talks about: urinary incontinence. One study showed that women who undertook a 6-week program of pelvic floor exercises during pregnancy had significantly less stress urinary incontinence.[23] In real world terms, these women were less likely to accidentally pee themselves when laughing, sneezing, or coughing. Aside from static pelvic floor exercises, like kegels, where you "lift inward," functional movements like squats are helpful at promoting normal pelvic floor function. According to biomechanist Katy Bowman, more is not always better when it comes to kegels. You don't necessarily want a tight pelvic floor; you want a *functional* one. A functional pelvic floor engages when needed and *relaxes* when it's not needed; in other words, it's not tight *all the time.*

During pregnancy and birth, your pelvic floor muscles are under significantly more load. It's both normal and necessary for these muscles to stretch during pregnancy to accommodate the baby (it's tight quarters in there) and yield during birth. Postpartum, it takes many months (often a full year) for them to return to pre-pregnancy strength and function.[24] If you understand how to properly engage *and relax* your pelvic floor muscles, postpartum recovery is significantly easier. If you're not sure how to do this, I highly recommend seeking the expertise of a women's health physical therapist. They specialize in helping women with pelvic pain, pelvic organ prolapse (if it feels like your insides are falling out), incontinence, and so much more.

In some countries, like France, all women are seen by a pelvic floor physical therapist postpartum. It should be the norm across the globe, but unfortunately, that's not the case. If you have any suspicion that things aren't "normal" down there, either now or after your baby arrives, ask for a referral from your primary healthcare provider. For more on postpartum recovery and exercise, see Chapter 12.

Note on Abdominal Exercises

Many doctors warn against abdominal exercise during pregnancy, citing an increased risk of diastasis recti, in which the rectus abdominus ("6-pack" muscles that run vertically from lower ribs to pubic bone) separate at the center, leaving a gap. However, some level of abdominal separation is a normal part of pregnancy. A gap often forms because the linea alba (the connective tissue that connects the two sides of your 6-pack muscles) has to stretch to accommodate your growing baby. Research shows that 66-100% of women have some degree of diastasis recti in the third trimester.[25] Interestingly, studies have found that women who regularly exercise are at a lower risk for having diastasis recti and if it does occur, heal quicker postpartum. In one study, women who did not exercise during pregnancy had a 2-fold higher risk of diastasis recti.[26] In another, inactive women had a 90% incidence of diastasis recti compared to only 12.5% among active women who were regularly performing specific core exercises during pregnancy.[27]

This means that engaging the appropriate muscles while doing abdominal exercises may actually *prevent* diastasis recti. Before starting any and *every* abdominal movement, pregnant or not (and even when getting out of bed), you should gently draw your navel towards your spine, then draw your navel up towards your rib cage. This engages the tranversus abdominus ("corset" muscles), the deep muscles in the lower back, and the muscles of the pelvic floor, thereby preventing the rectus abdominus from trying to do all the work. You essentially create a muscular brace around your midsection.

One research study sums up why this works: "transversus abdominis muscle activation could be protective of the linea alba and may help to prevent or reduce diastasis recti and speed up recovery, allowing women to return to their usual physical and social activities more quickly."[28]

Women who partake in exercise programs focused on transversus abdominus and pelvic floor activation report less back pain and pelvic pain.[29] The transversus abdominus is considered a primary stabilizer of the lower back and pelvis and works together with your pelvic floor muscles to maintain proper alignment of your torso.[30]

That said, not all abdominal exercises are right for pregnancy, especially in the second half. Exercises like crunches, "roll ups" in Pilates, and unmodified planks can put too much pressure on the abdominal muscles and pelvic floor.

If you notice any bulging at your midline while performing certain exercises, this is a sign that your body isn't coping well with that movement. You can try either engaging your tranversus abdominus more (bracing your abdominal muscles before exertion), modifying the exercise to reduce the load, or discontinuing that exercise altogether. I remember having to pay extremely close attention to my abdominal muscle activation during my third trimester, otherwise it would look like a two-by-four board was coming out of my abdomen. It was a sign I needed to modify my movements, so I did. Below, I share a few alternative exercises that more gently engage your core muscles.

Should you engage your core all the time?

In short, no. You want to engage your muscles when you need them, not all the time. They need a chance to relax. Would you walk around with your bicep flexed all day? Of course not! When you have a muscle group constantly engaged, it can't work properly when you really need it. It's already fatigued from being "on" all day long. Instead, focus your attention on your alignment as you go about your day, but only engage your abdominal muscles (by gently drawing your navel towards your spine "in and up" and bracing) before exertion, such as before lifting a bag of groceries, squatting down to pick something up off of the floor, twisting or turning (like unloading the dishwasher), or doing an exercise in Pilates class. Also, be sure your definition of abdominal engagement is not "sucking in," but rather tightening and bracing your abdomen. When your core is engaged appropriately, you should be still be able to breathe. It's a gentle and subtle activation, rather than the feeling of wearing a corset that is cinched uncomfortably tight.

Sample Exercises

Hip Stabilization

Lie on your back. If you are further along in your pregnancy and feel dizzy or faint while lying on your back, you'll want to perform this exercise on a slight incline (several towels or heavy blankets under your upper back may do the trick).

Put your hands on the pointy part of your hip bones. Imagine a rubber band hooked between the hip bones. From the inside, imagine tightening that rubber band and bringing your hip bones closer together, using your muscles to gently pull your hip bones towards the center line of your body. Hold for 10 seconds. Release all muscle tension with a few deep breaths. Repeat 5-10 times.

Abdominal Exercises

Abdominal exercises may help prevent or reduce back pain. All of the sample exercises here should be done while engaging the abdominal muscles, but this simple exercise specifically targets those muscles while also strengthening the low back. But don't think simple means easy! If you're not shaking, you're not doing this right.

Sit on a cushy mat with your knees bent, feet on the floor. Sit up as tall as you can and draw your navel to your spine and draw your lowest ribs backwards slightly (without changing your posture or the natural curve in your lower back). Bring the arms straight in front of you. Lean back about 30 degrees while maintaining a lifted spine. Do not let the low back "sink" down. Hold for a count of 10-15 seconds. Return to the starting position. Repeat 3-5 times.

You can progress this exercise by lifting the arms, opening the arms wide, or by making arm circles (try one at a time to challenge your obliques). Play around and have fun. You can also lean back further when you've developed the strength to do so without compromising your form. You want to avoid "doming" or "bulging" of your abdomen during this exercise. If you notice this occurring, you are leaning too far back.

Squats

Stand with your feet slightly wider than hips distance apart and feet parallel (or slightly turned out, if that's more comfortable for you). Engage your core muscles. Bend your knees and squat down, letting your butt stick out behind you. Keep your spine straight (not arched or rounded). Return to standing. Repeat 10-20 times. Bend as low as is comfortable for your knees. You may lift the arms as you squat to stay balanced. Add light weights and change up the arm movements if you want more of a challenge.

Cat & Cow Stretch

Start on your hands and knees with hands shoulder distance apart and knees hip distance apart. Ensure your hips are right over your knees and shoulders are right over your wrists, gently pulled away from your ears. Start with a flat back. Take an inhale. Exhale as you round your back by pulling your belly button towards your spine and moving your ribs towards the ceiling. Let your head drop. Inhale as you reverse your spine, allowing the belly to relax and the chest to open up. Lift your gaze slightly without craning the neck too much. Repeat 5-10 times.

Child's Pose

Kneel and sit back on your heels. Open up your knees wide. Place your hands on the floor in front of you and gently lean forward until your belly is resting between the knees. You can place your hands in front of the body and gently push into the floor (as you simultaneously draw your shoulders down and away from your ears) to better stretch your back. Or you may choose to rest here and release all muscle tension.

Side Lying Chest Opener

This stretch is great first thing in the morning when still lying in bed.

Lie on your side with your knees pulled towards your chest and your hands behind your head. Leaving your hands behind your head, bring your elbows together until they touch. Inhale as you open up the chest and allow the "top" elbow to draw towards the ceiling and behind the body. Pause to feel the stretch. Exhale as you return to the starting position. For a more intense stretch, ensure that your knees stay together as you open up the chest. Repeat 5-10 times on each side.

Side Leg Series: Circles, Lifts, Point Flex

Lie on your side with your legs straight at a 45 degree angle (slightly in front of your body). Use your bottom arm to prop up your head. Your other arm can rest on the mat to stabilize you. Position yourself so your hips are stacked on top of one another. Engage your abdominal muscles to stabilize your body. Imagine your top leg is longer than your bottom leg.

This series should be completed on both sides.

Circles

Begin by lifting the top leg to hip level and make small circles 10 times in each direction. Ensure that only the top leg is moving and the rest of your body is completely still. This requires strong engagement of the abdominal and oblique muscles.

Lifts

Lift the top leg about 2 feet from the bottom leg. Hold for a count of 3. Lower down. Repeat 5x.

Point/Flex

This is exactly like the "lifts" exercise above. This time point your foot before you lift the leg, then flex the foot as you lower the leg down. Repeat 3-5x. Then reverse the movement and flex the foot as you lift it up, then point as you lower down.

Wall Push-ups

There are 2 versions of this exercise: Regular Push-ups and Tricep Push-ups. If you are used to doing push-ups, you can do these on the floor or on your knees (instead of against a wall). Later in pregnancy, it's better to opt for knee or wall push-ups to reduce strain on the abdominal muscles and pelvic floor.

Regular Push-ups

Stand 1-2 feet away from the wall with your feet parallel and hip distance apart. Lift your heels 2 inches off the ground. Place your hands on the wall directly in front of your shoulders. Spread your hands about 2 feet apart. Do 10 push-ups, keeping your body in a straight line.

Tricep Push-ups

Place your hands on the wall directly in front of your shoulders, only about 1 foot apart. Bring your body towards the wall by bending your elbows, keeping them close to your body. Repeat 10 times.

Adjusting Exercise by Trimester

First Trimester

In general, there are no major changes you have to make to your exercise regimen other than avoiding the usual activities that jerk, bounce or risk abdominal injury. Also, be aware of your temperature and avoid overheating during exercise, which may be a concern if you live in a hot climate. If you practiced "hot yoga" preconception, now's the time to switch to non-heated yoga classes. Becoming overheated on a regular basis in early pregnancy may increase the risk for certain malformations and neural tube defects.[31]

You may experience more fatigue or nausea during the first trimester, so if your body does not allow you to exercise, don't worry. Many women temporarily exercise less in early pregnancy, but have a boost in energy in the second and third trimester.[32] Stay open to the possibility that a short 5-15 minute walk might help you feel better. Resistance exercises, like light weights or using resistance bands, have been shown to help combat fatigue and boost energy in pregnancy.[33] Gentle yoga or a short series of Pilates exercises, such as the side-lying leg series, is another great way to sneak in resistance exercise.

Second Trimester

Exercises done lying on your back may become uncomfortable at this stage in pregnancy, depending on how much weight you have gained or where the baby is positioned. This is because your baby's weight is pressing on the vena cava, a large vein that carries blood from your lower extremities back to the heart. This can make it difficult for you to receive enough blood and oxygen, leaving you light headed. There's no long-term harm if you experience this for a moment. Simply sit up, catch your breath, and avoid lying on your back for long periods of time from this point forward.

For this same reason, exercises where the hips go above your heart—such as bridge pose in yoga, pelvic tilts in Pilates, or any inversions—are generally avoided beyond 16 weeks. The exact timing, again, will depend on how much weight you have gained, the positioning of your baby, and other factors, so pay close attention to your symptoms and your body, modifying exercises for comfort. Some women happily continue these exercises without any adverse symptoms. Simply listen to your body when deciding what's right for you.

In general, short bursts of activity performed lying on your back, such as a series of abdominal exercises, are fine, depending on your symptoms. Some women will choose to prop themselves up at a slight angle on their elbows or with pillows, blankets, or bolsters for those activities.

Third Trimester

In the third trimester, feelings of joint laxity may become more noticeable as you're now carrying more weight from your growing baby and uterus. Take care to avoid over-stretching. Participating in joint stabilizing exercises, such as Pilates or using resistance bands, can help you cope with this. Hip and lower back pain are more common. You may find that movements like deep lunges more easily cause pain or make your hips feel out of alignment. Adjust your movements as needed to stay comfortable.

Make good posture a priority. Regularly reassess your posture and sit up straight, with shoulders gently pulled back and your chest open.

Your growing baby is also likely pushing up on your lungs, making it harder to catch your breath. Adjust the intensity of exercises as needed, being sure to never get too out of breath (remember the "talk test"). Baby is also compressing your stomach, so avoid large meals immediately before exercising.

At this stage you are also more likely to become overheated, so take rests when exercising to cool down and hydrate. Avoid exercising outside during hot or humid weather.

The third trimester is also the most common time for you to experience Braxton Hicks contractions, the unpredictable, but usually not painful, "practice" contractions that many healthcare providers believe prepare and tone the uterus for actual labor. When they happen, the uterus may tighten for 30-60 seconds or longer, then taper off. They generally are non-rhythmic and irregular in intensity. If you notice slight contractions during exercise (and especially if you're far from your due date), they might be Braxton Hicks. Just stop and allow the contractions to pass before resuming your activity. If they continue or become painful, call your provider. Braxton Hicks are more common when dehydrated, so be sure to always carry water with you when exercising (and don't forget to consume enough salt and electrolytes).

Summary

Exercise is safe, effective, and beneficial during pregnancy. If you're anything like me, you'll likely go through a lot of different phases with exercise depending on your stage of pregnancy. In early pregnancy, fatigue and nausea can make exercise a challenge some days. In later pregnancy, sometimes you have to get creative with what positions you can comfortably get into as you navigate your ever-growing bump and looser joints. There will always be excuses to not exercise if you look for them. Remember that prenatal exercise isn't about proving yourself to anybody, it's about keeping your blood flowing, getting outside, feeling strong, and connecting with your body that's doing the amazing feat of growing another human being.

Prenatal Exercise Cheat Sheet

Exercise 30 minutes or more every day.
Include strength exercises 2-3x/week.

Aerobic – walking, jogging, stairs, elliptical, dancing, swimming, stationary bike, low impact
aerobics, moderate hiking
Strength – arm and leg exercises, light weights, Pilates, prenatal yoga, resistance training
Flexibility – Pilates, prenatal yoga, stretching
Abdominal/pelvic floor exercises – Perform daily to help ease low back pain and prepare for
labor. Use your muscles to "hold the baby close" to your body; squats are ideal for this.

Benefits
- Prevents Complications – Lowers blood sugar and blood pressure, prevents excess weight gain, and prevents larger than normal babies. May ease bloating, low back pain, constipation, varicose veins, swelling in legs and feet.
- Strength – Improves posture, muscle tone, and endurance.
- Mental Health – Boosts your mood; eases stress, anxiety, and depression; improves sleep.
- Postpartum – Reduces postpartum weight retention; less chance of abdominal separation.

General Guidelines
- Take frequent breaks to prevent overheating; don't exercise in hot weather
- Drink plenty of fluids to prevent dehydration
- Eat before exercising
- Wear comfortable, supportive clothing (sports bra) and shoes
- After ~16 weeks, or when it becomes uncomfortable, avoid exercises lying on your back

Exercises to Avoid
Do not play contact sports. Avoid movements that jerk, bounce or risk abdominal injury: soccer, football, baseball, hockey, basketball, kickboxing, downhill skiing, gymnastics, etc.

Precautions
Check with your healthcare provider to see if exercise is safe during your pregnancy. Exercise with a partner if you can. Talk with your healthcare team if you take insulin or blood sugar medication, since your meal plan or insulin may need to be adjusted.

Signs to Stop Exercising
If you experience the following, call your healthcare provider:
- Contractions of the uterus
- Decreased fetal movement
- Dizziness, chest pains, headache, or shortness of breath
- Vaginal bleeding or leaking of amniotic fluid

Real Food for Pregnancy

Chapter 9:

Lab Tests

"The metabolic needs of the fetus peak in the third trimester during the phase of greatest growth. Maternal metabolism during early gestation is thus largely anabolic, in essence hoarding nutrients in preparation for the upcoming demands. Late in gestation, maternal metabolism becomes largely catabolic, shunting nutrients to the rapidly growing fetus."
- Dr. Zolt Arany, University of Pennsylvania

Some researchers describe pregnancy as a "stress test" for your body. Many organs and bodily systems are put to the test, like your thyroid gland, cardiovascular system, and pancreas. Your nutritional status coming into pregnancy and throughout pregnancy can play a role in how well your body adapts to these demands. Unfortunately, conventional prenatal care usually doesn't take a proactive approach and instead waits until obvious clinical signs of dysfunction arise. This leaves you vulnerable to pregnancy complications that could have been prevented.

When I was pregnant, I remember arriving for my first prenatal visit and asking which labs would be included in the preliminary first trimester blood work. I was shocked to learn what was *not* automatically included on the list. Things like my vitamin D levels or average blood sugar (hemoglobin A1c) or thyroid hormone levels that could, if out of balance, affect my baby's development or my risk of complications, were simply not on their radar. I had to specifically request these be added to my prenatal labs. I wanted to know if anything was "off," so I could address it *right then*, not months down the line—or worse—end up nutrient-depleted and with health problems postpartum.

I realized in that experience that I was probably in the 0.05% of pregnant mamas who had the medical background to ask the right questions and push for the right testing. From this first set of prenatal labs, I was able to see that my vitamin D levels were borderline low and make the informed decision to increase the dose of my vitamin D supplement (getting more sunlight was not feasible given the latitude where I was living and the time of year). I'll never know if maintaining sufficient vitamin D helped my pregnancy continue smoothly and helped me avoid complications, but I certainly didn't want to risk the alternative. I share my personal experience to illustrate the reality that many pregnant women face when it comes to lab tests—not being automatically screened for treatable or preventable conditions. My goal with this chapter is to fill the knowledge gap between pregnant women, their medical providers, and the research.

In this chapter, I'll go through several prenatal labs you may want to ask for and why. Some medical providers are on top of the latest research and some are not. It doesn't hurt to ask for these to be added to your list of labs. Plus, if your providers are resistant to heed your request, you'll have a pretty good sign that they are not as interested in preventative care as you are.

Each of the lab tests I'll go through are useful to request at your first prenatal visit. If any lab values are out of range, you can re-test later in pregnancy—per the discretion of your healthcare team—to fine tune your diet and/or supplement regimen. The primary labs I'll run through are nutrition-related tests that are easily ordered by any conventional doctor. There are always additional tests that can be done through a functional medicine practitioner, which I'll mention towards the end of the chapter. Please note that this chapter does *not* cover prenatal lab tests outside of the realm of nutrition.

Vitamin D

Deficiency in vitamin D is widespread in general, but even more common during pregnancy. In some areas of the world, vitamin D deficiency affects up to 98% of pregnant women.[1] At the same time, supplementing with this nutrient is effective at reversing deficiency and is incredibly inexpensive. It's perplexing to me that identifying and correcting vitamin D deficiency is not the norm, especially given that it puts you at higher risk for preeclampsia, having a low birth weight infant, and gestational diabetes (according to two major meta analyses).[2,3] Not to mention, vitamin D is an essential nutrient for your baby's development and can permanently affect things like bone development and immune function.[4,5]

It would be amazing if there was a one-size-fits-all quantity of vitamin D that every pregnant woman could supplement with and simply know she was getting enough, but unfortunately, that's not the case (though 4,000 IU is a good dose to start with).[6] As I explained in Chapter 6, your vitamin D levels are affected by everything from your skin tone, sun exposure, use of sunscreen or choice of clothes, latitude where you live, diet, supplements, and more. Getting your blood levels of vitamin D tested is the only way to know for sure if you're getting enough or if you need to supplement with a higher dose.

Ideally, ask to have your vitamin D levels measured several times during your pregnancy, starting with a baseline value during the first trimester (or pre-pregnancy). The test you should ask for is called 25-hydroxy vitamin D (or 25-OH vitamin D). Most labs suggest that normal vitamin D levels are at least 30 ng/ml, but numerous vitamin D experts suggest optimal levels are 50 ng/ml or more.[7] Interestingly, modern hunter-gatherer populations maintain vitamin D levels around 46 ng/ml, suggesting relatively higher vitamin D levels may be the true normal to strive for.[8]

When interpreting your lab results, be aware that vitamin D levels can be given in different units, typically either ng/ml or nmol/l. Check your lab printout to make sure you're interpreting it correctly (30 ng/ml is equivalent to 75 nmol/l and 50 ng/ml is equivalent to 125 nmol/l).

As a personal aside, I had my vitamin D levels measured each trimester of my pregnancy and was surprised to see that I needed to supplement with significantly more vitamin D (above the 4,000 IU dose) to maintain normal levels. At the time, I was living at a high latitude and the climate was cold, so sun exposure was not an option. Being able to fine-tune my supplement dose gave me peace of mind that I was doing what was best for my baby. By my third trimester test, I could see my levels had gone up and had reassurance that the dosage I had determined was right for me. I was also able to go into the postpartum time knowing what amount of vitamin D that I needed to take to pass enough through my breast milk. As you prepare for the postpartum period, know that breastfeeding mothers need a minimum of 6,400 IU of vitamin D per day to provide adequate vitamin D for baby (if your baby is exclusively breastfed).[9]

Iron

As I outlined in Chapter 6, iron needs go up during pregnancy by a factor of 1.5. Yet, deficiency in iron is fairly common and can lead to anemia, in which you have low levels of red blood cells and/or the iron-carrying protein, called hemoglobin. This can reduce your ability to transport oxygen to your tissues, leading to symptoms like fatigue, weakness, or difficulty concentrating.[10] However, many women have no obvious symptoms of anemia.

Iron plays a key role in normal fetal development and the prevention of pregnancy complications, which is why it's fairly routine to check iron status during pregnancy. Often, screening for anemia will happen in the first prenatal labs and again in mid-pregnancy. Iron-deficiency anemia in the first two trimesters of pregnancy is linked to a 2x higher risk for preterm delivery and a 3x higher risk for having a low-birth-weight baby.[11] Low iron can also impair your thyroid function, which can result in neurodevelopmental delays for your baby.[12]

At minimum, you should have your hemoglobin, hematocrit, and serum ferritin levels measured to accurately assess iron status during pregnancy.[13] Some practitioners will also check other markers of anemia, such as mean cell volume (MCV), which can help differentiate iron-deficiency anemia from folate or vitamin B12 deficiency, and serum transferrin receptor (sTfr), which is an indicator of tissue iron stores.[14] Be aware that some lab values, including hemoglobin, are affected by the natural fluid retention in pregnancy (called hemodilution), so be sure to take that into consideration when having your lab tests interpreted.

Thyroid

Your thyroid is a tiny gland located at the front of your neck that produces several hormones. Thyroid hormone levels are most widely recognized for their role in metabolism, however they influence many other systems in the body. During pregnancy, your thyroid gland must ramp up production of hormones by more than 50% to provide enough for both yourself and your baby.[15] Up until mid-pregnancy, your baby is entirely reliant on your thyroid hormones (it's only around week 16-20 that the fetal thyroid gland is mature enough to produce its own hormones).[16] Even then, maternal thyroid hormones are still transferred across the placenta throughout pregnancy and are essential to the normal development of your baby.

A recent research paper sums up the typical changes in thyroid hormones about as simply as possible:

> "Various physiological changes that accompany the normal pregnancy state increase the demands of the maternal thyroid gland. In response to the estrogen-stimulated rise in the transport protein, thyroxine-binding globulin (TBG), there is a concomitant rise in total T3 and T4 in the first half of pregnancy until a new steady state is reached. Also in the first trimester, there is a transient lowering of circulating TSH that coincides with peak human chorionic gonadotropin (hCG) concentrations. Due to the structural homology between hCG and TSH molecules, hCG binds to the TSH receptor and exerts a stimulatory effect—the increased hormonal output of FT4 results in the lowering of TSH levels via the negative feedback system. Following the initial increase in FT4 between approximately 6 and 10 weeks of gestation as a result of the high placental production of hCG during this time period, FT4 subsequently decreases over pregnancy."[17]

Did I mention the thyroid is complex? The above quote illustrates why it's so important to find a practitioner who understands how pregnancy impacts your thyroid function, especially when ordering and interpreting lab values.

The importance of identifying and treating thyroid problems cannot be understated and an underactive thyroid, called hypothyroidism, is the most common manifestation. As one study points out, "hypothyroidism may be associated with miscarriages, low birth weight, anemia, pregnancy-induced hypertension, preeclampsia, abruption placenta, postpartum hemorrhage, congenital circulation defects, fetal distress, preterm delivery, and poor vision development, in addition to the probable neuropsychological defect in the child."[18] In one study, the rate of fetal loss was 60% in women with overt, untreated hypothyroidism.[19] If you have a history of miscarriage, it's very important to have your thyroid checked.

Your baby's brain development is highly dependent on your thyroid hormone levels. Mild to moderate thyroid dysfunction can result in neurodevelopmental problems ranging from low intelligence, delayed verbal development, impaired motor performance, autism, and attention-deficit hyperactivity disorder (ADHD).[20]

Clearly, ensuring this tiny gland is functioning properly matters, *big time*. It begs the question why screening thyroid hormones is not routine. Many endocrinologists have been pushing for universal thyroid screening in pregnancy, but it has yet to be widely adopted. At the very least, the American Thyroid Association recommends routine screening for women over the age of 30, with any history of miscarriage or pregnancy loss, preterm delivery, infertility, autoimmune disease, obesity, family history of thyroid problems, or those residing in an area where iodine deficiency is common.[21] I'll go out on a limb here and say that a good portion of the women reading this book can identify with at least one of the above risk factors.

The challenge is that measuring thyroid function can be complex. There are several hormone levels that need to be measured and all are inter-related. Furthermore, hormone levels naturally fluctuate depending on which trimester you are in, and different methods for quantifying thyroid hormones can skew results. When having your thyroid checked, know that many conventional practitioners only measure one or two hormones (like TSH or T4), but it's ideal to have a full thyroid panel (as early in pregnancy as possible) to make a complete assessment, such as the following:

- Thyroid Stimulating Hormone (TSH)
- Free T4
- Free T3

- Reverse T3
- Thyroid Peroxidase Antibodies (TPOAb)
- Thyroglobulin Antibodies (TgAb)

Currently, there's a discrepancy between "normal" reference ranges and what's considered optimal. If you suspect or know you have a history of thyroid issues, it's worthwhile to seek the help of an experienced endocrinologist or functional medicine doctor who's familiar with the complex effects of pregnancy on thyroid hormone levels. Reference ranges for the above hormones shift during pregnancy and during specific stages of pregnancy. For example, TSH naturally drops in the first trimester, while T3 and T4 rise. According to one study, failure to use pregnancy-specific reference ranges could misinterpret upwards of 18% of thyroid test results.[22]

Thyroid antibodies are particularly important to measure (especially if your TSH is elevated), as this is an indication of an autoimmune thyroid condition that experts suggest "may ultimately prove the strongest risk factor for adverse outcomes" in pregnancy.[23] With an autoimmune thyroid condition, your body is actively attacking the thyroid gland, and given the demands your thyroid is already facing during pregnancy, it's very important to have this clinically managed during *and after* pregnancy. As pointed out in the American Thyroid Association's Pregnancy Guidelines, "When iodine nutrition is adequate, the most frequent cause of hypothyroidism is autoimmune thyroid disease (Hashimoto's thyroiditis). Therefore, not surprisingly, thyroid antibodies can be detected in approximately 30-60% of pregnant women with an elevated TSH concentration."[24] In other words, upwards of 60% of women who are hypothyroid are suffering from an autoimmune condition.

As with many health conditions, prevention is king, meaning if you're planning a pregnancy, get your thyroid screened prior to conception. If you're already pregnant, have your thyroid tested as soon as possible. Fully 70% of women with hypothyroidism have no obvious symptoms.[25] According to some research, lack of nausea or morning sickness in the first trimester can be a sign of underactive thyroid and/or iodine deficiency.[26]

Nutrition for Thyroid Health

Your nutrition and lifestyle impact the function of your thyroid gland. Adequate iodine intake is the most notable and clinically important since your body literally cannot make thyroid hormones without it, and yet 57% of pregnant women in the United States are deficient in iodine.[27] Dietary iodine requirements nearly double during pregnancy to 250 mcg per day (World Health Organization recommendations), though estimates of iodine needs are conservative, and those who are deficient may need higher levels for repletion.[28] In Japan, iodine intake is consistently higher than in other areas of the world, thanks to regular consumption of seaweed. Average intake in Japan is estimated at 1,000-3,000 mcg per day (though some seaweed-containing soups have up to 7,750 mcg *per 8 oz serving*), and yet no adverse effects on pregnancy outcomes have been observed from higher intakes.[29,30] For most of us, iodine deficiency is a bigger concern than getting too much.

Sadly, roughly half of all prenatal vitamins fail to include iodine altogether (according to a survey of 223 prenatal vitamins available in the United States).[31] To make sure you get enough, choose a prenatal vitamin that contains iodine and regularly consume iodine-rich foods, such as fish, seafood, and seaweed, as outlined in Chapter 3. For women who do not consume seafood, dairy products and eggs are the most important food sources of iodine.[32] Other foods that contain iodine include asparagus, beets, cranberries, and of course, iodized salt.[33] Be aware that the iodine from iodized salt declines with storage, especially in high-humidity areas, so it's not always a reliable source.[34]

One special note about iodine is that certain foods contain compounds, known as goitrogens, that block the uptake of iodine in the thyroid gland. It's wise to avoid soy products for this, and several other reasons, as outlined in Chapter 4. If you have known thyroid problems, you may also want to limit your intake of *raw* cruciferous vegetables (such as cabbage, kale, and broccoli), as these contain goitrogens. Luckily, cooking or fermenting cruciferous vegetables circumvents this problem.[35]

Other nutrients that are important to thyroid function include iron, selenium, zinc, and vitamin D. Iron is crucial because it acts as a cofactor for the production of thyroid hormones. Studies have found that low iron status is predictive of hypothyroidism in pregnant women.[36] Both selenium and zinc aid in the conversion of T4 to the more active form of thyroid hormone, called T3.[37] Selenium also helps to reduce thyroid antibodies and supplementation with this mineral during pregnancy may protect against postpartum hypothyroidism.[38] Adequate vitamin D levels may prevent or help treat autoimmune thyroid conditions.[39] Iron and zinc are both abundant in meat and seafood; selenium is highest in Brazil nuts, fish and seafood, liver and organ meats, beef, lamb, poultry, mushrooms, and eggs. There are other nutrients involved in thyroid health beyond those listed above, which is why a nutrient-dense, real food diet, as described in this book, is so crucial for thyroid health. For women who test positive for thyroid antibodies (in other words, have signs of an autoimmune thyroid issue), a diet that avoids gluten may be helpful.[40]

Beyond what you eat, exposure to certain chemicals can damage thyroid function. The thyroid gland is sensitive to the effects of many environmental toxins, from chemicals in plastics (plastic bottles, food storage containers, BPA from canned foods), tobacco smoke, flame retardants (on clothing, furniture, and household goods), bromine (which is added to many foods, like processed breads and certain beverages), chlorine (present in drinking water, household cleaners, and triclosan in antibacterial soaps/gels), fluoride (from toothpaste, dental treatments, and tap water), and non-stick chemicals that leach into your food (such as commercial food packaging and non-stick Teflon® pans).[41] This is not an exhaustive list, by any means. Every effort you make to reduce your exposure to unnecessary chemicals helps preserve your thyroid function and makes for a healthier pregnancy all around. Chapter 10 will explore this topic in more detail.

If you receive a positive diagnosis for a thyroid condition, your treatment may include replacement thyroid hormone and/or nutritional supplements. A lot of women want to avoid medication and go "natural," which is often my approach to health conditions, but thyroid issues—and especially thyroid issues *during pregnancy*—are a case where medication is often necessary and nothing to be ashamed about. Treatment now, however it looks for you, can help preserve long-term function of your thyroid gland (see Chapter 12) and ensure that your baby's brain develops properly. It's really that important.

Screening for Gestational Diabetes

Testing for gestational diabetes is a controversial topic. There are several approaches and none are perfect. When I worked in gestational diabetes public policy with the state of California and in clinical practice, I saw firsthand the complexity of this issue. We know that consistently elevated blood sugar is risky for both mom and baby, but some screening methods for gestational diabetes run the risk of "false positives" or "false negatives."

A lot of women don't want to do the traditional glucose tolerance test, where you drink a super sweet "glucola" and measure your blood sugar response. If you identify with this, I don't blame you. The drink tastes gross, it contains an ungodly amount of sugar, and it's often loaded with preservatives and food dyes. That said, it's how most research has differentiated between normal and abnormal blood sugar levels in pregnancy and remains widely used to this day. It's not that it's a bad test; it's just not the best test for every woman.

Luckily, the research on gestational diabetes has come a long way in the last 20 years. This section will address the various testing options and the pros and cons of each.

Hemoglobin A1c

Typically, gestational diabetes is screened for towards the end of the second trimester (24-28 weeks) under the assumption that insulin resistance is highest at this stage of pregnancy and therefore blood sugar problems only arise at this time. What we've now learned is that a considerable portion of so-called gestational diabetes is actually *undiagnosed prediabetes*, meaning many women come into pregnancy with preexisting insulin resistance. This is an important distinction to be aware of because when your body is insulin resistant, it has more trouble regulating your blood sugar since it does not respond properly to insulin. Screening average blood sugar levels in early pregnancy by way of hemoglobin A1c (also known as "A1c"), can offer a glimpse into what has been happening with your blood sugar over the past 3 months. This test shows how much hemoglobin, a protein in your blood, has been affected by the glucose in your bloodstream (in other words, what percentage of your red blood cells are sugar-coated).

A1c values are given in percentages in the United States. The higher your A1c, the higher your blood sugar has been, on average. A first trimester A1c of 5.7% or greater indicates prediabetes, which is treated the same as gestational diabetes.[42] Research has shown that an elevated first trimester A1c accurately predicts gestational diabetes in 98.4% of cases (meaning 98.4% of those women also failed a glucose tolerance test).[43] If you fall into this category, you can skip the glucose tolerance test and move straight to monitoring your blood sugar at home for the remainder of your pregnancy. If you have a normal A1c in the first trimester (5.6% or below), it means you're starting your pregnancy with good insulin sensitivity. However, because pregnancy causes changes in insulin resistance, you'll still want to read the rest of this section and decide what testing option to use once you get to the point in pregnancy where insulin resistance surges (typically between 24-28 weeks).

The benefit of having your A1c measured is that you identify blood sugar problems at the *beginning* of pregnancy and can be proactive about it rather than waiting until two-thirds of your pregnancy is over before realizing there might be a blood sugar problem. I believe all women should be screened with this test right alongside their other first trimester blood work. It's cheap, non-invasive, and gives you information you can act on right away.

The one caveat with using an A1c as a diagnostic measure is that it's not reliable at later stages of pregnancy due to the natural hemodilution of your blood and the more rapid turnover of red blood cells.[44] When your blood is more dilute and your red blood cells don't "stick around" as long, they are not in contact with glucose for as long, which results in a falsely low A1c reading. (In fact, if you happen to recheck your A1c in later pregnancy and it has *not* gone down, that's not a good sign.) If you're in your second or third trimester, you'll want to consider one of the other screening options outlined below.

Glucose Tolerance Test (Glucola)

Is it just me or does everyone hate the glucose tolerance test (also called a GTT, OGTT, or glucola)? There are several variations of the dreaded glucola and each involves drinking a specified amount of glucose and measuring your blood sugar response.

In the United States, many doctors use a two-step screening method for gestational diabetes, which involves a *screening test* with a smaller amount of glucose and a *diagnostic test* with a lot more glucose. The screening test involves drinking 50 grams of glucose and measuring blood sugar 1 hour after (it's not performed fasting). If a woman "fails" this, she moves on to the second test, which involves returning to the office fasted and drinking 100 grams of glucose and measuring blood sugar at fasting, 1 hour, 2 hours, and 3 hours. The problem with this method is that a fairly high percentage of healthy women "fail" the first test, while some women with excessive insulin production "pass" it and are never formally diagnosed. For those who go on to take the 3-hour test, diagnosis and treatment can be delayed for weeks, due to the time it takes to receive results and/or scheduling challenges. Finally, diagnostic criteria (the cut-off of what's "normal" or how many out-of-range numbers count as a positive diagnosis) arbitrarily varies depending on your care provider.

That's why the International Association of Diabetes and Pregnancy Study Group (IADPSG), the World Health Organization (WHO), and nearly all developed countries aside from the United States recommend the more reliable and accurate one-step method which involves drinking 75 grams of glucose and measuring blood sugar at fasting, 1 hour, and 2 hours. If any single reading is elevated, you have a positive diagnosis. Because the test is performed in a fasted state (unlike the 50-gram screening test), the results are far more accurate. The diagnostic criteria is more rigid (fasting <92 mg/dl, 1 hour <180 mg/dl, 2 hour <153 mg/dl), and this method more accurately identifies women at risk for "adverse pregnancy outcomes" associated with gestational diabetes.[45] Plus, it's just *one* test. The primary opposition to the one-step method is that, due to stringent diagnostic thresholds, more women would be diagnosed with gestational diabetes and that may increase healthcare costs. However, I believe that with low-cost interventions, like my real food approach, and the long-term health benefits to both mom and baby, these would be negligible or may even result in cost savings. If you're opting for the glucose tolerance test, I absolutely recommend the one-step method (75-gram, 2-hour test) over the outdated 2-step method.

What about the jelly bean test, juice, or a test meal?

Regardless of the method used for the GTT, many women simply don't want to drink the glucola. Some practitioners have offered jelly beans as a (less gross) alternative. The challenge with this method is that it's not standardized. In the one study that found the jelly bean test comparable to the glucola, researchers sent the specific brand of jelly beans to a lab for nutritional analysis and determined the amount needed to provide 50 grams of simple sugars, to ensure it was equivalent to the 50 gram glucola (it was 28 jelly beans, in case you're wondering).[46]

Most people assume you can just look at the nutrition facts label of a product and eat enough jelly beans to provide 50 grams of sugar or 50 grams of total carbohydrates, but in this instance, the required amount of jelly beans to yield 50 grams of simple sugars provided *72 grams* of total carbohydrates. Since every brand of jelly beans has a slightly different ingredient formulation and comes in different sizes, it's tough to know for sure if you're actually getting 50 grams of simple sugars or not. The authors of this study also don't endorse the use of the jelly bean test for anything other than the 50-gram glucola screening: "Because of their solid form and additional complex carbohydrates, however, jelly beans may create a different serum glucose response through the course of several hours. We therefore would not suggest substituting a "double dose" of jelly beans in a diagnostic 100-g glucose challenge test." To date, there have not been studies looking at the accuracy of the jelly bean test compared to the 75-g glucose tolerance test.

Fruit juice is another common stand-in for the glucola, but it poses similar problems as the jelly bean test. Juice is not 100% glucose, rather it's a combination of a variety of sugars, including glucose, fructose, sucrose, and others (the proportions of which vary from one fruit to another).[47] Each of these sugars has a different glycemic index, simply meaning that we can't expect the same blood sugar response to fruit juice as we would from pure glucose.

The third alternative is a test meal that contains 50-100 grams of carbohydrates (or more). Once again, the glycemic effect of a mixed meal that contains 50-100 grams of carbohydrates is not equivalent to 50-100 grams of pure glucose. Not all carbohydrates are broken down into glucose (like fiber), some resist digestion (resistant starch), and some have a much lower glycemic effect (like fructose). How quickly or slowly your body responds to the carbohydrates at a meal also depends on the quantity of protein, fat, fiber, liquid, and other nutrients eaten at that meal.

Attempting to recreate a glucose tolerance test with a whole meal, jelly beans, or juice is simply unreliable. The whole purpose of the glucola is that it's standardized. The "cut-off" points for a glucose tolerance test are set based on the average effect of consuming pure glucose and the resulting blood sugar peak that occurs afterwards. The varying composition of meals, varying size and formulation of jelly beans, and varying sugar types of fruit juice make them all somewhat imperfect stand-ins.

If you decide to opt for one of these anyways, please make sure your blood sugar is tested properly. When you do a glucose tolerance test in a lab, you have a formal blood draw (using blood from your veins) not a finger prick (capillary glucose). Studies that have compared the two note discrepancies of up to 25 mg/dl between results.[48] That's a *huge* range for pregnancy and could easily cause a false positive or a false negative.

In my opinion, if you're going to bother with a glucose tolerance test, do the *actual* test with a formal venous blood draw to get a reliable reading. If food dyes are a big part of your reason for declining, know that the lemon-lime flavor is often free of food dyes. If that still doesn't work for you, I've known several women to mix pure glucose (commercially sold as dextrose) with 8 oz of pure water to make their own flavorless, dye-free, preservative-free glucola with prior approval from their healthcare provider. You would need a gram scale to get the precise amount for the results to be accurate.

When a glucose tolerance test makes sense and when it doesn't

As I alluded to earlier, I don't believe the glucose tolerance test is right for every woman. I began to question the reliability of the GTT after observing several examples in clinical practice of healthy women "failing" the test; yet they were women who had completely normal blood sugar readings when testing at home (false positives).

What did all these women have in common? They were normal weight, ate a moderately low-carb diet, and were having uncomplicated pregnancies. In other words, they were healthy! We have to ask ourselves: who decided that it's normal (or ideal) to be able to clear 50 to 100 grams of sugar from your bloodstream quickly?

Interestingly, I found some animal research that put these findings into context. When pregnant horses are given a GTT, those that have been eating a natural diet of "fiber and fat" (grazing) versus those that are supplemented with "sugar and starch" (via a twice daily ration of grains) have completely different responses to the test.[49] The grazing animals consistently fail the test (high blood sugar), while the grain-fed animals pass with flying colors (normal blood sugar). But instead of veterinarians concluding that grazing animals have abnormal glucose tolerance, they recognize that the grain-fed animals are the ones exhibiting an abnormal metabolic response: "Feeding twice-daily grain meals rich in "sugar and starch" influenced glucose metabolism in horses to an extent that the natural adaptation of glucose metabolism to pregnancy was moderated. Feeding a diet rich in "fiber and fat" more closely mimics the natural grazing state of pasture and allows for adaptation of glucose metabolism to pregnancy and lactation." In other words, the horses fed grains had adapted by producing more insulin in an attempt to lower their dangerously high blood sugar levels as quickly as possible. The horses fed the normal diet of grass hadn't eaten an unnaturally high-carbohydrate diet for long enough to adapt (yet).

This finding is no different in humans. How quickly your body clears glucose from your bloodstream is related to how frequently you eat high-carbohydrate or high-sugar foods. It's well-known that a GTT is inaccurate if you eat a low-carb diet prior to the test. This has been documented in the scientific research since at least the 1960s.[50] When you don't regularly eat a lot of carbohydrates, your pancreas doesn't release large amounts of insulin at one time because it doesn't need to.

One study perfectly illustrates this: 325 Japanese pregnant women were given a 50-gram glucose tolerance test and those who ate a high-carbohydrate diet were significantly more likely to pass.[51] What's interesting about these results is that there was a very low rate of gestational diabetes (in all participants), the women were thin (average BMI of 19.6 and one third of participants underweight), and they had normal fasting blood sugar (average of 70 mg/dl). In this case, "moderately abnormal glucose tolerance" was an adaptation to a lower-carb diet, not a sign of an underlying blood sugar problem.

Decades ago, it was recommended that people increase consumption of carbohydrates prior to a glucose tolerance test to get an accurate result. This advice was eventually abandoned because most Americans already ate plenty of carbohydrates. If you do not make any attempt to limit your carbohydrate intake, regularly eat grains, potatoes or other starches, occasionally have juice, smoothies, or sweetened drinks, or enjoy sweets/desserts, you can expect a pretty accurate result from a GTT. If your body is truly well-adapted to a high-carbohydrate diet, your results should be well within the normal range. This represents the majority of pregnant women in the United States, and in these cases, I believe a GTT makes sense.

If, on the other hand, you're following a low-glycemic or low-carbohydrate diet (like the advice in this book), you may want to consider a different option.

Your three options are:

1. Take the GTT with the knowledge that you might get a "false positive."
2. Choose to eat a higher-carbohydrate diet (no less than 150 g per day) for a week prior to the test (this allows your pancreas time to adapt).
3. Simply decline the test and opt for home blood sugar monitoring.

Some doctors will also accept a fasting blood sugar (a venous blood draw) for further evidence of normal blood sugar levels, though this can leave up to 15% of women with gestational diabetes undiagnosed.[52] In general, fasting blood sugar is better at "ruling-out" than "ruling-in" gestational diabetes.[53] If your fasting blood sugar is less than 80 mg/dl, there's a very slim chance you have gestational diabetes.[54]

Some women prefer to just go forward with a GTT because they want a definitive diagnosis or are nervous about declining a "required" test. Remember, informed consent means that *any* test is optional, pregnant or not. Whatever you decide, go into it knowing the strengths and limitations of this method.

When I was pregnant, I personally decided to follow through with the 50-gram glucola as I was curious to see what my results would look like (I did it *for science!*). I started my pregnancy at a healthy weight, had gained weight within the expected range, had a normal first trimester A1c, and was eating a moderately low-carb diet (similar to the meal plans in this book). Per this office's protocol, they unfortunately would not do the one-step, 75-gram method. In other words, they used the two-step method with a 50-gram test followed by a 100-gram test. I did not carb-load in the week prior to the 50-gram test and not surprisingly, I failed that test (by a small margin, but a single point over is still "failing"). After discussing the results with my healthcare provider, I opted to monitor my blood sugar at home to determine if I truly had gestational diabetes in lieu of the 100-gram test. I tested my blood sugar 4x/day and by the end of 2 weeks, it was clear that my blood sugar consistently stayed in the normal range, even when trying out some higher carb meals. In other words, my response to the 50-gram glucola was a false positive, as is typical in people who eat low-carb.

If you're interested in doing a hybrid method, like myself, or opting entirely for home glucose monitoring, be sure you understand the pros and cons outlined below.

Home Glucose Monitoring

The final screening option for gestational diabetes, though certainly the most controversial, is to monitor your blood sugar at home. This involves using a blood sugar meter (glucometer) and blood sugar test strips to check your blood sugar 4x/day: first thing in the morning before eating (fasting), and 1-2 hours after each meal. After collecting 2 weeks of data, you and your healthcare provider can interpret the results by comparing your numbers to average pregnancy blood sugar levels and gestational diabetes cut offs. Most often, this is done between 24-28 weeks (the typical window for gestational diabetes screening and when insulin resistance often peaks), though it can be done at any point during pregnancy. Home glucose monitoring has both benefits and drawbacks, but overall, I think it works well for highly-motivated women, especially those who eat a lower-carb diet.

Considerations for home glucose monitoring:

For one, your diet impacts the results. This is both a good thing and a bad thing. On the plus side, you can learn what foods help sustain your energy levels without spiking your blood sugar and which ones do the opposite. You can see firsthand how your body responds to a meal with 75 grams of carbohydrates versus 20 grams, or a meal that has lots of vegetables versus a meal that doesn't. But the downside is that you can "eat to cheat." I've known women who will purposefully starve themselves or temporarily switch to a very low-carb diet to "pass" the test, then go back to their usual diet that includes cereal for breakfast, fruit smoothies, and large portions of starchy foods or sweets.

Remember that the goal of home blood sugar monitoring is to get an accurate picture of your blood sugar response to your *usual diet,* and you absolutely want to see if your blood sugar is running high. If you eat low-carb temporarily, then revert to a junk food diet and have high blood sugar, you're only hurting yourself and your baby. On the other hand, if you typically eat low-carb, or go back and forth, I recommend eating several high-carbohydrate meals to understand how that affects you. Most of us aren't "perfect" eaters all the time, so it's helpful to have data from both your typical meals and those that you consider less-than-ideal.

Second, you need to be motivated. Checking your blood sugar 4x/day for several weeks is cumbersome and takes planning. It's annoying to set alarms, to carry testing supplies with you, to track what you're eating, and to poke your finger all the time. Also, test strips can be expensive. Some feel the inconvenience is worth it and provides more useful, real-life information, but for others, it's easier to just go in for a glucose tolerance test and move on.

Third, the diagnostic criteria is poorly defined. How high does your blood sugar need to be and how many elevated readings does it take to trigger a positive diagnosis? That's a matter of clinical judgement and highly dependent on your healthcare practitioner's familiarity with gestational diabetes. In this way, home glucose monitoring is good at "ruling out" gestational diabetes, but leaves a bit of a grey area when deciding what counts as an official diagnosis. When it comes to blood sugar in pregnancy, there's absolutely a spectrum of severity. Given the current research, my opinion is that it's ideal to maintain blood sugar as close to the normal (optimal) range as possible.

Several decades of research show that healthy, non-diabetic pregnant women maintain blood sugar levels between 60-120 mg/dl (in other words, these are *normal* blood sugar levels during pregnancy):[55] Aside from the time immediately following meals, blood sugar stays below 100 mg/dl for the majority of the day. In fact, 24-hour average blood sugar is 88 mg/dl in healthy pregnant women. The following table shows the difference between normal blood sugar and the current targets for blood sugar in women with gestational diabetes.

Blood Sugar Levels in Pregnancy		
	Normal (non-diabetic)	**Gestational Diabetes Goals**
Fasting	70.9 ± 7.8 mg/dl	less than 90 mg/dl
1 hour post-meal	108.9 ± 12.9 mg/dl	less than 120-130 mg/dl
2 hours post-meal	99.3 ± 10.2 mg/dl	less than 120 mg/dl
	If you are outside of the United States, blood sugar is often measured in different units; mmol/L instead of mg/dl. You can convert blood sugar values from mg/dl to mmol/l by dividing by 18. For example, 90 mg/dl ÷ 18 = 5.0 mmol/l.	

You'll notice that there's a discrepancy between these values. The "goal" blood sugar for women with gestational diabetes is still 10-30 points higher than what's observed in non-diabetic pregnant women. For this reason, I defer to *normal* blood sugar levels when it comes to defining a positive diagnosis of gestational diabetes.

If your blood sugar is within (or below) the *normal* ranges, you most likely don't have gestational diabetes. However, if your blood sugar is above or hovering close to the target levels for gestational diabetes, you should keep an eye on it for the remainder of your pregnancy. Mild cases of gestational diabetes are often easily controlled with diet and lifestyle changes.

If you have borderline blood sugar readings, it doesn't hurt to continue to monitor it. Insulin resistance can change from week to week, so it's good to know if your blood sugar is trending up. There's absolutely no risk to having normal blood sugar levels, but there are known risks for high readings. Keep in mind, if you had opted for another screening method and got a positive diagnosis, you'd end up right in the same place: monitoring your blood sugar at home.

Take Home Message

No matter how you choose to be screened for gestational diabetes, it's helpful to understand the rationale—and caveats—behind each screening method. At the end of the day, normal blood sugar levels are what's best for you and your baby. If you get an abnormal result (from any testing option), know that home monitoring is ultimately the most helpful way to figure out how your diet and lifestyle impact your blood sugar and to be proactive about it. Even if you have an official "label" of gestational diabetes, know that if you maintain normal blood sugar levels, you have no higher risk of adverse outcomes than women without the diagnosis. Refer back to Chapter 7 for more and check out my book, *Real Food for Gestational Diabetes,* for full guidance on managing high blood sugar in pregnancy.

Advanced Testing

The above tests are a great starting point to help you fine tune your nutrition during pregnancy and any conventional doctor should be familiar with them. This is, of course, not an exhaustive list of tests. Other options for testing include comprehensive nutritional analysis, such as micronutrient analysis or levels of essential fatty acids (like DHA).

Certain genetic tests may also reveal differences in the way your body processes nutrients. For example, testing for the MTHFR genetic mutation can show you whether your body can process synthetic folic acid or not. If you're positive for MTHFR, you'd want to be especially certain that your diet is free of foods that are fortified with folic acid (like fortified cereals and breads) and that your prenatal vitamin contains L-methylfolate instead of folic acid.[56] It also means that you should focus more on methylation-supporting nutrients, such as choline, glycine, and vitamin B12. That said, I suggest all women— regardless of knowing this information—consume plenty of these nutrients. The study of how your genes influence your need for nutrients (called nutrigenomics) is still in its infancy. As research advances in this area, we'll hopefully have more insight into fine-tuning supplementation and/or dietary recommendations based on an individual's genetics.

Other than genetic testing, there are other specialty lab tests on the market that are frequently used by practitioners of functional medicine. Before you get sucked into the rabbit hole of ordering lab test after lab test, you'll want to ask yourself (and your healthcare provider) several questions:

- Are normal reference ranges for the test clearly defined for pregnancy (and for different stages of pregnancy)?
- What will change if the results come back abnormal? In other words, will the results be actionable?
- If so, will the treatment options be safe during pregnancy or breastfeeding?

There are so many metabolic shifts happening during pregnancy that it's controversial as to what to test or not. Many reference ranges are not accurate in the context of pregnancy; lipid and cholesterol levels are a perfect example. In virtually every pregnant woman, lipid levels change dramatically from early pregnancy to late pregnancy to postpartum. Total cholesterol can increase 25-50% and triglycerides often double, as the body preferentially burns more fat for fuel in late pregnancy.[57] If you were to identify "high" lipid levels, would you need to change anything, or is it just a variation of normal? (HINT: It's usually a variation of normal, and aside from eating well and exercising, conventional treatments, like statins, are contraindicated in pregnancy.)

Or, what if you have strange symptoms and lab testing reveals heavy metal toxicity? While pregnant, many of the treatments typically used are unsafe. In this case, even if you find out, you may not be able to do anything about it until you've had the baby (and perhaps not until you're done breastfeeding). At the end of the day, you'd end up going back to basics: food, lifestyle, and movement. In other words, the same foundational practices that every pregnant woman, regardless of test results, should be doing.

I could give several other examples, but this is really a case-by-case discussion to have with a practitioner of functional medicine/nutrition. If you have a certain health condition or concern that warrants extra testing, be sure it's clear what you will do with the results of the test and if knowing that information will influence your diet and lifestyle. If not, you might end up with anxiety over information overload and lack of treatment options.

With pregnancy, not everything is within your control, and sometimes simply laying the foundation, so to speak, with optimal nutrition is better than trying to nitpick a moving target. There's always the risk that we could pathologize something that's normal simply because there's a lack of data on pregnant women.

Note on Ketone Testing

Most women provide a urine sample at every prenatal visit and ketones are one of many markers that your healthcare provider may look at. Ketones are a byproduct of fat metabolism that circulate in your bloodstream and are excreted in your urine. Many clinicians have been taught that the presence of ketones in urine is a bad thing. However, as I'll explain below, having high *urine* ketones is not the same as having high *blood* ketones. High *blood* ketones, beyond a certain threshold, can indicate that your body is in an emergency state known as diabetic ketoacidosis (DKA) or that you are not consuming enough food (starvation ketosis) and therefore your body is utilizing your fat stores for fuel. These concerns are for good reason. Diabetic ketoacidosis has been linked to impaired fetal brain development.[58] Ketosis induced by starvation is also problematic, as this indicates a woman is not consuming enough energy or essential nutrients for her baby.

However, if you are *not* an insulin-dependent diabetic, have normal blood sugar levels, and are *not* starving yourself, the presence of ketones in your urine is usually nothing to worry about. During pregnancy, your body naturally has a tendency to go into a state called *nutritional ketosis* in which your body preferentially burns fat for fuel. This is even more common in late pregnancy, when your cells get energy "almost exclusively from burning fats."[59] Nutritional ketosis is more common in women who eat a diet limited in carbohydrates, and you're most likely to have ketones in your urine when you're fasted (first thing in the morning) or when it's been a long time since you last ate. Pregnant women naturally have urine ketone levels 3-fold higher than non-pregnant women after an overnight fast.[60]

The Institute of Medicine acknowledges that ketosis is a normal phenomenon of pregnancy, stating: "As part of the adaptation to pregnancy, there is a decrease in maternal blood glucose concentration, a development of insulin resistance, and a tendency to develop ketosis."[61]

How could a natural physiologic state be harmful? The short answer is: it's not. The presence of urine ketones typically *does not* mean that your blood ketones are high. In fact, urine ketones may increase by 50-100-fold while blood ketones will only rise 2-fold and remain below ketonemic levels (<1 mmol/L) in pregnant women. In other words, "large" urine ketones are rarely indicative of high *blood* ketone levels. Blood ketones in the case of DKA are 30-fold more than the *highest* level that's been recorded in pregnant women eating a low-calorie, low-carb diet—a diet that would be expected to cause high blood ketones.[62] Blood ketones, *not urine ketones,* are the only reliable way to check for DKA.

The low ketone levels observed in normal, healthy pregnant women is not problematic for the mom, nor is there evidence to show it harms fetal development. Only starvation ketosis (which involves extreme nutrient-deprivation) and ketoacidosis (involving extremely high blood ketone levels, acidic blood pH, and high blood sugar) have been proven harmful. Ketones present at physiologic levels, as is observed in the case of nutritional ketosis, actually provide 30% of fetal brain energy needs and are used in the synthesis of essential cerebral lipids.[63] Cord blood samples (fetal blood supply) indicate significantly *higher* ketone concentrations compared to maternal levels in healthy pregnant women in their second and third trimesters.[64] This means your body is actually *trying* to send ketones to your baby. A 2016 study of healthy, non-diabetic pregnant women and their infants found that placental tissue maintains high levels of ketones (average of 2.2 mmol/L—significantly higher than maternal blood levels) and that healthy newborns maintain elevated ketone levels during the first *month* of life.[65] In other words, low-level ketosis is both normal, and likely essential, to fetal development.

If you follow the dietary advice in this book, you may have ketones in your urine from time to time. I want you to be prepared if your healthcare providers try to tell you that something is wrong. Unless your *blood* ketones are elevated *and* your blood sugar is high (which could be an indication of DKA), there's nothing to worry about. Many in-the-know providers don't even check urine ketones anymore as they have virtually zero clinical relevance.

For those who want to learn more, a full analysis of the research and controversy surrounding ketosis in pregnancy can be found in Chapter 11 of my book, *Real Food for Gestational Diabetes.*

Summary

Hopefully, this chapter hasn't left you in the land of information overload. To summarize, it's ideal to have several labs checked in your preliminary blood work (typically in the first trimester): vitamin D, iron, thyroid hormones, and hemoglobin A1c. If any of the above come back abnormal, you can take action and/or have them re-tested later in pregnancy. If possible, I recommend testing vitamin D levels again in the second and/or third trimester to ensure you're supplementing with adequate amounts. Remember that if your hemoglobin A1c comes back normal in the first trimester, you'll still want to choose a screening option for gestational diabetes between 24-28 weeks, since insulin resistance naturally goes up in that stage of pregnancy. And finally, if you're considering additional lab testing, make sure you work with a knowledgeable provider and choose lab tests that will give you helpful and actionable information.

Real Food for Pregnancy

Chapter 10:

Toxins

"Exposure to various environmental pollutants induces synergic and cumulative dose-additive adverse effects on prenatal development, pregnancy outcomes and neonate health."
- Dr. Kaïs Al-Gubory, French National Institute for Agricultural Research

It's no secret that chemical exposure during pregnancy can be harmful. You probably intuitively know that, but you might not realize just how prevalent toxins are in your daily life. I always find it ironic that so much effort is spent telling women that certain foods, like sunny-side-up eggs or soft cheeses, are supposedly unsafe in pregnancy, and yet there's nary a mention that drinking water stored in plastic bottles or using certain cosmetics could be a far more serious threat. I truly wish those well-meaning, but often misguided, public health campaigns were spent informing women about the risks of everyday toxins instead.

Whether we like it or not, most of us are surrounded by potentially toxic exposures. From the pots and pans you cook with, to the containers you use to store water or leftover food, there are many places where unwanted chemicals can make their way into your body. But focusing on ingested chemicals doesn't go far enough.

You might be accumulating toxins from products that contact your skin, like cleaning products, soaps, shampoos, makeup, hair products, perfumes and lotions. A lot of people think you can't absorb toxins unless you ingest them or breathe in fumes, but that's not true. There's a reason certain medications can be delivered via patches; because a lot of what you put on your skin is absorbed directly into your bloodstream.

While it's true that some toxins are unavoidable, like air pollution if you live in a city, there are likely many avoidable toxins that make it into your daily life without your knowledge. This chapter will focus on the toxin exposure that you have some control over via the way you cook and store food, the products that furnish your home or are used for cleaning, and personal care products. After breaking down the research, I'll give you practical tips to help you minimize your exposure.

A little warning (and reassurance): a lot of the information in this section can be hard to swallow. Your first reaction may be anger: *Why in the world are these chemicals still used?* Or fear: *I've already exposed myself and my baby?!* Before you freak out, remember this: you are always doing the best you can with the information you have at the time. Your body has the blueprints for making a perfectly healthy baby, and avoiding toxins is just one of many areas of your life to continue to refine as research uncovers new information. Don't sweat the past. Focus on what you can do *now*.

Chemicals in Plastic (BPA and Phthalates)

During pregnancy, hormone levels are tightly regulated to guide normal growth of your baby. Chemicals that have estrogen-mimicking effects, widely known as xenoestrogens, encompass thousands of distinct chemicals that can throw off fetal development. A short list of xenoestrogens include: plastic chemicals (including BPA and phthalates), pesticides and herbicides (especially organochlorines), parabens, polystyrene (styrofoam), PCBs, perfume, and countless others.[1] For now, I'd like to focus on plastic.

There are several chemical compounds present in plastics that have hormone-disrupting effects, one of which is bisphenol-A, known more commonly as BPA. Exposure to hormone disruptors can be particularly harmful to development of your child's reproductive system (such as their genitalia and breasts). For example, in utero BPA exposure in pregnant mice, in the range currently being consumed by people, has been shown to alter reproductive development of their babies.[2] Pregnant mice also show abnormal breast tissue and impaired milk production, meaning it's possible that BPA could affect a woman's ability to breastfeed.[3] BPA can also impact blood sugar metabolism by interfering with normal insulin signalling, and causing dysfunction in the beta cells of the pancreas (the cells which produce insulin).[4] This may explain why offspring of BPA-exposed mice show early warning signs of diabetes.[5]

In humans, exposure to BPA may be a risk factor for miscarriage, premature delivery, and other "adverse perinatal outcomes."[6] Some research links prenatal BPA exposure to hyperactivity and other behavioral problems in children.[7,8] These are just a handful of studies demonstrating why scientists see the prenatal period as a "BPA window of vulnerability."[9]

BPA exposure is widespread and it's one of the highest volume chemicals produced worldwide. BPA is used in the production of polycarbonate plastics (like those used in hard plastic bottles and food storage containers), resins that line most metal food cans, water pipes, electronics, and a variety of consumer plastics, including kids' toys. More than 92% of urine samples from United States residents are positive for BPA and it's been detected in amniotic fluid, placental tissue, cord blood, and breast milk.[10] One study that compared BPA levels in urine and amniotic fluid found 5-fold *higher* levels in amniotic fluid, suggesting babies are being exposed to more BPA than previously thought.[11] The main source of BPA exposure appears to be food.[12] BPA more readily transfers to food and beverages when the containers/cans are heated, in instances such as reheating food in plastic containers in a microwave or leaving a plastic water bottle in a hot car.[13]

You might already be familiar with some of this information and purposefully buy BPA-free products, however that might be giving you a false sense of security. BPA-free plastics are good in theory, but what's used to replace them isn't necessarily any safer. After bad publicity about BPA came out, chemical companies scrambled to develop alternatives, one of which is BPS. Although it's less studied than BPA, research into its safety thus far has not been reassuring. Very low level exposure to BPS has been shown to disrupt hormone levels, embryonic development, and neurological development in lab animals in a similar manner to BPA.[14,15]

In addition to its use in plastics, BPA is used as a thin coating on thermal paper (like grocery store receipts or boarding passes at the airport). BPA readily transfers from receipts to other surfaces, including your skin. After handling receipts for even a few seconds, BPA levels spike in the blood. In general, the longer a receipt is held, the more BPA is absorbed into your bloodstream. In addition, the use of hand sanitizers prior to handling receipts enhances BPA absorption thanks to the presence of "dermal penetration enhancers" in these products.[16] This is important because many people use hand sanitizer when shopping or traveling.

Another group of potentially harmful chemicals used in plastics are phthalates, which contribute to flexibility, transparency, and durability of a variety of products (like vinyl flooring, shower curtains, plastic wrap, plastic bottles, and plastic bags). They are also added to many other products, including lotions, hair sprays, nail polish (phthalates help prevent brittleness and cracking), sealants, insect repellants, and fragrances (such as perfumes, scented candles, and air fresheners). In some cosmetics and perfumes, phthalates can be up to 50% of the product.[17]

The main way we're exposed to phthalates is through food products (via transfer from food packaging), however off-gassing of phthalates (inhalation) and direct absorption through the skin are also considerable sources of exposure.[18] In a study of phthalate exposure among two groups of pregnant women (in New York and Poland), 100% of participants had detectable levels of phthalates.[19] Think about that for a minute.

In studies on rats, exposure to phthalates results in hormonal changes and birth defects.[20] In both lab animals and humans, phthalates have anti-androgenic effects, meaning they can block the effects of certain hormones, like testosterone. This is particularly worrisome when it comes to genital development in boys. As one researcher explains, "Rodent studies indicate that prenatal exposure to some phthalates can disrupt normal male reproductive tract development, causing effects such as reduced anogenital (anus-to-penis) distance, undescended testicles, and testicular abnormalities affecting function."[21] Some of these abnormalities have been observed in human baby boys from prenatal exposure to "environmentally relevant levels of phthalates."[22] Brain development, particularly in boys, can also be affected by prenatal exposure to phthalates.[23] According to one study, these detrimental effects on mental and intellectual development persist into later childhood (even at age seven).[24] Exposure to phthalates is also linked to an increased risk of preterm birth.[25]

Clearly, exposure to BPA and phthalates is both common and carries health risks. Below are some tips to protect yourself from unnecessary exposure.

Tips to minimize exposure to BPA & phthalates:

- Avoid storing or heating food in plastic. Use glass, ceramic, or stainless steel containers for leftovers.
- Do not microwave food in plastic containers or covered in plastic wrap. The plastic chemicals can transfer into your food directly or outgas into the air upon heating.
- Do not let plastic wrap come in direct contact with your food. Opt for wax paper or parchment paper. (Aluminum foil is not a good choice; see the aluminum section later in this chapter.)
- Use a glass or stainless steel water bottle (ensure it is not lined or coated, as these often contain BPA or BPA-alternatives).
- When practical, bring a reusable glass or stainless steel mug when going out for coffee/tea (even paper cups are lined with plastic, plus the lids are usually plastic).
- Eat less canned food. Opt for fresh or frozen produce or prepared food sold in glass jars.
- Handle receipts as little as possible (grocery receipts, airline boarding passes, ATM receipts, etc.).
- Consume fewer drinks packaged in cans or plastic bottles (aluminum cans are lined with BPA—yet another reason to ditch soda!).

- Read ingredient labels on cosmetics and personal care products. Avoid products that contain phthalates. Phthalates often include the word "phthalate" in the name, like "diethyl phthalate."
- Stop using perfumes and scented products (air fresheners, home fragrances, laundry detergent, dryer sheets, scented candles, etc.). Avoid personal care products that list "parfum" or "fragrance" in the ingredients. If you're unsure, choose products that state "no synthetic fragrance" or "phthalate-free" on the label.
- Skip the nail polish and spend less time in nail salons.

Parabens

Like phthalates, parabens are common in personal care products and cosmetics. Parabens are a group of synthetic compounds that are often added to lotion, makeup, toothpaste, shampoo, deodorant, medications, and even certain food products to inhibit the growth of bacteria, fungus, and other microbes. On product labels, you may see them listed as methylparaben, ethylparaben, propylparaben, butylparaben or isobutylparaben. Typically, individual products contain very small amounts of parabens, but cumulative exposure can be problematic. Since women tend to use more personal care products than men, we are often exposed to higher levels of parabens, and this has serious implications in pregnancy: "The ubiquitous nature of these endocrine-disrupting compounds in female-directed cosmetic and personal care products places neonates at high risk for exposure."[26]

Parabens are known to disrupt hormone metabolism in the body by mimicking the action of estrogen.[27] Some studies have linked them to reproductive problems, which led the European Union to ban certain parabens in 2014.[28] In the United States and many other parts of the world, parabens are still widely used.

One way to estimate paraben exposure is to measure urine levels. Pregnant women who use lotion have urine paraben levels up to 216% higher than women who don't use lotion.[29] Shampoo, conditioner, and cosmetic use is also linked to higher paraben levels.[30] What's concerning is that some parabens can cross the placenta. In a study that measured parabens in urine and amniotic fluid at 3 separate times in pregnancy, 99% of urine samples came back positive for parabens.[31] Although amniotic fluid didn't test positive for parabens as frequently as urine did, certain parabens were found to readily cross the placenta. For example, 58% of amniotic fluid samples were positive for one paraben (propylparaben), suggesting direct fetal exposure. Worryingly, another paraben (butylparaben) was found in *higher* concentrations in amniotic fluid than urine.

Exposure to parabens in utero is linked to higher odds of preterm birth and growth restriction (both low birth weight and body length) in human infants.[32] It has also been found to affect sex hormone levels (like estrogen) and thyroid hormone levels in pregnant women.[33] This raises concerns for fetal brain development, given the key role of thyroid health on the developing nervous system. There has been very limited research into the effects of paraben exposure to long-term development of children, but one study looked at prenatal exposure to various chemicals and growth rate during pregnancy (via ultrasound) and after birth, all the way until the child's third birthday. Exposure to parabens in utero and in infancy was linked to higher body weight during early childhood (even after researchers adjusted for caloric intake), suggesting that the estrogenic effects of parabens may affect a child's metabolism and body composition long-term.[34]

The hormonal effects of parabens on both mother and baby (during and after pregnancy) are a clear sign that we need to get serious about reducing exposure. Fortunately, avoiding paraben-containing personal care products is effective. In one study, 100 girls were asked to refrain from using paraben-containing products to see if urine levels of the chemicals changed. After only 3 days, paraben levels in their urine dropped 44%.[35] Here are some additional ways to avoid parabens.

Tips to minimize exposure to parabens:

- Read labels on cosmetics and personal care products. Avoid methylparaben, ethylparaben, propylparaben, butylparaben, isobutylparaben, and other parabens. Search the Environmental Working Group (EWG) Skin Deep® database to find safe alternatives.
- Ditch deodorant or opt for a natural version (check your local health food store).
- Use natural oils as lotion, such as coconut oil, shea butter, tallow balm, etc.
- Use less makeup or opt for products that don't require preservatives, such as mineral-based powder foundation.
- Opt for preservative-free products.

Pesticides

It's often assumed that pesticides are only used in agriculture or to kill weeds, but they encompass a wide range of chemicals, including insecticides (kills insects), fungicides (kills fungus), herbicides (kills weeds), and rodenticides (kills rodents). The major classes of pesticides are organochlorines, organophosphates, carbamates, pyrethroids, and triazines. Although pesticides are a convenient solution to common pests, they can be dangerous to pregnant women. As a whole, "pesticides have been shown to impair female reproduction by targeting a variety of reproductive tissues and functions."[36] One researcher points out: "Every class of pesticides has at least one agent capable of affecting a reproductive or developmental endpoint in laboratory animals or people, including organophosphates, carbamates, pyrethroids, herbicides, fungicides, fumigants and especially organochlorines."[37]

Many pesticides interfere with hormone levels in the body and, like chemicals found in plastics, may alter reproductive development in utero. Maternal exposure to pesticides (in humans) has been linked to the following problems in their babies: urogenital malformations, infertility, semen quality impairment, and testicular, prostate, ovarian, and breast cancer.[38] For decades, it's been known that "parental involvement in agricultural work and/or parental exposure to pesticides has been associated with higher risk of a wide range of congenital malformations."[39] More recent studies continue to find evidence of harm. In one study, abnormal sex organs in human baby boys (like the urethral opening located underneath the penis instead of at the tip or undescended testicles) was linked to prenatal exposure to xenoestrogens. When their mothers' placentas were examined, they found higher levels of pesticides (especially organochlorines).[40] A separate study reported that sons of women exposed to pesticides have "a statistically significant decrease in penile length and a trend towards reduced testicular volume and serum concentrations of testosterone."[41]

In addition to the effects seen on reproductive organs, prenatal pesticide exposure can be harmful to the developing brain. Researchers note: "Children exposed to organophosphate pesticides, both prenatally and during childhood, may have difficulties performing tasks that involve short-term memory, and may show increased reaction time, impaired mental development or pervasive developmental problems."[42] This may be partially explained by the negative effects that pesticides have on thyroid function. One review article identified 63 pesticides that interfere with the thyroid system, which is concerning given that thyroid hormones are known to affect brain development, IQ, and behavior.[43] And yet, "the U.S. EPA has never taken action on a pesticide because of its interference with the thyroid system."[44]

Although some of the most toxic pesticides have indeed been banned, many persist in the environment and work their way up the food chain. A perfect example of this is DDT, which Rachel Carson revealed was adversely affecting reproduction in birds in her 1962 classic, *Silent Spring*. Sadly, these chemicals are so resistant to degradation and so toxic, that they continue to be found in the environment and our food supply to this day.[45] DDT and related pesticides (organochlorines) have been linked to fetal loss, even at very low levels of exposure.[46]

You'd think that modern pesticides would be safer, but that's not always true. Sometimes it takes decades for scientists to fully understand the health effects of these chemicals. One example of this is glyphosate. Initially, it was praised by the chemical industry for its supposed low toxicity, but after decades of research, scientists now say glyphosate is "probably carcinogenic to humans."[47] Glyphosate is the active ingredient in the most widely used pesticide, Roundup, and its use since the 1970s has increased 100-fold.[48] It is commonly applied in conventional agriculture, especially in the fields of genetically modified crops that are specifically engineered to withstand heavy applications of glyphosate. These crops are called Roundup-Ready because, unlike normal crops, they can survive when sprayed with this chemical cocktail (examples include Roundup-Ready corn, soy, and canola). Glyphosate is also used as a "crop desiccant," meaning it is sprayed on crops, especially wheat and other grains, to dry out the plants to allow for easier harvest. Unfortunately, both of these practices result in glyphosate residues accumulating in crops.[49]

Research into the toxicity of glyphosate suggests it can impair the function of a key enzyme in the liver involved in detoxification, called glutathione.[50] It also harms healthy gut bacteria and promotes the overgrowth of pathogenic bacteria in the intestines.[51] Pregnancy is a time when you want your liver and gut functioning optimally, to extract as much nutrition from your food while excreting waste products and toxins efficiently. Glyphosate appears to hamper both. Alterations in gut bacteria from glyphosate can also reduce your body's ability to absorb beneficial nutrients, especially minerals, like calcium, iron, magnesium, and zinc from your diet.[52]

Rats exposed to glyphosate in utero show signs of abnormal uterine development and a tendency to develop tumors.[53] Even more worrisome is that glyphosate—when tested both alone and as commercially available Roundup—is toxic to human placental cells at concentrations *100x lower* than the recommended use in agriculture. In fact, Roundup is exponentially *more toxic* than glyphosate alone. The researchers suggest that "the presence of Roundup adjuvants enhances glyphosate bioavailability and/or bioaccumulation."[54] This raises a number of concerns for people who regularly consume foods that are sprayed with Roundup (*non-organic* soy, corn, canola, grains and legumes) or those who use Roundup as a weed killer in their yard.

Soy is one food to be especially careful with, since the phytoestrogens it naturally contains may be even more harmful in the presence of Roundup. As one researcher explains: "[Roundup's] extensive use in genetically

Real Food for Pregnancy

modified soybean cultivation has raised concerns about possible synergistic estrogenic effects due to the simultaneous exposure to glyphosate and to the phytoestrogen "genistein," which is a common isoflavone present in soybeans and soybean products."[55] I don't recommend consuming much soy during pregnancy, as outlined in Chapter 4, but if you choose to consume it occasionally, be especially diligent to buy *organic* soy (glyphosate is not permitted on organic crops).

So, what can you do?

Whether we like it or not, pesticides are widely used. You can't avoid exposure entirely, but you can take steps to minimize it. First, choose foods that are grown organically and/or without harmful pesticides. An extensive review of over 343 studies found that conventionally-grown crops are 4x more likely to be contaminated with pesticide residues compared to organically-grown crops.[56] Plus, they found that organic crops routinely had higher levels of beneficial antioxidants. Studies that monitor pesticide levels in humans have found lower levels in those that eat primarily organic foods.[57,58] Whenever possible, seek food from small farms in your area, as they often don't spray with pesticides (or not as much as larger farms). Pesticides are expensive and small farms, even if they are not certified organic, usually try to minimize their use. Talk to your farmers and ask about their use of agricultural chemicals.

It's also helpful to learn which foods are commonly sprayed with high levels of pesticides, so you know what's most important to buy organic. Each year, the Environmental Working Group (EWG) analyzes pesticide residues of the most popular fruits and vegetables and publishes the "Dirty Dozen" list, which test the highest for pesticide residues, and the "Clean 15" list, which test the lowest. Although many believe you can simply wash produce to remove pesticide residues, this is often not the case, as many pesticides are systemic, meaning they are absorbed into the plant itself, not just on the surface. It's not a bad idea to wash your produce, but in most cases, it won't wash away pesticide residues.[59]

At the time of publishing this book, glyphosate residues are not routinely monitored in foods in the United States, so the best way to avoid exposure is to reduce your consumption of foods that are commonly sprayed and/or to purchase organic for these items. This includes cereal grains (like wheat, oats, and rice), corn, beans/lentils, and seeds (like sunflower seeds, canola, and cottonseed).[60] In a government-funded Canadian research study that measured glyphosate residues in over 3,000 food samples, fully one third tested positive.[61] Grains and legumes were among the most commonly contaminated (36.6% of grains and 47.7% of legume samples contained glyphosate). Also, other research has shown that animals fed genetically modified or conventionally-grown soy/corn have higher glyphosate levels than organic or pasture-raised animals, so be picky about the animal products you buy.[62]

You really have to take matters in your own hands here. As the EWG states, "The EPA's tolerance levels are too lenient to protect public health. They are a yardstick to help the agency's personnel determine whether farmers are applying pesticides properly. The levels were set years ago and do not account for newer research showing that toxic chemicals can be harmful at very small doses, particularly when people are exposed to combinations of chemicals." For example, strawberry growers may use a combination of up to "74 different pesticides in various combinations."[63] The problem with research on pesticides is that studies tend to look at pesticides one-at-a-time, however, "determination of "safe" levels of exposure to single pesticides may underestimate the real health effects."[64]

Tips to minimize exposure to pesticides:

- Buy organically-grown produce or purchase direct from local farmers who do not use pesticides (at minimum, buy organic/pesticide-free produce for the "Dirty Dozen" or items that you eat frequently and/or in large quantities). If you do not have access to—or cannot afford—organic or local vegetables, it's still better, from a nutritional perspective, to eat conventionally-grown vegetables than to not eat *any* vegetables.
- Local, small farms often use fewer pesticides than large operations even if they are not "certified organic." If in doubt, talk to the farmer.
- Avoid genetically modified foods, as these tend to have higher pesticide residues, especially for glyphosate (particularly corn, soy, and canola).
- Eat pasture-raised meat, eggs, and dairy (pesticide residues in commercial animal feed accumulate in the fatty tissue of animals fed corn/soy).
- If you drink coffee, buy USDA certified organic or Rainforest Alliance approved. Many harmful pesticides that are illegal in the United States are still used in countries that grow coffee.
- Buy organic grains and beans/legumes.
- Avoid soy, which has some of the highest allowable glyphosate residues.
- Steer clear of vegetable oils. See Chapter 4 for more about these oils.
- Do not spray pesticides in or around your home/garden.
- Avoid the use of chemical insect repellent and insecticides.

Non-stick Pans & Related Chemicals (PFCs)

Non-stick cookware is a modern convenience that most of us have in our homes. It exploded in popularity right alongside the low-fat dietary guidelines because almost nothing sticks to the pan even when you cook without added oils. Unfortunately, the chemicals that make up the non-stick surface on most of these pans are highly toxic. They are made of a chemical called polytetrafluoroethylene (PTFE) that, when heated beyond 325 degrees F or when scratched, begins to release another chemical called perfluorooctanoate (PFOA).[65] If you're searing a steak, your frying pan will easily reach 500 degrees F, practically guaranteeing the release of chemicals into your food and into the air you breathe, even if your non-stick pan is in perfect condition. Both PFOA and PTFE belong to a group known as perfluorinated chemicals (PFCs), all of which are man-made. In fact, nowhere in nature will you find fluorine and carbon bound together. These chemicals are incredibly resistant to breakdown. Once they get in your body, they are there to stay for quite a while. It's estimated that it can take up to 4-5 years for your body to metabolize and excrete PFCs.[66]

Researchers note that PFCs are detectable in the blood of nearly all pregnant women.[67] Like so many other chemicals, higher levels of exposure increases the odds of certain pregnancy complications. Pregnant women with high blood levels of PFCs are at higher risk for having a low birthweight baby.[68,69] PFCs may also impact the growth of your baby's organs and bones, resulting in smaller abdominal circumference, birth length, and head circumference.[70] Higher rates of preeclampsia have been observed in women who are highly exposed to PFCs.[71] These chemicals are known endocrine disruptors, affecting both reproductive hormones and thyroid hormones.[72,73,74] Data from Inuit and Chinese populations show that PFCs can depress thyroid hormone levels during pregnancy.[75,76] Even more worrisome is that thyroid function of newborns can be disrupted from prenatal exposure to PFCs.[77] I've mentioned this several times, but it bears repeating: Impaired thyroid health can interfere with your baby's brain development.

If you already avoid the use of non-stick pans, you may assume you're ok. But, it turns out that PFCs are used in a wide range of products including stain-resistant and water-resistant coatings (for carpets, clothing, and upholstery), paint, and even food packaging (to keep food from sticking to the container). Needless to say, we're in contact with a lot of PFCs, most often from food, contaminated water, or consumer products. Researchers note, "Human biomonitoring of the general population in various countries has shown that, in addition to the near ubiquitous presence of PFOA in blood, these may also be present in breast milk, liver, seminal fluid, and umbilical cord blood."[78] Of all food products, PFCs are particularly high in microwave popcorn because they are transferred from the coating on the popcorn bag into the corn kernels upon heating. Other common dietary sources are canned meat, hot dogs, chicken nuggets, French fries, and chips.[79]

Clearly, limiting exposure to PFCs is wise during pregnancy. Here are some practical ways to do it.

Tips to minimize PFC exposure:

- Avoid the use of non-stick pans and kitchen utensils (opt for cast iron, stainless steel, glass, or ceramic cookware). Remember to check bakeware as well, such as cookie sheets and muffin tins. Strictly avoid Teflon® cookware.
- Eat less microwave popcorn, prepackaged food, microwave dinners, and fast food, as the packaging often transfers PFCs into the food.
- Avoid the use of stain-resistant or water-repellent sprays (decline optional stain treatment on new carpets and furniture).
- Buy clothing without the Teflon®, Scotchgard™ or Gore-Tex® tags. (If you live in a rainy climate, this may simply be unavoidable. Pick your battles.)
- Don't use household chemicals or personal care products with the words "fluoro" or "perfluoro" or "PTFE" in the ingredients list. Computer cleaners are common offenders (which often use 1,1-difluoroethane).

- Check with your local water source to ask about contamination with PFCs. Some water filters, like Berkey® filters, can remove PFCs.

Fluoride

Fluoride is a non-essential mineral, meaning your body has no nutritional requirement for it. This might come as a surprise, since it has been added to water supplies and dental products for decades as a means to help prevent cavities. Interestingly, a 2015 Cochrane review of over 155 studies on water fluoridation found that there wasn't enough evidence to show it was effective at preventing cavities.[80] Nonetheless, debating the effects on cavities is not the purpose of this section. Rather, I want to focus on the effects of fluoride on pregnancy outcomes.

There are several systems in the body that are highly sensitive to fluoride, namely the bones, thyroid, kidneys, and brain. This raises concerns during pregnancy because fluoride is known to cross the placenta, meaning your fluoride exposure predicts your baby's fluoride exposure.[81] Several studies have looked at prenatal fluoride exposure from drinking water to determine how it impacts children's health. Children conceived and raised in areas with low levels of fluoride in the drinking water have significantly higher IQs when compared to children from areas with high levels of fluoride in the drinking water.[82,83] A study from Mexico echoes these findings, noting lower scores on cognitive tests in children up to age 12 if their mothers had high fluoride exposure during pregnancy. What's frightening about this study is that these effects were seen even when fluoride levels in the water were "in the general range of exposures reported for other general population samples of pregnant women and nonpregnant adults."[84] A separate study concluded that "cognitive alterations in children born from exposed mothers to fluoride could start in early prenatal stages of life."[85]

Childhood associations are one thing, but there's strong evidence that fetal development is affected by fluoride. Due to China's former one-child policy, there's actually fairly extensive human data on unborn fetuses from mothers who resided in areas with differing levels of fluoride in the drinking water. This data reveals how fluoride directly affects fetal tissues. Taken together, these studies found high levels of fluoride in fetal bone and brain tissue, and "major pathological damage" to a variety of cells if mothers lived in areas with fluoridated water.[86,87,88,89,90] One of these studies concluded that, "accumulation of fluoride in the brain tissue can disrupt the synthesis of certain neurotransmitters and receptors in nerve cells, leading to neural dysplasia or other damage."[91]

Furthermore, a study on otherwise "healthy" newborns found that the level of fluoride in drinking water where the mothers resided during pregnancy consistently correlated with neonatal neurological assessments. Those from highly fluoridated areas scored significantly lower on neurological, behavioral, visual, and auditory tests, leading the authors to conclude that "fluoride is toxic to neurodevelopment and that excessive fluoride intake during pregnancy can cause adverse effects on neonatal neurobehavioral development."[92] Since fluoride is chemically similar to iodine, it's suspected that disruption to thyroid hormones may be one way that brain development is affected. Rat studies have found that brain development, learning, and memory are particularly impacted in rats born to mothers that are both deficient in iodine *and* exposed to fluoride.[93]

Finally, skeletal development can be influenced by fluoride exposure: "Excessive fluoride ingestion in pregnant women may possibly poison and alter enzyme and hormonal systems in the fetus causing disturbances to osteoid formation and mineralization. Knock-knees, bowlegs, and saber shins develop when walking begins."[94] There's actually a name for the syndrome: skeletal fluorosis.

The most common way we're exposed to fluoride is through fluoridated water and dental products, like toothpaste, mouthwash, and fluoride treatments at the dentist's office. Over 95% of toothpastes contain fluoride and "a single strip of toothpaste covering the length of a child's brush contains between 0.75 to 1.5 mg of fluoride," which exceeds the level of fluoride used in many prescription fluoride treatments.[95] It's important to continue to see your dentist during pregnancy for regular cleanings, since hormonal changes can worsen plaque buildup, but you'll want to ensure you're not exposed to fluoride in the process. Simply ask your dentist or dental hygienist to perform cleanings with fluoride-free products.

There are two other common sources of exposure, which may seem unusual. One is non-organic grapes, thanks to the popular use of a fluoride-containing pesticide called cryolite, and the other is tea. Black, green, white, and oolong tea all come from the "tea plant" (camellia sinensis), which is known to accumulate fluoride from the soil and concentrate it in the leaves. Studies have found that lower quality tea made with mature leaves tends to have higher fluoride levels, so if you're a tea drinker, opt for the best quality you can afford.[96] Higher quality teas often use the young, tender leaves, which contain significantly less fluoride. There are case reports in the literature of fluoride poisoning in people who consume extremely large quantities of tea on a daily basis for years (more than a gallon a day), however there are no reports to suggest that moderate tea consumption is harmful.[97] Of all teas derived from the tea plant, white tea has the lowest levels of fluoride (and is also the lowest in caffeine). On a somewhat related note, red tea (rooibos), which is not from the camellia sinensis plant, is very low in fluoride and is caffeine-free.[98]

Tips to minimize fluoride exposure:

- Use fluoride-free toothpaste, mouthwash, and dental products.
- Avoid dental procedures that use fluoride (fluoride gels, varnishes, or rinses). Continue to see your dentist during pregnancy, however request fluoride-free products be used for dental cleanings.
- Filter your tap water using a water filter known to remove fluoride, such as a Berkey® filter.
- Opt for organically-grown grapes, since many vineyards use a fluoride-containing pesticide called cryolite.
- If you drink tea (black, green, white or oolong tea), go for the highest quality available. Consider switching to white tea, which has the lowest fluoride levels of the above varieties, or try rooibos tea (red tea).

Aluminum

You might be thinking that aluminum is an odd addition to the list of toxins to avoid in pregnancy, but exposure to aluminum is common and the implications important enough that I had to discuss the research. For many of us, aluminum is a regular part of our lives without us even thinking about it. Found in aluminum foil, aluminum cookware, anti-perspirant deodorants, antacids, and even baking powder, it might be something you come in contact with or ingest on a daily basis.

That's not exactly a good thing, given that "there is no known physiological role for aluminum within the body."[99] Aluminum is known to cross the placenta and is toxic to placental and uterine cells in studies on mice.[100] Decades of research have shown that aluminum can accumulate in the brain and can cause a range of neurological problems (such as Alzheimer's disease in adults).[101] Since your baby's brain is being formed in utero, exposure to aluminum during this sensitive period of development could be especially problematic. "Aluminium can act as a powerful neurological toxicant and provoke embryonic and fetal toxic effects in animals and humans after gestational exposure."[102] Simply put, you don't *need* aluminum in your body, nor do you *want* it there.

For ethical reasons, we don't have human studies on women intentionally exposed to aluminum during pregnancy, however, as mentioned above, mouse studies have been performed. In mice exposed to aluminum via their mother's diet during pregnancy and through lactation, researchers note "significant and dose-dependent disturbance in the levels of neurotransmitters," including serotonin and dopamine. These pups also had deficits in sensory motor reflexes, movement behaviors, and weight gain. The researchers concluded: "Aluminum exposure during pregnancy has potential neurotoxic hazards to the in utero developing fetus brain."[103]

A separate study, which reviewed the available data on aluminum exposure during pregnancy, concluded that "oral exposure during pregnancy can produce significant changes in the tissue distribution of multiple essential trace elements, with possible consequences on fetal metabolism."[104] Of all age groups, unborn babies are the most vulnerable to the toxic effects of heavy metal exposure, including aluminum.[105] Researchers note that "Human embryos and fetuses are at higher risk of developing aluminum storage, particularly in the developing osseous [bones] and nervous tissues [brain]."[106]

So what are the biggest contributors to aluminum exposure?

Some researchers point the finger at antiperspirants as "arguably the most important single contributor to the body burden of aluminium as their use involves applying about 2 g of aluminium to the skin every day."[107] Others contend that "over-the-counter antacids are the most important source for human aluminium exposure from a quantitative point of view."[108] One warns that "caution should be taken with common anti-reflux medications such as antacids that contain aluminum and other aluminum-containing drugs during pregnancy to protect the newborn from a possibly dangerous aluminum overload during gestation."[109] Either way, the use of aluminum-containing antiperspirants and antacids is not a good idea.

Certain vaccines are another route of exposure, in which "up to a milligram of aluminium is injected along with an antigen or allergen."[110] As pharmaceutical companies continue to phase out mercury from vaccines, higher amounts of aluminum adjuvants are being used.[111] Topical and injected aluminum are significant contributors to overall body aluminum given that they bypass your digestive tract, which normally prevents a significant amount of it from being absorbed, and instead enter your bloodstream directly. In fact, "only 0.25% of dietary aluminum is absorbed, while aluminum hydroxide (the most common form of aluminum used in vaccines) when injected may be absorbed by the body at nearly 100% efficiency over time."[112]

Although many claim that aluminum from vaccines is inert, concerns about its safety have arisen after it was was found to have "unexpectedly long-lasting biopersistence within immune cells in some individuals."[113] Since then, rodent studies have tested the effects of aluminum adjuvants to hopefully glean a better understanding of adverse vaccine reactions observed in some people. Interestingly, when multiple doses of aluminum were tested, the *lowest* dose proved most toxic, with mice showing decreased activity levels, altered anxiety-like behavior, and accumulation of aluminum in certain areas of the brain 180 days after injection.[114] The researchers noted that the neurotoxicity of aluminum adjuvants do not follow the typical "dose makes the poison" rule commonly accepted in the field of chemistry. A separate rodent study on the safety of aluminum adjuvants came to a similar conclusion, stating, "contrary to popular assumptions of inherent safety of aluminum in vaccines, there is now compelling data from both human and animal studies which implicates this most widely used adjuvant in the pathogenesis of disabling neuroimmuno-inflammatory conditions."[115] To date, safety studies specifically on the effects of aluminum vaccine adjuvants on pregnant women (and potential effects on their babies) have not been completed.

When I first started writing this chapter, I did not set out to talk about vaccines. However, as I continued my research into the sources of heavy metal exposure, I discovered that vaccines are one of them, and I felt that it would be wrong for me to intentionally leave this information out of the book simply to avoid controversy. There are many practitioners who feel that the risks of contracting a disease outweigh the risks associated with heavy metal exposure. While I do not disagree with this line of thinking, knowledge of the ingredients in vaccines, including heavy metals, is a fundamental part of informed consent.

Contamination of food items with aluminum during cooking, storing, or processing are yet another possible way you may be exposed to aluminum. The use of aluminum cookware, utensils and aluminum foil is a considerable source of exposure, as aluminum can readily leach into your food. For example, when fish is wrapped in aluminum foil for cooking, aluminum concentrations increase by a factor of 2 to 68 after heating (yes, up to 68x more aluminum).[116] In this study, acidic ingredients and longer cooking times significantly increased the amount of aluminum that accumulated in the fish. Other studies have found similar results, noting that "the use of aluminum foil for cooking contributes significantly to the daily intake of aluminum through the cooked foods."[117] The amount of aluminum in some of the food samples from this study exceeded the World Health Organization's upper intake limits.

Lastly, soy products may contain high levels of aluminum, believed to be leached from the aluminum tanks in which soybeans are acid washed/processed, or in certain instances, from the addition of mineral salts (often aluminum chloride). Most commercial tofu, for example, is pressed in aluminum boxes (in place of the traditional wooden boxes), which leaches aluminum into the final product. Aluminum exposure can come from many sources, but luckily, these are often within your control.

Tips to minimize aluminum exposure:

- Ditch aluminum foil—both for cooking and storing leftovers. If you must use it while cooking, prevent it from coming in direct contact with your food by placing a sheet of parchment paper in between the foil and your food. Be especially cautious with acidic ingredients (such as tomatoes, lemon, vinegar, yogurt, etc.), as these increase the amount of aluminum that transfers to your food.
- Avoid the use of aluminum pots and pans, including those cute stovetop aluminum espresso makers. Many cookie sheets and cake pans are made of aluminum. Recycled metal pots of unknown

quality, like you might find at a thrift store, may contain high levels of aluminum.

- Check ingredient labels on deodorants/antiperspirants, buffered aspirin, sunscreens, makeup (especially primers), and facial scrubs. Search for the word "alum" or "aluminum salts" in the ingredients.
- Do not use aluminum-containing antacids (see Chapter 7 for tips on managing heartburn).
- Eat fewer soy products.
- If aluminum is relevant to your decision on prenatal vaccinations, review the vaccine package insert to determine which ones contain aluminum.

Mercury

Mercury is widely known to be a neurotoxin and virtually every pregnant woman I've met is aware that it should be avoided. Mercury readily crosses the placenta, so your exposure to this heavy metal is predictive of your baby's exposure. In fact, some research has found that mercury "accumulates in fetal tissues resulting in fetal blood concentrations that typically exceed maternal levels."[118] This is a major public health concern because prenatal mercury exposure is linked to neurodevelopmental problems and lower cognitive performance during childhood.[119]

Decades of industrial use have resulted in mercury contamination across the globe. This has had the unfortunate result of contaminating oceans and waterways with mercury, where it continues to work its way up the food chain and accumulate in certain species of fish and seafood.

But before you swear off fish entirely, remember that a) only certain types of fish are high in mercury and need to be entirely avoided (namely: swordfish, shark, king mackerel, tilefish) and b) just because fish may contain mercury doesn't mean you'll necessarily absorb it. This is because most fish contains high levels of selenium, which can help counteract the toxicity of mercury, as discussed in Chapter 3. This, along with omega-3, iron, vitamin B12 and iodine content, may explain why higher fish intake in pregnancy, despite the mercury exposure, is associated with better child cognitive scores at age 3.[120] Plus, these benefits last far past toddlerhood. In a study of nearly 12,000 women and their children, those who ate more than 12 oz of seafood per week (not less) during pregnancy had children with better cognitive outcomes from birth through age 8.[121] These researchers concluded that the "risks from the loss of nutrients were greater than the risks of harm from exposure to trace contaminants in 12 oz seafood eaten weekly." Simply put: although there's nothing you can do at this moment about mercury contamination in oceans, the benefits outweigh the risks for eating most types of fish.

Interestingly, while everyone obsesses over fish, studies have found that amalgam fillings (commonly called silver fillings) may be a stronger contributor to mercury levels in pregnant women than fish.[122] That's because amalgam fillings are roughly 50% mercury. The more amalgam fillings in your mouth, the higher the mercury levels in your bloodstream and in cord blood.[123] When it comes to dental work in pregnancy, be picky. Dentists in Austria, Germany, Finland, Norway, the United Kingdom, and Sweden have been specifically instructed to avoid placing amalgam fillings during pregnancy.[124] However, not all countries and not all dentists heed this advice. If you need dental work while pregnant, insist against the use of amalgam. If you already have amalgams, please know that removing fillings during pregnancy or even while breastfeeding is not a good idea, since that exponentially increases your mercury exposure, at least for a short period of time. Wait until you're done breastfeeding to explore the option of amalgam removal (and only under the care of a highly experienced holistic or biological dentist who specializes in this area).

Finally, another potential route of exposure is from mercury-containing vaccines in the form of thimerosal, and some researchers are pushing for it to be phased out of vaccines entirely. As one researcher explains: "The problem with thimerosal is that it contains 49.6% mercury by weight which may cause neurotoxicity in humans, especially in fetuses, neonate and infants whose brains are still developing."[125] Some scientists are particularly concerned with mercury exposure in pregnancy due to the "risk of adverse neurodevelopmental effects in the unborn child."[126] If you choose to get vaccines in pregnancy, request mercury-free and read the package insert to confirm at the time of your appointment.

Tips to minimize mercury exposure:

- Avoid eating swordfish, shark, king mackerel, and tilefish (these are high in mercury, but low in selenium). But, continue to enjoy other fish and seafood. Limit tuna to 6 oz per week.
- If you require dental work during pregnancy, do not get amalgam fillings or crowns.
- If you choose to get vaccines in pregnancy, opt for mercury-free (also, read the above section on aluminum).
- Since some mercury exposure is inevitable, be sure to incorporate the lifestyle tips at the end of this chapter to minimize its impact on your body and your baby.

Other Chemicals to Avoid

The chemicals reviewed above are not the only chemicals that are potentially harmful in pregnancy; rather, they represent those that can be minimized by informed lifestyle choices. In other words, you have *some* control over your level of exposure.

Numerous other chemicals are implicated in reproductive problems, though limiting exposure to some of these can be a challenge, thanks to widespread environmental pollution and other factors. This includes heavy metals, persistent organic pollutants (like PCBs and dioxins), bromine, formaldehyde, flame retardants, antibacterial chemicals, and many others.[127]

For example, exposure to flame retardants is "associated with reproductive toxicity, thyroid hormone disruption in pregnant women and newborns, and poorer mental and psychomotor development including decrements in IQ and poorer attention in children."[128] Antibacterial chemicals, especially triclosan, have been linked to hormonal disruption and gut bacteria imbalances in lab animals and certain adverse neonatal outcomes in humans, including slower fetal growth and reduced head circumference.[129,130,131,132]

The following might not apply to you nor be an easy fix, but I still want to highlight a few key areas that may further reduce chemical exposure during your pregnancy.

Tips to minimize exposure to other chemicals:

- Reduce time spent in high-pollution areas, if at all possible.
- Do not smoke and avoid exposure to secondhand smoke.
- Use a high-quality water filter, such as a Berkey®, to remove contaminants from your cooking and drinking water.
- If buying furniture, choose items that are made without flame retardants.
- Wash your hands often, especially before meals. Hand-to-mouth transfer of household dust or contaminated soil are a major source of exposure to a wide range of chemicals and heavy metals.
- Regularly clean your home with a vacuum cleaner fitted with a HEPA filter, which is more efficient at trapping small particles and dust than standard filters.
- Avoid exposure to paint, varnishes, epoxy, sealants, industrial glues, solvents, and other common products used in construction and woodworking. These products off-gas harmful chemicals.

- Swap out home cleaning products for natural alternatives. For example, try white vinegar in a spray bottle for wiping down counters or mopping floors in lieu of chlorine bleach or antibacterial products.
- Weather permitting, and based on air pollution in your area, open windows to air out your home whenever possible. Multiple building materials and home furnishings outgas for years, and some studies indicate indoor air pollution can be higher than outside for this reason.
- Get a houseplant. The NASA Clean Air Study helped identify numerous houseplants that remove common chemicals from the air. Among them are: Boston ferns, peace lily, spider plant, and aloe vera.
- Do not take herbal supplements without first knowing the quality of the supplement (and of course, the safety of that specific herb during pregnancy). Many have been found to be contaminated with heavy metals.[133]
- Avoid the use of products that contain antibacterial chemicals (especially triclosan), such as soaps, wipes, hand gels, and toothpaste. Certain cutting boards and plastics can also contain them. Preserve your microbiome and use plain ol' soap and water.
- Do not smoke and avoid secondhand smoke.
- Cook with high-quality pots and pans. Low-quality cookware, especially those made from recycled metals, can transfer heavy metals into your food (like lead and aluminum).
- Be cautious about cooking or storing food in ceramics/pottery, as some have lead-containing glazes. The FDA advises using lead-testing kits (check online or at a hardware store) to ensure your ceramic cooking vessels or dishes are food-safe.[134]
- Do not incinerate your garbage. Burning plastics and metals releases chemicals into the air, many of which become more toxic after burning.
- If you work in an industrial job, among machinery, in farming, or with chemicals, talk to your employer about ways to minimize your exposure to chemicals.

Tips to help your body gently and safely eliminate toxins

Aside from reducing exposure, another strategy to avoid the harmful effects of chemicals is to enhance your body's natural ability to detoxify. Let me be clear: a full-blown "detox" is absolutely not recommended during pregnancy. By design, the process of "detoxing" liberates toxins that are stored in your body and releases them into your bloodstream to be processed by your liver and kidneys. Since your blood supply is ultimately your baby's blood supply, and because many toxins cross the placenta, a "detox" could actually *increase* your baby's exposure to toxins. Also, many of the popular methods touted as "detoxes" are not safe in pregnancy. For example, going on a juice fast, which deprives your body of countless essential nutrients, or loading up your body with a bunch of herbal laxatives, is entirely contraindicated while pregnant (and frankly, not the best method to detox even when you're *not pregnant*).

However, several everyday practices can assist in eliminating toxins gently and safely. Providing optimal nutrition and prioritizing certain foods/nutrients can help promote normal liver function. A healthy, functioning liver is more efficient at transforming chemicals to less toxic substances that can then be excreted through your digestive system (stool) and kidneys (urine). Below are several lifestyle tweaks to gently and safely enhance your body's innate detoxification systems.

1. **Drink plenty of filtered water.** Your body naturally eliminates chemicals through urine, sweat, and bowel movements. Consume adequate water (100 oz or more per day) to help these systems operate efficiently.
2. **Eat more vegetables, especially greens.** It seems too simple to be effective, but studies have found that eating green vegetables enhances your body's ability to excrete various persistent organic pollutants.[135] This is likely due to a combination of the high levels of fiber, chlorophyll, vitamin C, magnesium, and antioxidants found in fresh greens. In addition, eat more cruciferous vegetables, like broccoli, cauliflower, kale, cabbage, and Brussels sprouts. Cruciferous vegetables have been shown to boost the liver's ability to detoxify.[136] Garlic and cilantro have also been shown to aid in detoxification.[137]
3. **Consider taking a supplement of chlorella or spirulina.** These two edible algaes are an extremely rich source of the green pigment found in all plants called chlorophyll, as well as iodine, selenium, iron, and other micronutrients. In rat studies, chlorophyll has been shown to prevent absorption of a common pollutant, called dioxin, from the digestive tract.[138] This effect has also been shown in humans. Pregnant women given chlorella supplements (6 g per day, taken in split doses of 2 g after each meal) during their 2nd and 3rd trimesters end up with significantly lower dioxin levels in their breast milk (40% lower, in fact), suggesting that chlorella helped them gradually detoxify during pregnancy.[139] In the above study, no adverse effects of chlorella supplementation were noted in mothers or their infants. Chlorella may also help reduce mercury levels in the

body.[140] Consider having chlorella (or chlorophyll-rich green veggies) alongside foods that are commonly contaminated with dioxins and mercury (such as fish) to get the "best of both worlds," allowing you to benefit from the nutrients in fish with less risk of toxin exposure. Another form of algae called spirulina is also beneficial, particularly to protect against fluoride toxicity. In a study of pregnant rats exposed to fluoride with or without spirulina supplementation, offspring in the fluoride-only group had brain damage, thyroid dysfunction, and behavior problems; however, the group that received spirulina had offspring who were protected from these effects and did not experience "fluoride-induced depletion of thyroid hormones."[141] The authors suggest that spirulina be used as a prenatal supplement in areas with high fluoride levels in the water to minimize the risks of neurodevelopmental disorders. Spirulina may also protect against lead poisoning and inhibit the transfer of lead from mother to baby in utero.[142] If you're curious about taking it yourself, know that spirulina supplementation of 1500 mg per day has been shown to be safe in pregnant women (and also reduces the rates of anemia).[143]

4. **Get plenty of selenium.** This trace mineral is required for optimal function of your liver and thyroid, and is also known to help your body bind and safely eliminate heavy metals, including mercury, cadmium, and thallium.[144] Selenium-rich foods include Brazil nuts, fish and seafood (especially oysters), liver and organ meats, pork, beef, lamb, poultry, mushrooms, and eggs. Note that wild-caught salmon is higher in selenium than farm-raised.[145] Check that your prenatal vitamin contains selenium (a minimum of 60 mcg and up to 200 mcg) and if not, consider a separate supplement.

5. **Consume enough glycine.** As reviewed in Chapter 3, glycine is required for the production of your liver's major detoxification enzyme, glutathione. Your body's need for glycine increases exponentially during pregnancy, meaning you may have to go out of your way to consume enough. Foods rich in glycine include bone broth, slow-cooked meats/stews (especially tough cuts of meat that have a lot of connective tissue), chicken skin and pork rinds (or any animal skin), and collagen or gelatin supplements.

6. **Include more fiber-rich foods.** Fiber helps alleviate the harmful effects of chemicals in several ways: by binding to toxins so they can be excreted in your stool; by encouraging regular bowel movements, so waste products don't have a chance to be reabsorbed in your intestines; and by feeding beneficial bacteria in your gut, which play a role in detoxifying harmful chemicals all on their own. The best

sources of fiber are chia seeds or flaxseeds, non-starchy vegetables, berries, shredded coconut, legumes, and nuts/seeds.

7. **Eat more vitamin C.** This vitamin is a powerful antioxidant that can prevent damage from numerous chemicals. For example, vitamin C is protective against the harmful effects of fluoride, PCBs, and mercury.[146,147,148] Foods rich in vitamin C include bell peppers, broccoli, Brussels sprouts, strawberries, pineapple, oranges and other citrus fruits, kiwi, and kale.

8. **Move your body.** Exercise and stretching not only improve blood flow, but also help stimulate your lymphatic system—a key part of your circulatory and immune system. Your lymphatic system plays a significant role in the removal of toxins and waste products from your body. To put it simply, the more you move, the more efficiently your body can detoxify. Make it a habit to exercise regularly, even if it's only for short amounts of time. See Chapter 8 for advice on prenatal exercise.

Summary

Reading this chapter has probably felt a bit "doom and gloom." I felt the same way while researching and writing all of this. It's disheartening and frankly scary to read how your baby could be affected by chemical exposures, many of which were either unknown to you previously or may simply be out of your direct control. What I find frustrating is that no one is warning you about this.

I included a thorough discussion on toxins because although food and exercise are the cornerstones of a healthy pregnancy, they aren't a cure-all. You can eat all organic foods and take the best prenatal vitamins money can buy, but if you're cooking your food in non-stick pans and using perfume everyday, you're missing an important piece of the puzzle. I know we agree on this: you want to do the best for your baby.

Exposure to many of the chemicals highlighted in this chapter *are* within your control, at least to some extent. You can't control what you're gonna breathe outside, but you *can* control what you eat and what products you put on your body. Every little lifestyle change you make adds up. If you noticed numerous ways that you are exposed to chemicals, choose one or two habits to work on this week. For example, swap out your laundry detergent for fragrance-free and start using glass containers to store leftovers (instead of plastic containers or aluminum foil).

In most cases, chronic exposure is the big concern. So, take one thing at a time to focus on. Gradually clean up your household cleaning supplies, get picky about the quality of food you buy, think about the personal care products you rub on your skin, and know that with each of these little tweaks, you're protecting your baby. You can't *eliminate* exposure, but you can *lessen* it, and that's the most important point to focus on. Plus, these practices are not just important during pregnancy. Infants and young children are still highly vulnerable to chemicals, so cleaning up your household now will protect your family for years to come.

Chapter 11:

Stress & Mental Health

"Human neurodevelopment requires the organization of neural elements into complex structural and functional networks called the connectome. Emerging data suggest that prenatal exposure to maternal stress plays a role in the wiring, or miswiring, of the developing connectome."
- Dr. Dustin Scheinost, Yale School of Medicine

We all experience stress, but it's often exponentially higher during pregnancy. Suddenly, it seems like every decision you make is going to make or break the health of your baby. There are so many questions, unknowns, and fears that spring up.

Is my baby moving enough today (or maybe too much)?
What is childbirth gonna be like?
Are my lab tests abnormal?
What if I have complications?
Can we *really* afford a baby?
How will my work/career be affected?
Will my body ever go back to normal?
Will my partner still love me?
Is my baby growing properly?
Am I prepared for the postpartum period?
Will I be able to breastfeed?
What if something goes wrong?
Will I be a good mom?

And that's just a *short* list! Know that experiencing these fears and anxieties is, at least to some extent, a normal part of pregnancy. As one researcher puts it, "Although pregnancy is often portrayed as a time of great joy, that's not the reality for all women... anxiety during pregnancy can change pregnancy into an agonizing and unpleasant event of women's life span."[1]

Depression during pregnancy is also common, affecting up to 25% of women.[2] While the discussion of postpartum depression has gained a lot of attention in recent years, *prenatal* depression is not as widely discussed.

There's no magic pill that will erase these worries, but you can find ways to manage your feelings and support your mental health during this time. Pregnancy *can* be enjoyable, even if you're dealing with some complications. And finding ways to process tough emotions and anxiety is crucial for your health, your birth outcomes, and the long-term health of your baby. Although this book focuses primarily on prenatal nutrition, it isn't the only thing that affects your baby's development.

Research has revealed strong ties between emotional and mental health during pregnancy and numerous pregnancy outcomes. I share the following information not to overwhelm you with scary statistics, but to make it clear that a healthy pregnancy relies on more than just good food and exercise. You need to take care of *all of you*.

Side Effects of Stress

One of the most widely accepted side effects of stress during pregnancy is preterm birth. In fact, pregnant women with high levels of stress have a 25-60% higher risk for preterm delivery even after accounting for other known risk factors.[3] Stress, anxiety or depression may also directly or indirectly affect your blood pressure and can lead to preeclampsia in some cases.[4] Your baby's growth and development can be affected by stress experienced in utero. Chronic anxiety may "cause changes in the blood flow to the baby, making it difficult to carry oxygen and other important nutrients to the baby's developing organs," which may explain why moms with high anxiety tend to have smaller babies.[5] High levels of stress hormones are also directly associated with decreased growth of the placenta, and researchers suggest this may pre-program your child's ability to handle stress later in life.[6]

Furthermore, brain development and risk for neurobehavioral disorders are affected by prenatal stress.[7] This is most likely a result of exposure to cortisol, a hormone that's released in times of stress. Cortisol crosses the placenta and women who are overly stressed tend to have high cortisol in their amniotic fluid. In one of the few studies that simultaneously assessed cortisol levels and birth outcomes, it was found that high cortisol levels in amniotic fluid was predictive of several infant outcomes, including low birthweight and both infant fear and distress at 3 months of age.[8] A separate study linked high cortisol in pregnancy with reduced brain growth during baby's first 6 months of life.[9] Women who report depression during pregnancy tend to have high cortisol levels.[10] This raises important questions about how prenatal stress can affect infant psychological health, and makes it clear that stress management and mental health should be a high priority while pregnant.

It's also likely that moms who are overly stressed or depressed may not have the time or energy to eat as healthfully, exercise regularly, or have consistent sleep habits. In other words, it may not always be the stress itself that's to blame, but the self care that doesn't happen when we're overwhelmed or consumed by our mental state. For example, think of what constitutes "comfort food" for you. It's often refined carbs or sugars that'll give you a quick dopamine surge, and thus offer a temporary distraction from whatever is making you feel down. And when you're super anxious, it's nearly impossible to turn off the mental chatter in your brain and go to sleep (or stay asleep). Then sleep deprivation further fuels high cortisol levels and cravings for comfort foods. One thing feeds into the other.

Tips to Reduce Prenatal Stress

So what can you do about it? Like I said, there's some level of prenatal stress and anxiety that simply comes with the territory; that's normal. It's when stress is chronic and prevents you from taking care of yourself that it becomes problematic.

Simply noticing that you're stressed is the first step to finding the best solution(s) for you. Get curious about what areas of your life are contributing the most. Is is a hectic schedule? Not feeling connected to your partner or support systems? Feeling worried about birth? Anxiety about the world of parenthood? Is it your physical health: complications, aches/pains, or your changing pregnant body?

It can honestly be anything. Even if it sounds silly verbalizing it, try. Once you give it a name, you'll have more power to work through it. Then, consider what would help you the most. For example, is there a way to simplify your schedule, such as working fewer hours? Is there a way to carve out more "me time" in your week? Can you reach out to your partner or loved ones to express your concerns and ask for support? Can you work with a therapist? The benefit of formal therapy is that you have an objective person to help you process your thoughts.

Curiosity is key. Stay open to whatever comes up for you and know that there are countless ways to manage stress and relieve anxiety. Sometimes tackling these feelings head-on is the way to go. Other times, heightened stress is simply a result of being pulled in too many directions, and the solution is more about consciously *doing less* than it is about doing anything extra.

Although anxiety, depression, and stress are experienced differently, effective lifestyle treatments share a lot of similarities. In one study, pregnant women were given just one piece of advice: *"Eliminate things that are stressful and/or participate in things that increase your level of relaxation."* Even that vague advice was effective at reducing depression, stress, and cortisol levels.[11] In other words, your approach to stress reduction and self care doesn't need to be anything fancy.

Mindfulness

One specific practice that I want to highlight is mindfulness. Mindfulness is simply being aware of your feelings, thoughts, and body sensations in the moment and accepting them without judgement. Many people think mindfulness is something that's only done while meditating or while relaxing, but in truth, it can be incorporated to all areas of your life, from the way you eat, to the way you walk, to the way you wash dishes, to the way you approach conversations with others. Mindfulness is not about relaxing, clearing your mind, or getting rid of negative thoughts; rather it's about noticing and accepting where you are at this moment. So often I hear women talk about how they think they *should* be feeling rather than acknowledging that the way they feel right now is valid. This undertone of judgement only adds to pre-existing worries and stressors. The antidote is mindfulness and unconditional acceptance. "Negative" emotions have less power when we accept them at face value and know that they are just one more thing in life that is transient, like clouds that float across the sky.

Studies have shown that practicing mindfulness during pregnancy leads to significant reductions in pregnancy-related anxiety, worry, and depression.[12] It's amazing how simply noticing things like your heartbeat, breath, or kicks in your belly, can help you feel so much calmer and more connected with your baby. This is a practice that will also serve you well during birth since mother-directed pushing, something that absolutely requires mindfulness on your part, is associated with fewer perineal tears, less maternal fatigue, and higher APGAR scores in infants.[13,14]

Self Care Practices

Whether you opt to try mindfulness or something else, the below list should get your wheels turning about what to consider when it comes to stress management and self care. Many women have found one or a combination of the following approaches helpful:

- Spend time outdoors. Walk in the park, go on a hike, sit by a river, work in your garden, etc.

Real Food for Pregnancy

- Practice deep breathing. There are numerous methods, but consciously slowing down your breath while silently thinking "breathe in, breathe out" is enough.
- Incorporate mindfulness. The way you eat, walk, communicate, and simply go about your everyday life are all opportunities to practice mindfulness. Become aware of how you feel in different situations, allow yourself to feel the feelings, and observe your reaction without judgement.
- Call a friend or trusted family member. Get a fresh perspective or just let go and vent to someone who's a good listener.
- See a therapist, psychologist or other licensed mental health practitioner. Maternal mental health is a highly specialized field. If possible, seek a provider who is trained in maternal mental health and has experience serving pregnant women. A list of providers can be found on the Postpartum Support International website *(www.postpartum.net/)*.
- Meditate. If you're new to meditation, try a short guided meditation to get started. There are numerous free or low-cost apps, videos, and recordings available. Even 1-5 minutes counts. You don't need a special cushion or outfit or even a set amount of time for meditation to be beneficial.
- Visualization. I know it sounds woo-woo, but imagining the ideal outcome as if you're living it, whether that's feeling baby develop perfectly or having a calm birth, is surprisingly helpful. Even though it's literally "all in your head," placebo effect is a proven phenomenon.
- Hypnotherapy. I consider this similar to guided meditation and visualization. There are several hypnotherapy programs specific to pregnancy and birth, which often include a recording (or several). Simply turn on the recording before bed or while relaxing on the couch.
- Yoga nidra. This is also known as "sleep yoga." It involves no formal postures, rather you lay in one place and draw attention to your breath and to various areas of your body, one by one.
- Sleep. Getting adequate rest is important to overall mental health and can affect levels of neurotransmitters. It can be challenging to get enough sleep as you get further along in your pregnancy, thanks to hormonal changes, trouble finding comfortable positions, and having to pee more often. A few things may be beneficial: aim for a similar bedtime each night, stay off electronics in the last 1-2 hours before bed, use blackout curtains in your room (even small amounts of light interfere with your melatonin levels, a hormone that helps you sleep), and try a pregnancy body pillow to make sleep more

comfortable. Yoga nidra, mentioned above, is a wonderful addition to your bedtime routine.

- Tapping/EFT. Emotional Freedom Technique, also called tapping or EFT, helps reduce the emotional impact of memories or incidents that trigger emotional distress by tapping on various acupressure points with your finger. Studies have found it effective at lowering stress and cortisol levels.[15] There are countless videos online that walk you through this simple practice step by step. You can also talk through what's bothering you somewhat "stream of consciousness" style while you tap on the specific EFT acupressure points.
- Massage. Make sure your practitioner is aware of your pregnancy and knowledgeable about appropriate positioning. In later pregnancy, massages can be performed on your side or on a special pregnancy pillow, which allows you to lay face down (for the first time in months—it feels amazing!). Massage therapy has been shown to help alleviate prenatal depression, even when a woman's partner is the (not-formally-trained) masseuse.[16]
- Acupuncture. Studies have found it an effective tool to help manage stress and anxiety.[17] It's also specifically been shown to reduce prenatal depression.[18]
- Laugh out loud. Watch a silly comedy movie.
- Journal. Some find it easier to process emotions while writing versus talking. Allow yourself to "free write" whatever comes to mind without judging what comes out on paper or worrying about grammar. This is an exercise in letting it all out.
- Engage in spiritual practice or your faith community.
- Move. All forms of movement tell your body to release more feel-good endorphins. Choose your favorite.
- Listen to music. Play an instrument. Dance. Sing. Give yourself permission to let go.
- Gratitude. What are you grateful for in this moment? If you're especially overwhelmed, start with the very basics: "I'm grateful for the air I breathe... for the bright sun or cleansing rain... for honoring my body's need to slow down right now..." It's great to make this a daily habit by writing down a list every morning or evening (or both!). You'll be surprised how much is going "right" in your world, even on the most awful of days.

Can you think of anything else that makes you feel more relaxed, connected with your baby, and at ease with life? *Do it.*

My list is not all-inclusive and there's plenty of room for you to explore other avenues for self care and stress management. Remember the study I mentioned earlier: even the simplest of advice, to "avoid stress and relax more," is effective. You just need to make the conscious choice to try. If you do this to the best of your ability and still struggle, now is time to reach out to a mental health professional.

Professional Help

There's absolutely, positively no shame in asking for help in navigating your thoughts and emotions, especially when you're living in a sea of ever-changing pregnancy hormones. Pregnancy often triggers reactions that are complex and hard to wrap your brain around, even if you've previously felt like you have a handle on your mental and emotional state.

Be aware that prenatal depression, anxiety, and other mental health concerns may not be on your doctor's radar, so you may have to specifically request a mental health screening or a referral. It can be hard to get the help that you need in some health systems, which means that you may have to ask several times, advocate for yourself, and follow up, follow up, follow up. It may not be easy, but if you think you are having a mental health issue, it can take persistence to get appropriate care (unfortunately). As mentioned above, you'll want to find a provider who's trained in maternal mental health and who regularly serves pregnant women. A list of providers who specialize in this area can be found on the Postpartum Support International website *(www.postpartum.net/)*.

Nutrition Connection

Last, but certainly not least, eating a nutrient-dense diet provides your body with the raw materials to support overall brain health. (Yes, of course, I have to bring it back to food.) This is not to discount the power of self care and specific practices that you use to address stress, but food is an important piece of the mental health puzzle that's often overlooked. Researchers note that "Women are particularly vulnerable to the adverse effects of poor nutrition on mood because pregnancy and lactation increase nutrient requirements."[19] Studies show that micronutrients including iron, zinc, folate, vitamin B6, B12, calcium, selenium, choline, vitamin D, and omega-3 fats (DHA) affect maternal mental health and well-being.[20,21]

This may explain why some women notice such a profound difference in their mood after eating certain foods. For example, anemic mothers who supplement with iron have improvements in depressive symptoms.[22] Also, women with prenatal depression (and postpartum depression) tend to have significantly lower levels of omega-3 fats, like DHA, and higher levels of omega-6 fats in their bloodstream.[23] If you're not already regularly eating seafood, like wild salmon, or supplementing with fish oil, make it a priority.

Lastly, imbalances in the microbiome can affect mental health (via what's known as the "gut-brain axis") and emerging research suggests that probiotics may help lessen depression and anxiety.[24,25] Fermented foods, such as yogurt, kefir, sauerkraut, and/or a probiotic supplement are wise choices to support your mental health. Circle back to Chapters 2 and 3 for more details on prenatal nutrition and nutrient-dense foods. In times of stress and emotional upheaval, it's sometimes hard to want to eat healthy, and yet right now it's more important than ever. Pay close attention to how you feel after eating by applying the mindful eating techniques discussed in Chapter 2. Some women notice an almost immediate positive or negative mental reaction to certain foods, which can help further guide your food choices.

Summary

Remember, managing your stress is just as important as all the other lifestyle choices you make each day, like eating nutrient-dense foods and moving your body. Finding ways to take care of your mental and emotional health is vital. There's more than one way to approach this, but I have consistently found mindfulness, in one form or another, to be effective.

Practicing mindfulness allows you to be fully present for the ups and downs of pregnancy, the challenges and rewards of birth, and the whirlwind that is caring for a newborn. When you are aware and accepting of your feelings, you'll be better equipped to enjoy the special moments and milestones and carry on through the tough points unphased. That said, if you feel you need more help than the self care tips in this chapter, do not hesitate to reach out to your healthcare provider to explore other options, which may include a referral to a specialist in maternal mental health or other avenues.

Chapter 12:

The Fourth Trimester

"The postpartum period is a time of transition for a woman and her new family, when adjustments need to be made on physical, psychological, and social levels."
- Dr. Elizabeth Shaw, McMaster University, Hamilton

O ur busy, modern world seems to pretend that once you give birth, you're good to go. Everyone wants to pamper pregnant women, but postpartum? After a few weeks, it's as if people expect you to carry on with business as usual.

These unrealistic expectations lead a lot of women to ignore the absolutely crucial period of rest and recovery in the early postpartum months. And yet this time is vital to your emotional well-being, your physical recovery, and of course, for bonding with your precious baby. I've known too many women who have pushed too hard, too soon, to get back to everything they were doing before pregnancy, only to end up exhausted, depressed, and physically suffering. This is not something you want to mess around with. Traditional cultures had specific instructions on what activities were encouraged or discouraged for new mothers in the early weeks; these practices are strikingly similar across the globe, as I'll explain in the following section. For the most part, your job was simply to recover, rest, eat food (that was cooked *for you*), and feed your baby.

Nowadays, many women feel compelled to "do it all" and be the supermom who exclusively breastfeeds, returns to work quickly, and bounces back to her pre-pregnancy body in no time. Though this is theoretically possible, it's not common, nor is it without consequences. The reality is that life with a baby is uncharted territory. Once you have a baby, you enter the "4th trimester," an adjustment period of several months in which baby needs near constant attention, day and night. Some theorize that a newborn's brain is not yet developed enough to understand that he or she is a separate being from you. There will be days when having even 5 minutes to yourself without an interruption is a miracle. Writer Olivia Campbell put it well in an essay on postpartum recovery: "The myth that once baby and mother are separate entities, I will immediately revert back to feeling like myself again leaves me blindsided by the continued sense of symbiosis postpartum."[1] It doesn't last forever, but when you're "in the thick of it," it's no joke. The fewer demands you can place on yourself during this phase, the better. Your body and your baby *need* you to rest and recover.

That's why this section is *not* going to tell you to enroll in "baby body bootcamp" or any other unrealistic (and potentially harmful) practices. This is not about "bouncing back" quickly or fitting into your jeans right away. Rather, I want to focus on the ways you can slow down, take care of yourself, heal from pregnancy and birth, replenish your nutrient stores (for your own health, and also so you can prepare for a future child if you choose), set yourself up for success with breastfeeding, and restore your physical self through safe, gentle movements. I will be specifically highlighting traditional postpartum practices from around the globe and how you can apply this wisdom to optimize your own recovery. My hope is that you are empowered and prepared for a smooth transition into your new role as a mother.

A Traditional Approach to Postpartum Healing

There's a lot we can learn from traditional cultures when it comes to the postpartum period. Although they all have their own quirks, postpartum traditions have many similarities country to country. This includes several weeks of rest to recuperate, establish breastfeeding, replenish nutrient stores with special foods, and ease up on physically demanding activities. This section is a compilation of information from women I interviewed directly and what's available in the published research on these customs and the rationale behind them.

In many cultures, the immediate postpartum period is considered a vulnerable time and it's customary for new moms to observe upwards of 40 days of "confinement" to rest and recover. Confinement has a slightly negative connotation, but I think the word used in the Amazon, *resguardo*, which derives from the Portuguese verb *resguardar*, meaning "to protect," is a more accurate description of the goals of these first few weeks: to protect mother and baby. Though the exact number of days/weeks can vary slightly, it's fascinating that the time frame is similar in Jordan, Lebanon, Egypt, Palestine, Mexico, China, Southeast Asia, Eastern Amazon, and many other parts of the world.[2,3] Even in Western medicine, 6 weeks seems to be a significant marker that closes out the initial postpartum healing phase.

In China, the customary practice is called *zuo yuezi*, which loosely translates to "sitting the month" or "doing the month," during which time female relatives do all of your housework and cooking. They specifically prepare warming *yang* foods to boost your *chi* (life force or energy). You are also restricted from reading or watching movies (to avoid eye strain and to encourage rest) and from showering or washing your hair (to avoid getting cold; warm sponge baths, however, are permitted).[4] Similar practices are common in Korea and Thailand.

In Korea, for example, a new mother's only duties are to "eat and sleep to restore her health" while her mother (the baby's grandmother) cares for all of her needs.[5] In some areas of Japan, it's customary for women to return "to her family home at 32-35 weeks gestation to be cared for by her mother until approximately 8 weeks postpartum." Similarly, Himba women in Namibia return to their mother's compound in the last trimester of pregnancy and stay there for several months after giving birth.[6] Organized support for new moms are also commonplace in parts of Jordan, Nigeria, Guatemala, India, and numerous other countries.[7]

In Cambodia, women practice *ang pleung* (also called mother-warming or roasting) for a minimum of 3 days, during which time a mother stays in her bamboo bed that has a small fire underneath. This practice is thought to increase blood flow in the uterus, prevent blood clots, and be a crucial part of postpartum recovery.[8] After mother-warming, woman are encouraged to stay in bed for the remainder of the month. Heavy lifting, standing for long periods, and exposure to cold, rain, or dew are avoided.

In Mexico, women practice "la cuarentena," in which they move back in with their family or have their mother/mother-in-law come to live with them for approximately 40 days. Being in an intergenerational setting means there are plenty of helping hands to prepare food, care for you during recovery from birth, and assist in day-to-day needs. Regular massages and abdominal wrapping with a "faja" are believed to help prevent uterine prolapse, support "loose" or "open" bones, encourage abdominal organs to go back into place, and protect against cold/wind.[9]

In Ayurveda, an ancient form of medicine from India, women are encouraged to take up to 6 weeks of rest at home, have daily massages, and eat "warming" foods (prepared by others, of course), including plenty of warm fluids believed to encourage milk production. In addition, visitors are kept to a minimum, mother and baby remain indoors as much as possible, and exposure to harsh lights or drafts is limited.[10]

In Tanzania, Maasai women reportedly remain in their homes (called bomas) for three months postpartum to recover from birth and to care for their newborns.[11] In the Amazon, women are expected to stay close to or inside of their homes for 40-41 days, with special rules early on. Specifically, "During the first week postpartum, women were seen as being especially fragile and spent almost the entire day in a reclined position in their hammocks."[12]

Adapting Traditions for Modern Life

Admittedly, there are some practices that may seem extreme nowadays, but understanding their origins and possible applications can be helpful. For example, discouraging women to bathe or wash their hair for a period of time is noted in several cultures and may stem from concerns about clean water or getting too cold after bathing. Limiting baths could be viewed as a way to prevent infections in mother or baby. Concerns over a mother or infant getting cold or being exposed to harsh weather (wind, rain, and snow) are common themes. Maternal and infant mortality are legitimate considerations in developing countries, especially those without access to modern medicine, so the focus on staying warm and protected are logical. These, however, may be less relevant if you live in a developed country with clean water, reliable shelter, adequate clothing, and heat.

Similarly, most of us do not live in villages or even in an intergenerational home where around-the-clock support is easily accessible, so some traditions have to be adapted to work within our lives. For those of us who live hundreds or thousands of miles from our families, having our mother/mother-in-law live with us is often not feasible (and perhaps, not something you want to entertain, even if they *do* live around the corner).

What is clear, though, is that women in traditional cultures are not expected to "do it all" alone and are actively *discouraged* from doing so in the early weeks after giving birth. This is the polar opposite to modern expectations. A review of traditional postpartum practices from over 20 different countries found one thing to hold true across them all; that these practices "allow the mother to be 'mothered' for a period of time after the birth."[13]

In contrast, Western countries seem to expect women to return to their normal activities rather quickly after birth. A Korean woman who married into an American family and gave birth in the United States shared her confusion:[14]

> *"Approximately 7 days after I gave birth to our baby daughter, my husband's family gathered to celebrate her arrival. I felt that all their concern was for the baby, rather than for me, the new mother. In Korea, very elaborate consideration and attention is granted to the new mother after birth. As a Korean, I also looked forward to enjoying the role of a patient until my full recovery, usually lasting 1 month... his family treated*

me as a healthy person who could resume normal activities almost immediately. For example, my husband expected me to drive to the pediatrician's clinic for the baby's first physical checkup 7 days after giving birth."

From my own experience and that of my American friends, I can say most of us wished we had taken it slower in the early weeks, and even months, postpartum. Our culture seems to push new moms to try to get back to life as usual and resume all normal activities rather quickly. You're praised for going on a walk in the first week postpartum, for getting out for a date night with your partner, and for hitting the gym mere weeks after you've given birth. Magazine covers of celebrities "doing it all" with a newborn in tow only stoke the fire. For many of us, career demands make it all the more challenging to truly take time off. The lack of adequate maternity leave (and paternity leave) in America only highlights this gross oversight.

But being a supermom, at least in the early months, can come back to bite you later on. Many cultures view inadequate recovery time (or failure to comply with traditional practices) as the root of health problems later in life. Though this sounds like an old wives' tale, it's not entirely superstition. In my own nutrition practice, I've observed more challenges with breastfeeding, adrenal fatigue, and thyroid problems among mothers who pushed too fast, too soon and didn't allow adequate time to truly recover.

How Will You Rest, Recover, and Receive Support?

My challenge to you is to envision how you will be supported after the birth of your child. If this is your first child, it'll be hard to imagine not being able to care for your own needs. You might be blindsided by how hard it is to walk even the 10 steps to the bathroom during the first days after birth, how much time it takes to feed a baby, and how frustrating it is to never have two hands to eat a meal (why babies are always hungry right when your meal is ready is beyond me).

Planning for Postpartum Support:

- Who can you rely on to help you during these intense few weeks/months?
- If you don't have family or friends to help, can you consider hiring a postpartum doula or a housekeeper (or both)?
- Can someone arrange a meal train for you, in which friends or family sign up to deliver a meal to your house each day for several weeks?
- Or can you pack your freezer with meals in the last few months of your pregnancy, so you're prepared with easy, nutritious meals?

- If you have other children, is it possible to have additional childcare for a time?

I know how hard it is to ask for and accept help. We're raised to be self-sufficient and independent women, but I promise you that reaching out or pre-arranging help does not make you any less strong or competent. *It means you're smart.* And it means your recovery from birth and transition to new motherhood will be much, much smoother. We put so much emphasis on planning for birth, but very little on planning for the postpartum phase (I was guilty of the same thing, by the way). This desperately needs to shift.

The following sections highlight additional insights we can glean from postpartum practices around the globe and what modern scientific research has to say, starting with nourishing foods.

Real Food & Postpartum Nutrient Repletion

A lot of women assume that nutrition during pregnancy is what matters most; once baby is born, you're off the hook and can eat whatever you want. You might be surprised to learn that nutrient needs in breastfeeding moms are *higher* than while you were pregnant. Technically, you're still growing a baby. Your baby is just outside of the womb. That means nourishing yourself should remain a huge priority.

Plus, depending on the circumstances of your labor and delivery, it may feel like you've run a marathon (or two). You absolutely need to replenish your energy and take in additional nutrients to account for blood loss and wound healing (particularly if you've had a perineal tear or a surgical birth). Even in an uncomplicated delivery, your body undergoes significant changes as your uterus shrinks down to its pre-pregnancy size, your connective tissues adapt, your breasts begin producing milk (whether or not you choose to breastfeed), and your skin regains elasticity.

Across the board, traditional cultures put a heavy emphasis on postpartum nutrition. Though there are clear regional differences in cuisine, one thing is clear: animal products are a mainstay. From rich bone broths to organ meats, from seafood to eggs, our ancestors understood that the nutrients found in these foods were extremely important for healing and milk production in new moms. The second commonality is that "warming" foods are encouraged. Yes, this includes steamy broths, herbal teas, and porridges, but it also includes recipes with warming spices, like cinnamon and ginger. Some cultures have differences of opinion on which foods are warm or cold (it's not always temperature or spiciness), but I'll do my best to highlight the commonalities.

In China, *yang* foods are considered warming, while *yin* foods are cooling. In the immediate postpartum period, a woman is considered to be in a *yin* state and must rebalance her system by eating more *yang* foods. Rich bone broths made from pig's feet or chicken and enriched with seaweed, ginger, and vinegar might grace the table.[15] In addition to the heavy emphasis on broths and soups, foods that encourage milk production and healing include pork, chicken, organ meats, rice, eggs, sesame seed oil, ginger, ginseng, herbal teas, and rice wine.[16] Animal foods are central: "Meat is served every day, usually rotating between chicken, pork, pig liver and kidney."[17] According to some reports from Southwest China, women are encouraged to eat 8-10 eggs per day to enhance milk production and boost brain development of her infant.[18] At the same time, cooling *yin* foods are discouraged, especially raw vegetables and fruits, cold liquids, and even plain water (warm herbal tea is given instead). Some cooked vegetables are permitted, such as Chinese kale, mushrooms, carrots, and string beans (though this varies based on the report).[19]

In India, emphasis is also placed on warming foods including whole milk (heated before serving), ghee (clarified butter), nuts, ginger, and jagerry (unrefined sugar).[20] Among Malaysian Indians of South Indian descent, dishes made with shark, sting-ray, chicken, and salted fish are emphasized as well as spicy curries. At the same time, cold foods, such as tomatoes and cucumbers, are avoided.[21]

In Mexico, soups and warming beverages are also on the menu. Brothy chicken soup with onions, garlic, and cilantro is a common postpartum recovery meal. Hot chocolate and *atole*, a thick, sweetened beverage made with masa (corn), milk, and cinnamon are given to encourage milk production.[22]

In the Amazon state of Pará, the ideal food for the first week postpartum is boiled chicken; after this week, a broader variety of foods are permitted, including game meat, certain fish, acai berries, manioc (a starchy tuber), rice, and beans.[23] Aside from acai berries, fruit is strictly avoided for the first 40 days.

In Korea, new mothers are often served a special seaweed soup called *miyuk-kuk*.[24] In Cambodia, warm rice porridge and a rich dish called *khaw* is served, which is braised beef, pork or fish with salt, pepper and palm sugar. Warming beverages are served (like herbal tea and homemade wine), while cold, sour, and raw foods are avoided.[25]

In Northern Nigeria, women eat a porridge made of groundnuts (peanuts) and rice that's enriched with local salt. Spicy foods are also emphasized.[26] In

South Africa, high-protein foods are encouraged, while cold foods are avoided as they are believed to reduce milk production.[27]

Nutritional Rationale Behind Traditional Healing Foods

In many ways, the foods emphasized in traditional cultures make perfect sense. When you're recovering from pregnancy and birth, there are tremendous shifts going on internally. Healing tissues that have been stretched, torn or cut (to put it bluntly) require plenty of protein, especially the amino acids glycine and proline, which your body uses to make collagen. These are found in abundance in the connective tissues, bones, and skin of animal foods. Electrolytes and fluids are crucial to replace those lost during labor. All of these nutrients are found in bone broth and any slow-cooked stews, soups, and curries that incorporate animal foods.

If you've lost a significant amount of blood, replenishing with red meat and organ meats, especially liver and heart, would provide high amounts of easily absorbed iron and vitamin B12. Foods such as eggs and seafood would provide additional protein along with iodine, B-vitamins, zinc, choline, DHA and a variety of other nutrients that help speed healing and also enrich breast milk.

Furthermore, energy needs go up during recovery from birth. Attention given to easy-to-digest foods, like cooked vegetables, slow-cooked meat, and starchy porridges is both intentional and logical; your body can more readily extract calories from cooked foods compared to raw foods. Lastly, traditionally-emphasized foods are often widely available in that area (hence why they vary region to region), provide necessary calories for recovery, and often fall into the category of comfort foods. On a nutritional and emotional level, these are exactly the foods your body wants *and needs* during this vulnerable time.

What Should You Eat?

For the most part, you can continue eating the way you did during pregnancy through the postpartum phase with just a few modifications. As mentioned above, you'll need more calories, which means more food all around. Breastfeeding mothers, especially, find themselves ravenously hungry in the early weeks. It's estimated that exclusively breastfeeding mothers burn an additional 500 calories per day for the first 6 months postpartum. If you're listening to your hunger cues (and have enough help to bring food to you when needed), you'll be just fine.

I remember the morning after giving birth, my husband brought me breakfast. It was a typical-sized breakfast that I was used to eating during pregnancy, but it was nowhere close to the amount of food my body needed. I was like a bottomless pit for weeks. I remember saying to him, "For future reference, I'm gonna need *triple* the amount of food from now on." It was shocking how hungry I was!

It's actually quite easy to accidentally undereat during this phase, especially if you don't have someone preparing food for you (did I mention newborns are demanding of your time and attention?), so I can't emphasize enough the importance of arranging help preparing meals, having pre-made freezer meals at the ready, and also stashing snacks around the house where you plan to feed your baby and rest.

Foods to Enhance Postpartum Recovery:

- Soups, hearty stews, and curries made with bone broth. These warming comfort foods supply collagen-building amino acids, electrolytes, and many micronutrients. See the Recipe Appendix for bone broth, chicken & vegetable soup, coconut chicken curry, and carnitas.
- High-iron foods, such as slow-cooked meat (think pot roast or pulled pork) and organ meats, such as liver, kidney, and heart. Remember that you can hide liver in many recipes, as I do in chili, meatloaf, shepherd's pie, and meatballs. See the Recipe Appendix for those recipes as well as a tasty liver pate.
- High-fat foods, like pork, butter/ghee, fatty fish, nuts/seeds, etc. My nutty "granola" bars, spinach dip, and maple pots de creme in the Recipe Appendix make great postpartum snacks.
- Foods rich in omega-3 fats, such as seafood, eggs, and grass-fed beef. Try the grilled salmon, salmon cakes, and spinach quiche in the Recipe Appendix.
- Iodine-rich foods, such as seafood or seaweed-infused broths (this can be as simple as adding a piece of dried kombu to your batch of bone broth). Roasted nori "seaweed snacks" are a convenient option.
- Soft-cooked vegetables (instead of raw veggies or salads). Any of the vegetable recipes in the Recipe Appendix are appropriate, as are the vegetables included in soups and stews.
- Well-cooked grains/starches, such as oatmeal, rice, or sweet potatoes (eaten alongside plenty of fat and protein to provide enough energy and stabilize your blood sugar). See my comments about carbohydrates in the following section.
- Plenty of warm liquids, like broths and teas (such as herbal lactation teas). A good rule of thumb is to aim for 1 oz of fluids per ¾-1 pound of body weight (110-150 oz per day if you weigh 150 lbs). If you're nursing, have a glass of water or some tea every time you nurse.

A Note About Carbohydrates

As mentioned above, you can continue to eat the same nutrient-dense prenatal diet during the postpartum phase, as long as you eat bigger portions and honor your hunger cues. The meal plans in this book (Chapter 5) are nutritionally adequate and well-balanced for postpartum healing. Some of you may be eager to drop the baby weight and be tempted to cut back on carbohydrates more than what you see in my meal plans, however you want to do so with caution.

It's no secret that I'm a proponent of lower-carbohydrate eating, however, *if you are breastfeeding,* the immediate postpartum period is not the best time to severely decrease your carbohydrate intake. Rather, the early weeks are a time to focus on bonding with your baby and establishing your milk supply. In some women (certainly not all), making a sudden shift to a very low-carb diet can lead to a drop in milk supply. It's unclear what the underlying cause is and research is scarce in this area, but there are several plausible explanations:

1. Lower-carb diets naturally reduce hunger levels and may result in undereating. Inadequate calorie intake is known to reduce milk supply.
2. Lower-carb diets result in water loss and make dehydration more common. That's a problem since extra fluids are required to produce breast milk.
3. Lower-carb diets may deplete electrolytes, which are also excreted in breast milk.

Although these theories have yet to be rigorously tested in *human* moms, research from dairy cows offers some insight. The dairy industry, which has a clear incentive to keep milk production up, has found that milk production drops when cows don't consume enough energy and therefore go into the fat burning state known as ketosis.[28] For this reason, dairy farmers actively try to keep their milking cows *out of ketosis,* to keep milk output high. A low-carb diet makes ketosis more likely, as does not eating enough calories in general. Since many women choose to eat low-carb as a means to lose weight, undereating is often the reality. Also, ketosis is more common when your carbohydrate intake is minimal.

It's hard to know whether the blame should be placed on inadequate calories or inadequate carbohydrate intake—or both—but it's important to recognize that breastfeeding requires fuel, and your body rapidly uses blood glucose, to make milk. Metabolically, most women can "get away with" eating more carbohydrates in the short term, or at the very least benefit from maintaining the level they consumed during pregnancy. Even in women with type 1 diabetes (in other words, those who produce no insulin), insulin needs drop dramatically in the first week following birth and the body becomes more insulin sensitive.[29] Once you birth the placenta and say goodbye to placental hormones, insulin resistance plummets. It's an innate survival mechanism that favors quick access to glucose to fuel on-demand, round-the-clock milk production. This means that extremely low carbohydrate intake during this time may not be necessary or ideal.

Now, this is not to say that you can *never* taper down your carbohydrate intake while breastfeeding, but I personally suggest waiting until your milk supply is well established (typically several months) to make significant changes. Even then, you'll want to do so gradually and with keen awareness that you still need to keep your calorie intake up to continue to produce the same quantity of breast milk. Also, you'll need to account for the natural diuretic effect of this way of eating by drinking plenty of fluids and liberally salting your foods (remember, salt is an electrolyte). In the single study done on low-carb diets in breastfeeding women (performed at 8-12 weeks postpartum), milk output was compared from women who ate a higher-carb or a low-carb diet with equal calories. There was no difference noted in milk output on the low-carb diet, however, carbohydrates were only limited to 137 g per day in the low-carb group (the high-carb plan provided 265 g).[30] In other words, it was a *moderately* low carb diet, much like my recommendations in this book, not necessarily a ketogenic or low-carb, high fat (LCHF) diet. Since breastfeeding increases your energy needs, you may have a higher intake of carbohydrates (gram-wise) while the proportion of carbohydrates stays the same (percentage of calories from carbohydrates). Some women find it helpful to look at it in this context.

In my professional experience, I find that most breastfeeding mothers who have a well-established milk supply need a minimum of 50 g of carbohydrates per day to maintain their supply. Yes, there will be exceptions to this rule, so please experiment and gradually find your own sweet spot for carbs.

We know there are cultures that thrived on very low-carbohydrate diets, such as the Inuit of Alaska, Canada, and Greenland. They were clearly still able to breastfeed and their bodies were adapted to a diet extremely limited in carbohydrates. That's the key, though. Their bodies were *adapted* to this way of eating. If going low-carb or *much* lower-carb means a sudden shift in the way you usually eat, you need to allow plenty of time for your body to adapt. In other words, don't go from something like 200 g of carbs/day to less than 20 g overnight and expect your milk supply to stay the same. Plan ahead and track your food intake for a week or more to get a baseline for your usual carbohydrate and calorie intake *before* you begin the gradual process of decreasing your carbs.

Breastfeeding

If you've made it this far in my book, I'd wager you're the type of person who has read (ad nauseum, no doubt) about the benefits of breastfeeding. There are innumerable immune, digestive, cognitive and metabolic benefits of nursing (for both you and baby), but this section is not about that. Other authors and researchers have already done an amazing job sharing that information. Instead, I want to share about oft-neglected topics, including the realities of breastfeeding, how to set yourself up for success, and the nutritional demands that breastfeeding places on your body.

If your goal is to follow the World Health Organization's recommendation to exclusively breastfeed for the first 6 months and "continue breastfeeding along with appropriate complementary foods up to two years of age or beyond," you'll want to be prepared for the journey ahead.

Learning to breastfeed is like learning a new language, especially if you run into challenges. There's a lot of lingo: *let down, football hold, side lying nursing, breastsleeping, galactogogues, tongue ties, lip ties, foremilk, hindmilk, latch, thrush, block feeding, power pumping, cluster feeding, nursing pads, nursing bras, nursing pillows, breast pumps, nipple cream...*

And please notice my choice of the word "learning." Breastfeeding, although natural, doesn't always come naturally. It's something that takes time to learn, both for you and your baby, even among women who have breastfed several babies. The first few weeks are often the most challenging as you adjust to a new routine, figure out the best positions, help your to baby latch properly, and frankly, get used to spending hours upon hours stuck on the couch with a baby on your boob each and every day.

Our public health campaigns about the benefits of breastfeeding seem to do a great job at informing people of the benefits of nursing, but fail at showing the realities of day-to-day life as a nursing mom. Most women attend a breastfeeding class to help prepare, and don't get me wrong, I absolutely encourage you to take a breastfeeding class while pregnant, but I found the best preparation for me was actually spending time with new moms. Why? Because you see how often babies actually nurse. It's a lot. It's no doubt a full-time job (in the early months, anyways).

It's easy to get overwhelmed, question your supply *("There's no way she could be hungry again. She just ate!"),* and find yourself frustrated by how time consuming it is to nurse a baby. This is why having support during this time is crucial. If and when you run into nursing challenges, you want to have a trusted resource (or several) to turn to. At minimum, you'll want to have a lactation consultant who you can call—ideally, an International Board Certified Lactation Consultant (IBCLC)—and a fellow breastfeeding mom or "peer counselor."

I was personally shocked at how much nuance there is to breastfeeding. Things like nipple pain can have dozens of possible causes and if it's happening, you can't wait—you need help immediately, not a week from now. I was fortunate to have a good lactation consultant on call to help me when I needed it. Simply getting reassurance that your experience is normal or affirmation that something's off and needs troubleshooting is huge. With early breastfeeding, sometimes even one or two nursing sessions with a strange latch can turn what was an OK thing into misery. I can't stress the importance of having a well-trained lactation consultant at the ready if challenges arise. Additionally, the website KellyMom.com is an excellent evidence-based resource, and your local La Leche League may also prove invaluable. Ask around in your community as there may be other resources right at your fingertips.

Nutritional Demands of Breastfeeding

Breastfeeding is also nutritionally demanding. When I was first making notes on what to write about breastfeeding, I jotted down *"Eat lots of food, all the time. Drink lots of water, all the time."* When it comes to nursing, the term *hangry*—the love child of the words hungry and angry—takes on a whole new meaning. If there's one piece of advice to take with you during the early weeks, it's this: "try to remember to eat." If you manage to pull that off, you're already doing an amazing job.

Simply eating and drinking *enough* is crucial to establishing and maintaining your milk supply. Often, this common sense advice is taken to mean that "what you eat doesn't affect your milk" and that's partly true and partly not. I'll start by saying that it's always been taboo to discuss how diet affects the quality of breast milk because there are already so many barriers to breastfeeding. As a breastfeeding mother (at the time of writing), I completely understand this hesitation.

So let me be crystal clear: Women who are unable to eat a nutrient-dense diet *still* make the best food for their baby. It's *still* a superfood, rich in immune-boosting antibodies and easy-to-digest proteins, fats, and carbohydrates. The information in this section is *not* meant to discourage mothers from breastfeeding because their milk "isn't good enough" or imply that breastfeeding moms need to eat "perfectly" to make nutritious breast milk.

Rather, I simply want to encourage new mothers to eat as much nutrient-dense, real food as possible, so you can both replete your nutrient stores after pregnancy *and* produce the most nutritious milk for your ridiculously hungry, rapidly growing baby. This is about self care and nourishment for *both of you*. It's about ensuring that you have the ability to heal from childbirth and handle the stresses of motherhood without burning out, while your baby gets optimal nutrition to develop and thrive.

Why a Nutrient-dense Diet is so Important While Breastfeeding

With that lengthy disclaimer in mind, let's dig into the research for a bit. The whole process of breastfeeding is nothing short of a miracle, designed to help babies survive even if a mother is facing dire nutritional circumstances. This survival mechanism means that certain nutrients are relatively unaffected by maternal diet and nutrient stores. Calories, protein, folate, and most trace minerals are sufficient even in breast milk of undernourished women. However, adequate intake is still important to keep *your* nutrient stores topped up. Take folate, for example. As one researcher describes, "as a consequence of maintaining the level of folate secretion in milk, women with low intakes will become more depleted as lactation progresses."[31]

For other nutrients, maternal diet *does* affect the concentrations in breast milk. This includes vitamins B1, B2, B3, B6 and B12, vitamins A, D and K, choline, fatty acids (such as DHA), and certain trace minerals (such as selenium and iodine).[32,33,34,35] Many of these nutrients are vital to brain development. At the time of birth, a baby's brain is only about 25% developed, and goes on to double in size in the first year of life.[36]

B vitamins

When it comes to B vitamins in the diet, all except folate directly impact milk concentrations. Research that has examined B vitamin content of breast milk and compared it to infant requirements during the first 6 months of life has found that breast milk of nutrient-depleted mothers supplies only 60% of the required thiamine, 53% of riboflavin, 80% of vitamin B6, 16% of vitamin B12, and 56% of choline needs for a young infant. The author comes to the following conclusion: "The overall picture that emerges is consistent across nutrients and points to an urgent need to improve the information available on breast milk quality."[37] Again, this message is rarely discussed outside of academia for fears of discouraging women from breastfeeding.

One B vitamin of particular concern is vitamin B12. Women who consume diets lacking in animal foods are at high risk for vitamin B12 deficiency and for having low B12 levels in their breast milk.[38] Infants that fail to receive enough vitamin B12 often present with "irritability, anorexia, and failure to thrive, marked developmental regression and poor brain growth."[39] Several case reports highlight the problems associated with strict vegan diets (meaning those that exclude all animal products, including meat, fish, eggs, and dairy—and thus all food sources of B12).[40,41,42] "A summary of case studies indicates that symptoms appear around 4-7 months of age and include severe growth stunting (length, weight, and head circumference) and cerebral atrophy [brain shrinkage] and a large number of muscular, behavioral, and other developmental problems, some of which are not reversed by treatment in 40-50% of cases."[43] Yes, not consuming enough vitamin B12 can *cause your baby's brain to shrink*. In all of the above cases, the infants were exclusively breastfed.

In one 9-month-old infant of a vegan mother, "dystrophy, weakness, muscular atrophy, loss of tendon reflexes, psychomotor regression and haematological abnormalities" were observed as well as profound vitamin B12 deficiency.[44] In fact, as early as 6 months of age, this child had lost the ability to even roll over herself. The mother had been vegan for 10 years and both her blood levels and breast milk vitamin B12 concentrations were extremely low. After just 2 days of supplementing the infant with vitamin B12, she regained the ability to roll over and became interested in her environment again, and by 10 days, the infant was showing signs of normal muscular movements. This infant was lucky; as stated above, up to 50% of these cases result in *irreversible* damage to the child.

Though vegan diets pose the greatest risk for B12 deficiency, it's important to note that even lacto-ovo vegetarians (those who abstain from meat and fish, but include eggs and dairy) consistently have lower vitamin B12 levels in their blood.[45] Thus, both vegetarian and vegan women are at risk for vitamin B12 deficiency. To ensure you get enough vitamin B12—and can transfer enough to your breast milk—inclusion of animal foods and/or consistent supplementation is essential.

Choline

Choline needs are at an all-time high during lactation, as this nutrient is indispensable for brain development. The estimated daily need for choline is 550 mg in breastfeeding moms (compared to 450 mg during pregnancy), which is higher than at any other stage of your life. While even this goal is tough to meet for most women, studies have shown that intakes of more than double that amount (930 mg per day) significantly increase choline levels and other beneficial metabolites in breast milk, including glycine.[46] Adequate choline intake during early development "increases memory capacity and precision of the young adult and appears to prevent age-related memory and attentional decline."[47] High demands for choline may explain why eggs, organ meats, and other choline-rich foods are emphasized in many traditional cultures during postpartum healing. Also, many women find that supplementing with lecithin, which is rich in choline, helps prevent clogged ducts.[48] Whether or not that's related to the choline content of lecithin is not known.

Fatty Acids and DHA

Fatty acid levels are also reflected in breast milk. In other words, the quality of fat you eat directly affects the fat composition of your breast milk. This is true for all fats, including omega-3 fats, omega-6 fats, trans fats, saturated fats, and monounsaturated fats.[49,50] Total *quantity* of fat in breast milk is also higher in women who eat more fat, which may explain the anecdotal reports of infants being more content and less colicky when a mom shifts her diet to include sufficient amounts of fat.[51] Since fat is relatively slow to digest, it's possible that babies stay fuller for longer in these cases.

Perhaps of most importance is the brain and vision-boosting omega-3 fat, DHA. Studies have found that the "concentration of DHA in human milk varies more than 10-fold and depends on the mother's dietary DHA intake."[52] Furthermore, infants of mothers with high DHA concentrations in their milk have better neural and visual development.[53] Women who eat a vegan diet have milk concentrations of DHA of only 0.05%, while fish-eating, omnivorous women (eating an average of 4.5 oz of seafood/day) have DHA concentrations of 2.8%.[54] That means it's still very important to consume seafood, grass-fed beef, eggs, and/or your DHA supplement while breastfeeding. As discussed in previous chapters, plant-based omega-3 supplements (aside from algae-based DHA) are not sufficient. For example, researchers have found that supplementing women with flaxseed oil does *not* increase DHA in breast milk.[55]

In addition to boosting DHA levels, consumption of animal fats improves the overall fatty acid profile of breast milk. In women who eat more animal fats, higher levels of beneficial medium chain fats are noted.[56] Medium chain fats are known to rapidly convert to energy (they are "ketogenic") and have a calming effect on the brain. This seems advantageous to young infants, who appear to stay in ketosis during at least the first month of life.[57,58] Some medium chain fats also have antibacterial and immune-boosting properties, which may be important for an infant's developing digestive system.[59] In addition, the quality of animal foods you consume can further enhance your breast milk. In a study out of the Netherlands, women who adhered to an organic diet (>90% of meat and dairy from organic sources) had significantly higher levels of a type of fat called CLA in their milk.[60] This fat has beneficial effects on metabolism, may improve immune function, and may lower the risk of allergies and asthma in infants.[61]

In contrast, a diet that's high in omega-6 fats or trans fats results in higher milk concentrations of these less-desirable fats.[62,63] For trans fats, in particular, researchers note a "highly significant linear relationship" between maternal intake and trans fats levels in the blood of their breastfed infants. Trans fats may have harmful effects on infant development by interfering with essential fatty acid metabolism (such as DHA) and disrupting normal cell membrane structures where they take the place of healthy fats.[64] Studies on rodents have raised concerns that trans fat intake during pregnancy and lactation may have long-term negative effects on insulin signaling and hormonal disruption in offspring.[65,66] In simple terms, it's possible that trans fats may predispose your child to obesity and diabetes later in life. This makes it especially important to avoid processed vegetable oils and any products made with "partially hydrogenated oil" including margarine and shortening. Be aware that bakery products, breads, snacks and fast foods account for nearly 60% of total trans fat intake.[67] If and when you consume these foods, triple check the labels to ensure there are no "partially hydrogenated oils" in the ingredients.

Vitamin A

Like fats, levels of fat-soluble vitamins in breast milk are affected by a mom's diet. Vitamin A is crucial to infant growth, immune system development, and prevention of infections. Perhaps it's by design that the first milk an infant receives, called colostrum, is especially high in vitamin A. In the first 6 months of life, it's estimated that your baby will receive "60 times the amount of vitamin A that they received during the 9 months of pregnancy."[68] Unfortunately, women who don't eat enough vitamin A have low levels in their breast milk.[69] Women who avoid animal fats are at particularly high risk for deficiency, as this serves as the only source of preformed vitamin A outside of supplements (as described in Chapter 3). You want to be careful if you rely heavily on supplements to meet your vitamin A needs, as not all contain the most bioactive form. In one study that compared vitamin A levels in breast milk, women who took a prenatal vitamin that contained only beta-carotene (no preformed vitamin A) had vitamin A-deficient breast milk 40% of the time compared to only 4% in women whose prenatal vitamin contained retinol (preformed vitamin A).[70] These prenatal vitamins contained equal amounts of "vitamin A," just in different forms. Given the importance of vitamin A on infant development, it makes sense that traditional cultures emphasized high-fat animal foods that are rich in this key nutrient. Butter, ghee, lard, tallow, organ meats and fish are all wise additions to your postpartum diet.

Vitamin D

Vitamin D levels also vary widely in breast milk, with lower levels noted in women who do not consume enough vitamin D (from diet or supplements) or do not get regular sun exposure. Since this describes the average woman, breast milk has long been regarded as "vitamin D deficient" and exclusively breastfed infants are recommended a separate vitamin D supplement of 400 IU per day. In fact, "vitamin D deficiency is almost universal among solely breastfed infants not receiving oral vitamin D supplementation."[71] However, recent research has shown that by providing moms with sufficient vitamin D, she will also transfer enough into her breast milk to meet her infant's needs. A very well-designed study tracked the effects of a maternal vitamin D supplement on vitamin D levels in maternal blood, breast milk, and in breastfed infants. Interestingly, vitamin D levels in breast milk are measured as "antirachitic activity" since vitamin D is known to prevent rickets. This study found that women receiving 6,400 IU of vitamin D per day had higher vitamin D levels and passed enough vitamin D into their breast milk to meet the demands of their babies (without the need to directly give the baby a separate infant vitamin D supplement).[72] If you've been supplementing with vitamin D during your pregnancy, continue to do so and check the dosage to ensure you're taking at least 6,400 IU per day.

Iodine

Like the other nutrients already discussed, your intake of iodine predicts milk levels. In geographical areas with a high prevalence of iodine deficiency and goiter (an enlarged thyroid gland), breast milk concentrations of iodine are very low. In addition, iodine levels tend to decline in milk over the first 6 months as a mother becomes more deficient herself (this occurs even in women who supplement with 150 mcg/day).[73] Studies have found insufficient iodine levels in breast milk from women residing in France, Germany, Belgium, Sweden, Spain, Italy, Denmark, Thailand and Zaire.[74] This is important because the "small iodine pool of the neonatal thyroid turns over very rapidly and is highly sensitive to variations in dietary iodine intake."[75] In simpler terms, this means you need a consistent and reliable source of iodine to ensure your baby gets enough. As you may recall from previous chapters, iodine is key for thyroid, brain, and metabolic health. Researchers note that "adequate breast milk iodine levels are particularly important for proper neurodevelopment in nursing infants."[76] Worryingly, some environmental pollutants that interfere with iodine metabolism seem to also preferentially take its place in breast milk and may increase the demand for iodine above current recommended levels.[77] Avoidance of the toxins mentioned in Chapter 10 is equally important to adequate iodine intake.

Regular consumption of seafood, seaweed, eggs, dairy, and a prenatal vitamin that contains iodine (or a separate iodine supplement) are wise choices while nursing. Perhaps this explains the Korean tradition of serving iodine-rich seaweed soup to new mothers.

A Nutrient-dense Diet Means Nutrient-dense Breast Milk

As you can see, your diet *does* affect your breast milk. We know that the nutrients in breast milk can *and do* vary based on what a mom eats and her nutrient stores, but not many people openly talk about it. Of course, not every nutrient is affected, and your body will certainly sacrifice your own nutrient stores whenever possible to make the best milk for your baby. However, to suggest that "diet doesn't matter" during this time is clearly not an evidence-based message.

We need to honor the fact that *your* body needs to be replenished during this time as well. Nutrient stores are already at an all-time low following pregnancy. Now's the time to build them back up. The same foods that will speed along your recovery from childbirth are the ones that enrich your breast milk, so take a moment to review those foods in the preceding pages.

Let me reiterate that this is not about eating "perfectly." I fully recognize that choosing nutrient-dense real food is not always easy, nor is new motherhood. There will be many weeks and months ahead that will challenge you physically and emotionally as a mother, especially with sleep deprivation. There will be times when you have to make food choices simply for convenience and practicality. It's always better to simply *eat* than to go without food or stress about your dinner not being "good enough." This is not about feeling guilty for those days. The key message here is *inclusion* not *exclusion;* Include more nutrient-dense foods in your diet as often as you can. It's your overall diet quality that's most important, not day-to-day variations.

I also want to acknowledge the reality that breastfeeding is a full-time job for the first several months. I had several nicknames for myself during that time, including "Sow Cow" and "Mobile Milk Unit" (which conveniently shortens to MMU or "Mooooo"). We are mammals after all, and I found solace in the fact that most mammals nurse round-the-clock and on-demand, just as I was doing. I had to rely heavily on family members and friends to keep me well-fed during this time. Remember, new mothers need to be "mothered" as well.

It's a humbling experience to be the sole source of food for an infant (for the first 6 months, anyways). Life, by necessity, slows down. A lot. I remember looking at my son at a few months postpartum and just marveling at the fact that this little guy was growing entirely from my milk. Yes, my body grew him during pregnancy, but until you introduce solid foods, that baby is entirely relying on *you*. It's both amazing and daunting to think about. My point in sharing this is to be gentle with yourself. Yes, your nutrient intake influences your breast milk, but just the fact that you're breastfeeding in the first place (for any duration—whether that's a few weeks of a few years) is an irreplaceable gift to your baby.

Supplements

As you know, I take a "food first" approach to nutrition and encourage you to get the majority of your nutrients from food. That said, we're all human and there are days where you may fall short, especially given the high nutrient needs for postpartum replenishment and breastfeeding. In addition, some nutrients are more reliably obtained from supplements, like vitamin D. Below are some supplements to consider taking.

Prenatal Vitamin

As previously mentioned, nutrient needs go up following pregnancy, particularly for nursing moms. This explains why most health professionals encourage you to continue taking your prenatal vitamin for the duration of breastfeeding. Even in moms who choose not to breastfeed, it's wise to continue your prenatal for at least 6 months postpartum to replenish nutrient stores. If you're almost out of your prenatal vitamin, consider choosing one of the comprehensive formulas that I recommend. Get the list at **www.realfoodforpregnancy.com/pnv/**.

DHA

The omega-3 fat, DHA, continues to be important postpartum. For nursing mothers, a DHA supplement ensures your milk contains enough. But even for women who are not nursing, replenishing DHA that was preferentially transferred to the baby during pregnancy is key. Data from animal studies shows that brain levels of DHA decline by 18% after a single "reproductive cycle" and this same phenomenon is believed to happen in humans.[78] In other words, pregnancy depletes your brain of DHA. Since low levels of DHA have been linked to reduced cognitive function, depression, and greater susceptibility to stress—and since we know that pregnancy and breastfeeding increase demands for this special fat—it's crucial to consume enough DHA during *and after* pregnancy. If you want to keep "mom brain" at bay and nutritionally protect against postpartum depression, keep taking your DHA supplement.

Vitamin D

For nursing mothers, vitamin D needs are increased during this time compared to during pregnancy in order to provide sufficient vitamin D in breast milk (as detailed in the previous section). Since the majority of women either do not get regular sun exposure without sunscreen in midday hours, or live at a latitude where it's not even possible to make vitamin D from the sun year round, a supplement is a wise choice. If you are breastfeeding, a minimum of 6,400 IU per day is recommended. Even non-breastfeeding mothers should continue to take a vitamin D supplement at similar levels. Researchers suggest that the RDA for vitamin D should be somewhere near 7,000 to 8,000 IU per day, but your dosage can be fine-tuned by having your blood levels of 25-hydroxy vitamin D measured by your doctor.[79,80] Although your prenatal vitamin contains some vitamin D, most contain far too little, which makes a separate supplement necessary. When choosing vitamin D supplements, opt for vitamin D3, which is also called cholecalciferol, in lieu of the less-potent vitamin D2.[81]

Iodine

Compared to all other age groups, iodine needs are highest among postpartum and breastfeeding women. Aside from the benefits of iodine supplements on iodine levels in breast milk (discussed in the above section), iodine is also crucial for *your* well-being. Adequate iodine intake now could help prevent postpartum thyroid dysfunction, which is shockingly common. If you tested positive for thyroid antibodies during pregnancy, your chances of having postpartum thyroid issues are upwards of 50%.[82] This is important since a properly functioning thyroid gland ensures you have enough energy, are able to manage the inevitable stresses of new motherhood, can lose the baby weight, and preserve your fertility, should you choose to have another baby. Iodine is also specifically beneficial for breast health, and some reports show that the breast is even more effective at taking up and storing iodine than the thyroid gland.[83] Since most prenatal vitamins either fail to include iodine or don't include enough, you may need to take a separate iodine supplement. Check your prenatal vitamin first. If it doesn't include at least 290 mcg/day—or you don't regularly consume seaweed and seafood—you may want to take a separate iodine supplement.

Probiotics

Inclusion of probiotics, whether from supplements or from regular consumption of fermented foods, is just as helpful postpartum as it was during pregnancy. This is particularly important if you received antibiotics during/after labor or had a C-section. Use of antibiotics is well known to disrupt normal gut flora and increase the likelihood of yeast overgrowth, which could manifest as problems for yourself or your infant. The last thing you want to deal with while healing from birth is a vaginal yeast infection, chronic diarrhea, or oral thrush in your infant. It's now widely recognized that your baby's microbiome, which governs everything from immune and digestive health to lifetime risk of obesity, are affected by the way you birth and how your baby is fed. Breast milk naturally contains beneficial bacteria (including lactobacilli and bifidobacteria), but their levels are lower in women who have received antibiotics in pregnancy or while breastfeeding.[84]

Even if you did not receive antibiotics, probiotics may serve as somewhat of an insurance policy. In one study, women given probiotic supplements (*Lactobacillus rhamnosus* at 20 billion CFU per day) during the last 4 weeks of pregnancy and throughout lactation produced breast milk with fully double the levels of immunoprotective compounds. Plus, the rates of eczema in their infants during the first 2 years of life showed a clear benefit of probiotic supplementation: only 15% in the probiotic-supplemented group had eczema, compared to 47% in the group that did not receive probiotics.[85] A separate study found that a high-dose, multi-strain probiotic (900 billion CFU per day; that's quite high!) given during the last 4 weeks of pregnancy and continued while nursing was protective against infant colic, regurgitation (spitting up), and overall digestive discomfort.[86] Also, the mothers in this study had lower levels of inflammatory biomarkers in their breast milk, which may have other long-term benefits to their infants. For tips on choosing a probiotic supplement and information on probiotic-rich foods, see Chapter 6.

Gelatin or Collagen

The role of gelatin and collagen in healing connective tissue and skin explain why foods such as "pig trotters soup" are encouraged for women healing from childbirth in China. A separate supplement of either gelatin or collagen protein may be helpful if you don't happen to enjoy or regularly consume things like bone broth, slow-cooked meat/stews, chicken skin or pork rinds. Even if you *do,* a little extra nutritional support can't hurt to encourage your belly skin to regain elasticity, to speed healing of your perineal tissues, and to help your uterus to return to its former size. I made a habit of adding a tablespoon of collagen powder to almost every cup of herbal tea I drank postpartum to ensure I consumed enough. I also kept Tart Cherry Gummies on hand for a quick and nutritious snack (see Recipe Appendix).

Other Supplements

The above list is by no means comprehensive. Depending on the circumstances of your birth and health history, there may be numerous other supplements to consider taking. I recommend seeking the advice of your healthcare practitioner if you want a more individualized supplement plan.

For example, if you lost a lot of blood during childbirth or were already anemic during pregnancy, you may consider an additional iron supplement, spirulina, and/or dessicated liver (in addition to eating plenty of iron-rich foods). If you have a perineal tear or surgical wound to heal, having extra vitamin C, zinc, and vitamin A (along with collagen/gelatin) may help speed healing. If you're feeling sore, bruised, or swollen, the homeopathic remedy, *Arnica montana,* is extremely helpful for reducing inflammation. If you have postpartum constipation, which is very common in the first week or two, additional magnesium, a stool softener, or even short term use of herbal laxatives may be helpful. (I'm usually opposed to herbal laxatives, but the first few bowel movements postpartum can be scary to pass because the same tissues that just stretched—or maybe tore—during birth need to stretch again. Having softer bowel movements makes it far easier to pass.)

Some women choose to consume their placenta, as it's a rich source of nutrients (in a lot of ways, it's similar to liver) and advocates say it helps ease the hormonal shifts that occur after pregnancy, may improve postpartum mood, and may boost milk supply. That's a personal decision, and although conventional medicine finds it rather controversial to do so, it's common practice among other mammals. Overall, there are few studies on "placentophagy," and often women make the choice based on personal anecdotes from other moms who found it beneficial. However, there is one small, well-designed study worth mentioning. This was a randomized, double blind, placebo controlled trial in which 27 women were given a supplement containing either their dehydrated placenta or a similarly prepared placebo (dehydrated beef) with the goal of determining whether placenta capsules improved postpartum mood and recovery.[87] Placenta samples were also evaluated for nutrient content. Overall, the women receiving the placenta supplement "experienced a postpartum decrease in depressive symptoms and fatigue that was not experienced by those taking the placebo supplement." Nutritional analysis of the placenta capsules showed "modest concentrations of some micronutrients and hormones." One analysis showed that placenta capsules could provide 24% of a woman's daily iron needs (when taken in a dosage of 3,200 mg of dehydrated placenta per day).[88] If you choose to consume your placenta, ensure that it's handled and prepared hygienically, as there have been case reports of some becoming contaminated with harmful bacteria.

Other supplements commonly used during postpartum recovery are herbal remedies, especially lactation blends, designed to boost milk supply. In general, these "galactogogues" are well-tolerated, though I want to remind you that no herb is a replacement to a nutritious diet. In other words, consuming adequate calories and enough fluids is most important when it comes to maintaining your milk supply; herbal galactogogues are secondary. Common galactogogues include chamomile, fennel, nettle, fenugreek, goat's rue, blessed thistle, milky oats, and many others.[89] In addition to boosting milk supply, chamomile may improve sleep quality and help reduce postpartum depression.[90,91] Lecithin is also commonly taken by nursing mothers to prevent or treat clogged ducts. Since it's a naturally rich source of choline with no clear contraindications, it's not a bad choice to add to your supplement regimen or to have on hand just in case. I recommend sunflower lecithin, which is sourced from sunflower seeds instead of soy.

Beyond galactogogues, many cultures emphasize the use of herbs that help with hormone balance, adrenal health, and mental health. For example, adaptogenic herbs are extremely helpful during the postpartum phase and are generally considered safe while breastfeeding. As the name suggests, adaptogens help your body adapt to the physical, mental, and emotional demands of motherhood. *Rhodiola rosea* is one of the most commonly used adaptogens, though every culture has their own adaptogens unique to their climate and herbal traditions (this includes, but is not limited to, ashwagandha, holy basil, reishi, maca, and eleuthero).

When it comes to postpartum mood, St. John's wort is commonly used. A case study of a breastfeeding woman taking St. John's wort found that extremely low levels transfer into breast milk and no adverse effects were noted on her infant, however the authors cautioned that long-term studies are lacking.[92]

As the above study highlights, some herbal compounds can pass into breast milk, so it's wise to consult an herbalist if you're unsure. Though many herbs can increase milk supply, some can have the opposite effect. Sage and mint, when taken in sufficient quantities, can lower milk supply. Unfortunately, like the research into herbs in pregnancy, studies are lacking on the use of herbs in breastfeeding women, so I'm not able to offer much evidence-based information here. I suggest you defer to a well-trained herbalist, midwife, or healthcare practitioner for personalized guidance.

Lab Testing

With advances in functional medicine, there are seemingly endless lab tests that you can order these days. For the purposes of this section, I want to focus on just a few labs you can easily order through any doctor or midwife to assess some basic parameters. Most healthcare providers schedule a follow-up appointment at 6 weeks postpartum, which is an ideal time to request several lab tests (often, these are not routine practice).

Vitamin D

As discussed previously, vitamin D is essential to numerous systems in your body. Deficiency is extremely common in pregnant and postpartum women. For example, fully 69% of American women, 65% of Canadian women, 77% of German women, 91% of Chinese women, 96% of Indian women, and 67% of Iranian women have inadequate vitamin D levels.[93] Aside from aforementioned effects on the breastfeeding infant, some research has found a relationship between low vitamin D and postpartum depression.[94] Getting your vitamin D levels assessed allows you to fine-tune your supplement dosage. The test to ask for is "25 hydroxy-vitamin D." Most labs suggest that normal vitamin D levels are at least 30 ng/ml, but numerous vitamin D experts suggest *optimal* levels are 50 ng/ml or more.[95] When interpreting your lab results, be aware that vitamin D levels can be given in different units, typically either ng/ml or nmol/l. Check your lab printout to make sure you're interpreting it correctly (30 ng/ml is equivalent to 75 nmol/l and 50 ng/ml is equivalent to 125 nmol/l).

Iron/Anemia

Following pregnancy, anemia and iron deficiency are fairly common. Iron transfer to the baby in utero coupled with blood loss during/after birth reduce maternal iron stores. Since iron helps carry oxygen in your blood to fuel every cell in your body, it's no coincidence that low iron levels tend to result in fatigue. Many women can avoid anemia by consuming plenty of iron-rich foods, however if you're experiencing any of the following common symptoms, it's wise to get it checked out: fatigue, loss of color in your skin (especially the face), shortness of breath, feeling faint or lightheaded, dizziness, and fast heartbeat. At minimum, ask for hemoglobin, hematocrit, and serum ferritin levels. Discussion of the best-tolerated and best-absorbed forms of iron, as well as food sources, can be found in Chapter 6.

Thyroid

As your body readjusts after birth, hormone levels can take some time to find their equilibrium. Often, the focus is just on female hormones, but your thyroid gland—and all of its hormones—must also find a new normal. Sometimes this process is relatively uneventful, and other times, thyroid problems develop. Thyroid abnormalities that appear within a year of giving birth, collectively known as "postpartum thyroiditis," are surprisingly common. In fact, "up to 23% of all new mothers experiences thyroid dysfunction postpartum, compared with a prevalence of 3-4% in the general population."[96] That's almost a *quarter* of new moms!

If you had abnormal thyroid labs during or before pregnancy, you'll want to be on high alert. Researchers note that the "vast majority of women who develop postpartum thyroiditis are thyroid antibody positive prior to pregnancy."[97] In other words, these women already had signs of autoimmune thyroid disease before having a baby, and the stresses incurred on the thyroid during and after pregnancy triggered full-blown thyroid disease. It's estimated that 10-17% of women have thyroid autoimmune disease during pregnancy (meaning they are positive for thyroid antibodies but have otherwise normal thyroid hormone levels).[98] In these women, fully *one third* will develop postpartum thyroid problems within the first year after delivery.[99]

Having a properly functioning thyroid is important for maintaining your energy levels (obviously necessary when trying to keep up with a baby or toddler), supporting your fertility (if you want another child, this is crucial), promoting normal postpartum weight loss, and for your mental health. Postpartum thyroid dysfunction is a known risk factor for postpartum depression.[100] Simply put, your thyroid function is a quality of life issue.

Common signs of postpartum thyroiditis include:

- Anxiety, irritability, or depression
- Rapid heartbeat or palpitations
- Difficulty losing weight (hypothyroidism) or unexplained weight loss (hyperthyroidism)
- Increased sensitivity to heat/cold
- Fatigue
- Tremor
- Insomnia
- Constipation
- Dry skin
- Difficulty concentrating

A surprisingly small percentage of clinicians run thyroid labs at postpartum check ups, and when they do, it's often not a full panel; reasons for this lack in screening are beyond my comprehension. Ask your doctor to run a full thyroid panel, including thyroid antibodies, at your postpartum check up(s). A full panel may include:

- Thyroid Stimulating Hormone (TSH)
- Free T4
- Free T3
- Reverse T3
- Thyroid antibodies: Thyroid Peroxidase Antibodies (TPOAb) and Thyroglobulin Antibodies (TgAb)

Be aware that postpartum thyroiditis can appear in a "triphasic" pattern in which, depending on the timeframe, your lab tests may show hypothyroid, hyperthyroid, or a normally functioning thyroid.[101] If your lab tests show that everything is fine, but you're still not feeling quite like yourself, it's worth it to get retested in another month or two to reassess. Treatment for thyroid disease would depend on your lab values and symptoms, but may include nutritional support and/or medication (replacement thyroid hormone). Refer back to Chapter 9 for a deeper discussion of thyroid testing and nutritional support for the thyroid. Many nutrients are involved in thyroid function, but one thing to note is that women with postpartum autoimmune thyroid conditions are often vitamin D deficient, and supplementing with vitamin D has been shown to improve thyroid function.[102]

Additional Lab Tests

If you had any preexisting health conditions or newly developed ones during pregnancy (such as high blood pressure or high blood sugar), ask your provider about any relevant postpartum tests. For example, women with gestational diabetes are at a lifetime higher risk for prediabetes or type 2 diabetes, so postpartum blood sugar screening is recommended at your postpartum check up (typically 6-12 weeks). In an ideal world, a full panel on micronutrient status would be fantastic and could help guide targeted supplementation (or focus your food choices), however this is something you'd likely need to order through a healthcare practitioner who practices functional medicine/nutrition.

Exercise & Physical Recovery

After months of carrying around extra weight and being physically hindered by a big belly, many women are eager to get back to their usual exercise routine. Your motivation may be to lose the baby weight, tone your muscles, or simply to "feel like yourself" again. Whatever the reason, and they are all valid, I urge you to approach exercise with a bit of caution. The physiological changes that your body goes through during pregnancy and birth are significant and your connective tissue, abdominal muscles, and pelvic floor require time to heal—probably more time than you think. Jumping into a high intensity "get your body back" bootcamp, going running, or lifting heavy weights just weeks after giving birth is usually not a good idea.

At minimum, most exercise physiologists recommend a 6-week rest period after birth before resuming exercise beyond walking and strategic rehabilitative exercises (such as gentle pelvic floor or abdominal activation).[103] In other words, less is more in the early postpartum phase. Ignoring this crucial healing period can contribute to injury, pelvic organ prolapse, worsening abdominal separation (diastasis recti) and incontinence.

Take it Slow

Some research has found that it takes a full year for your pelvic floor to return to normal function following birth.[104] Engaging in high impact activity that puts excessive pressure on your pelvic floor too soon in your recovery is a recipe for incontinence or prolapse. Incontinence is when you unintentionally leak urine or poop. Prolapse, or more specifically pelvic organ prolapse, is when one or more of your pelvic organs descend downwards and may even protrude out of the vaginal canal. Pressure, dragging, or fullness in the pelvic region, sensations of bulging, or the feeling of "sitting on a ball" are common symptoms of prolapse.

Any of the above symptoms—or worsening of them—experienced within a few days of exercise is a signal that your body is not ready for that type of exercise, at that intensity, and at that duration yet. Your pelvic floor needs a bit of "babying" to regain normal strength and function. Remember, for those of you who had a vaginal birth, those muscles had to stretch to 2-3 times their normal length; they don't go back to normal immediately. Your ligaments, which suspend your pelvic organs and were stretched by your uterus, also do not immediately return to normal length; this is true for all mothers, whether you delivered vaginally or by C-section. That means these muscles and ligaments cannot handle the same pressure and load in the early months postpartum that you may have been accustomed to pre-baby.

Similarly, your abdominal muscles have also been stretched and weakened during pregnancy. The majority of women experience diastasis recti as a normal part of pregnancy, which is when you have a vertical separation of your abdominal muscles (specifically your rectus abdominus). For some, this heals on its own, but many women benefit from rehabilitative exercises to help "close the gap" and (re)learn to properly brace their abdominal muscles again. Some women choose to wear an abdominal binder for a bit to help provide additional stability and support for their torso in the early weeks. In Mexico and some parts of Asia, abdominal binding is a routine postpartum practice.[105]

In general, it's wise to avoid abdominal exercises that involve crunch-like movements, such as sit ups, or those that put too much pressure on the abdominal wall, such as full planks, for a period of time. You need to build up strength *before* you go back to these exercises. Even rolling to the side when getting out of bed, rather than sitting straight up, is helpful in the early weeks, as this reduces strain on the abdominal muscles and pelvic floor. If you had a C-section, your body has the additional task of healing all the layers of abdominal tissue that were compromised from surgery—and that takes time.

As Marika Hart, a physiotherapist who specializes in prenatal and postpartum exercise says, "You want to find your Goldilocks level of exercise." She suggests that postpartum women approach exercise in a similar manner as if they were recovering from surgery (and if you had a C-section, you *are!*). That means starting with gentle exercises and very gradually progressing to more challenging exercises on *your own timeline* based on how well you're recovering.

Seek Professional Help

Monitoring your recovery, learning to reactivate your abdominal and pelvic floor muscles, and deciding which exercises are safe to try (and when) is surprisingly nuanced. Although your 6 week postpartum visit with your doctor or midwife is typically when you are cleared to resume exercise, it's important to realize that you are not having a pelvic floor assessment in terms of muscle function. That is simply not their specialty; that's what a women's health physical therapist does (also called a pelvic floor specialist or women's physiotherapist, depending on where you reside).

On that note, I highly recommend you seek the professional opinion of a women's health physical therapist *before* you resume your usual exercise routine. Even if you're not sure you need one, meaning you think you feel "fine" down there or don't think you have abdominal separation, ask for a referral at your postpartum check up anyways. It's good to at least have the option available to you. Simply having the reassurance that everything is A-ok is good for your peace of mind. Being careful and proactive during these early months, by allowing your body to heal on its own timeline, can prevent problems decades from now.

Symptoms of prolapse may not show up for some time after birth. Across the globe, up to *half* of all mothers have some degree of pelvic organ prolapse and it's estimated that up to 20% of those women will opt for surgery by the time they are 80.[106,107] Those statistics are so high that it's anyone's guess why prolapse is not more openly discussed.

As mentioned in Chapter 8, some countries include pelvic floor physical therapy as part of all women's recoveries, whether or not they complain of pain or dysfunction. They understand that the musculoskeletal strain of birth, and even pregnancy itself, necessitates a period of rest, recovery, and specific rehabilitative exercises. Unfortunately, this is not the case in the United States.

Pain with sex, incontinence, prolapse or feelings of abdominal weakness or separation are all clear signs that you should get an assessment by a women's health physical therapist. Plus, learning (or re-learning) how to properly engage your pelvic floor and abdominal muscles is not something everyone can easily do on their own. About 25% of women perform pelvic floor exercises, such as kegels, incorrectly even if they've been instructed on how to do them properly.[108] Working with a specially trained physical therapist ensures that you get it right. Studies have shown up to 70% improvement in symptoms of stress incontinence (where you accidentally pee when you sneeze, cough or laugh) in women who practice pelvic floor exercises under the direction of a physical therapist that specializes in pelvic floor health.[109]

Though it may be tempting to simply do a lot of kegel exercises, in which you lift and squeeze your pelvic floor muscles, know that this is not always enough, nor is it even advisable. Proper pelvic floor function is a balance between learning to contract and relax those muscles. It is also dependent on the alignment of the rest of your body (i.e. your posture). For example, if you sit or stand with your tailbone tucked under, your pelvic floor muscles tend to shorten and weaken over time. Or, if you constantly tighten your pelvic floor muscles without ever allowing them to relax to normal length (like doing hundreds of kegels a day), those muscles are actually less able to yield and support the load of your body, especially under force. This can result in pelvic pain, spasms, prolapse, or incontinence. Think about it for a moment. If you're training your biceps to be strong, you both bend and extend your elbow. You don't keep it bent all day long.

This is why most physical therapists incorporate full body functional movements to strengthen the pelvic floor after initial therapy. Exercises that involve squats, glute activation (your butt muscles) and balance/stabilization tend to promote involuntary contraction of your pelvic floor. Ultimately, that's the goal—that you don't have to think about activating your pelvic floor muscles, but that they engage when they need to (like when you sneeze or lift something heavy) and they relax when you don't need them (like when you're sitting on the couch or laying down). Keep it mind that it may take many months to get to that point, though.

Reality Check

For me, as a former Pilates Instructor who was active throughout my pregnancy and experienced with postpartum rehab, the early postpartum healing phase was a humbling time. I knew I would need time to heal, but I assumed that I would somehow be spared from diastasis recti and that my pelvic floor muscles would bounce back ahead of the usual timeline. I fell victim to the idea that everything would go back to normal quickly after having a baby. After the initial healing of my perineum and my postpartum bleeding had ceased, I felt pretty good and figured I would be able to do most of the things I had done before pregnancy. I had already been walking and felt fine. When I went out on a moderately intense hike at about two months postpartum, I begrudgingly had to turn around only a mile in because of discomfort in my pelvic floor. I had to back off from the hiking and do shorter, gentler hikes for another month or two before I was ready for that. At the time, it was crushing because all I wanted to do was get out and hike a mountain after so many weeks stuck inside nursing all day!

I was also disappointed that I had abdominal separation, despite doing "all the right things" during pregnancy (I hadn't realized how common it is). I went to see a women's health physical therapist, and after a full assessment, she reassured me that everything was healing up just fine, but that it would likely take a year for my pelvic floor and abdominal muscles to fully heal. Yes, a *full year*. So, even though my pelvic floor was healing fine, I didn't have incontinence, my abdominal gap was closing up, and I was doing all the right rehabilitation exercises, I still wasn't back to "normal" for a while. Looking back, the physical therapist was spot on. By about 10 months postpartum, I could do most of the same exercises that I was doing pre-pregnancy, but still … that took *10 months*. I believe I was able to avoid incontinence, prolapse, and a worsening abdominal gap because I listened to my body and slowed down.

Instead of going to a bootcamp style class, I went on gentle hikes and walks at my own pace (while babywearing or while my husband carried our son). Instead of doing high intensity workouts, I did modified Pilates and yoga exercises on the floor while my infant napped or did tummy time. Instead of lifting heavy weights, I relied on carrying my son as my "weight lifting." I also noticed that carrying my baby in my arms, as opposed to always babywearing, took a lot of pressure off my pelvic floor and back—and as a bonus, I got super strong arms.

Your postpartum healing may take a different path. You may feel ready for more intense exercise earlier than I did, or you may need to take it easy for a lot longer. It's hard to know how quickly your muscles and connective tissues will "bounce back," but it's helpful to assume that you'll need close to a year. If you take just one thing from this discussion, remember this: it is crucial to stay mindful of how your body feels during and after exercise. If things get worse, it's a clear sign your body is not ready for that activity *yet*. Don't take it personally or think you've done anything wrong. Simply give your body more time to heal and try it again in a few weeks or months down the road.

Weight Loss & Loving Your Body

In addition to the pressure a lot of women face in getting back into an exercise routine soon after baby is born, many also feel like they need to lose the "baby weight" quickly. Remember though, it took 9 months to grow a baby and for your body to make all the necessary accommodations. Why would we expect the weight to "fall off" quickly? Now, there are some women who *do* lose the weight rather quickly, don't get me wrong, but many find it takes longer than they expected. There's a huge variation in the rate of weight loss postpartum. The mantra "9 months on, 9 months off" is a good one to repeat if you're feeling frustrated.

Immediately following birth, most women lose 10 or more pounds simply from the weight of the baby, loss of amniotic fluid, and the uterus shrinking down. The remaining weight that you gained during pregnancy may come off gradually or quickly depending on a lot of factors, like how much weight you gained in total during your pregnancy and whether or not you're breastfeeding. Keep in mind that not every aspect of weight loss is within your direct control. Hormonal changes, a ravenous appetite spurred by breastfeeding, less physical activity, disrupted sleep, thyroid or adrenal problems, lack of time to cook, and postpartum mood changes are all potential contributors.

Even for women who lose the weight relatively quickly, the shape and function of their bodies can take a long time to recover. You may have stretch marks, your belly button may look different, you might have loose skin, your breasts will have changed, and your joints may feel different. Some of these will evolve and change over time. Some may be here to stay. I think one area that's particularly ignored is the fact that we, as women, need time to mourn the loss of our old selves—of our old bodies. We may have spent two or

Real Food for Pregnancy

three or more decades without kids and suddenly after having a baby, everything is different.

A 1985 research paper on pregnancy and postpartum body image sums it up well:

> *"The idealized female body is valued in our society. However, the changes that occur to the body due to pregnancy reflect that the woman is perhaps further from the ideal body than she ever has been. After delivery, the woman's body still appears pregnant. This is a very dissatisfying experience for many women. This dissatisfaction with the body has been identified as one of the factors which contribute to the critical nature of the postpartum period."*[10]

Though a lot has changed since the '80s, these words are just as relevant today as they were decades ago. Recognizing that your feelings are normal and giving yourself space to experience them is part of getting to a place of love and acceptance. Start by finding a few things about your body that are amazing and that you can appreciate. The fact that your body was able to create a new life from scratch is pretty miraculous, isn't it?!

In terms of weight loss, I encourage you to focus on internal healing for the first 3-6 months before you even entertain the idea of actively trying to lose weight. This is especially important for breastfeeding moms, since you want to remain well-nourished to maintain your milk supply and to provide the most nutrient-dense milk possible. Remember: restricting your food intake also restricts your *nutrient* intake.

If you *do* choose to actively pursue weight loss, focus first on your food. Rather than restrict total calories, take a close look at the *quality* of foods in your diet. For many women, the craziness of new motherhood means more take-out or fast food, more snacks, and more desserts. Quick pick-me-ups, like sweetened caffeinated drinks, might be sneaking in more than you realize. Bringing in healthier items to naturally displace the less healthy ones is a good start—and it may be all that's needed. Swapping out processed snacks for more satiating, nutrient-dense options, such as nuts or beef jerky, might help. In addition, ensuring you get a protein-rich breakfast can help regulate your appetite and blood sugar throughout the day, ultimately leading to less cravings for sweets. Although cutting back on carbs often helps with weight loss, breastfeeding moms may need to take a few precautions. Be sure to read the section titled "A Note About Carbohydrates" earlier in this chapter for more on this topic.

Another area to consider is mindful eating. It's easy to slip into overeating— or *mindless* eating—in the early months "just in case" you get stuck on the couch nursing a sleepy baby for 3 hours. This is not necessarily a bad thing when your baby is very young; breastfeeding uses up a lot of energy. However, once your baby is older, your body will expend less energy to make breast milk and you will have more frequent and longer breaks between tending to your baby. You may not necessarily *need* to eat as much or as frequently at 9 months postpartum as you did at 1 month postpartum (or maybe you will; we're all different). Bring awareness back to your hunger and fullness cues during this time to help cut down on mindless eating.

It may sound too good to be true, but mindful eating has been shown to be a more effective—and "less arduous"—way to lose weight postpartum when compared to programs that require you to strictly weigh, measure, and record every morsel of food you eat.[111] Mindful eating is more realistic and more sustainable in the long run, so whenever you're ready, revisit Chapter 2 for a refresher. Whatever strategy you take, it's wise to aim for no more than 1-2 pounds of weight loss per week.

Mental & Emotional Health

It's unclear to me why there's so much stigma around experiencing and expressing true postpartum emotions. New mommyhood is not all sunshine and rainbows, yet so many depictions of this time are all cutesy photos of sleepy newborns (probably thanks to social media). I think if we still lived in proverbial villages and spent quality time with new moms (not just 1-3 hour visits midday, but saw a full 24-hour picture), we'd have more realistic expectations of this time. We'd see the 4th trimester firsthand and understand that young infants are constantly attached to mama (or want to be). We'd see that most infants don't sleep through the night consistently for a long, long time. We'd see that breastfeeding is a full-time job. We'd see that full recovery from birth can take quite a while. We'd see that caring for a baby is amazing and exhausting and emotional all at the same time. Plus, we'd have a heck of a lot more help available to handle the day-to-day challenges of motherhood.

Taking care of your emotional well-being during this time is hard, and yet so important. It's normal to go through highs and lows, called "baby blues," especially in the early months. The huge hormonal shifts that happen along with sleep deprivation can make you feel a little "all over the place" for a while. You may have tears of joy one minute as you gaze into your newborn's eyes, followed by tears of frustration and exhaustion just hours later. Rest assured that this is a normal part of adjusting to motherhood.

That said, persistent feelings of depression or anxiety that interfere with your daily life or make it challenging to take care of your baby absolutely warrant your attention. It's estimated that 30% of women experience some degree of postpartum depression (PPD) in the year following birth.[112] This figure is likely an underestimate, given that many women feel uncomfortable expressing their feelings or may subconsciously worry about the stigma attached to PPD. If you think that's you, don't hesitate to seek help.

Leave all avenues open to explore—from nutrition, time for self care, simplifying your schedule or lifestyle, formal therapy, to pharmaceuticals. See Chapter 11 for specific recommendations, including how to find a specialist in maternal mental health. If you had a traumatic birth, getting counseling or therapy for PTSD is especially helpful.

Some research suggests that "depletion of nutrient reserves throughout pregnancy and a lack of recovery postpartum may increase a woman's risk for maternal depression."[113] Choline, vitamin B12, iron, vitamin D and DHA are of utmost importance during this time for your mental health and for all the reasons discussed elsewhere in this chapter. As one research paper notes, "During the last three months of pregnancy, the fetus accumulates an average of 67 mg/day of DHA through the placenta, and then through breast milk— a situation that would favor depletion and the risk of postpartum depression."[114] Also, thyroid problems have been linked to postpartum depression, so if you have not had your thyroid checked, now's the time to talk with your provider about lab tests.[115]

One of the biggest complaints I hear from new moms is the lack of time for self care. When all attention is on baby, sometimes you can barely sneak away for a few minutes to even shower before you hear that little cry to be picked up or fed or changed. It takes a little creativity to fit in the usual things that keep you mentally grounded, whether that's a warm bath, a walk outside, meditation, or something else altogether. I found that aside from having someone to hand the baby to for a bit (admittedly, the only way I was able to take a decent shower for months), listening to mindfulness meditations while I nursed or went on a walk (while babywearing) was one way to take time for *me* and to process my emotions. What's one way that you can sneak a little more self care into your week?

Another commonly overlooked factor in postpartum mental health is the fact that motherhood can be isolating. Maybe it's hard to leave the house because your baby hates the car seat. Perhaps going out to dinner, something you used to love doing with your partner, feels impossible now. Maybe you don't have family nearby, or friends who have kids, that can relate to what you're going through. I experienced all of the above. The most helpful thing for me was to find other moms who I could talk to and vent my emotions. Online forums of moms with common interests is a good start. Or, if it's possible, finding an in-person group can help. Your local library, YMCA, pediatrician's office, or community center may offer specific meetups for moms. You might look up a mama-baby yoga class or stroller walking club. Some women find their mom friends through prenatal classes and manage to stay connected after they've had their babies. It may take some time and effort find mom friends, but it goes a long way in normalizing the ups—and especially the downs—of motherhood. It's helpful to have the reassurance that this is a season of life, and gradually, month by month, you'll feel more like yourself again.

Pregnancy Spacing

I hesitated to include information on pregnancy spacing in this book. Why would a dietitian give you advice on family planning? But then I thought, given the nutritional toll that pregnancy and breastfeeding puts on your body, how could I *not* cover this topic? Since many women are delaying children until later in life, having closely spaced children is often the only way to have a larger family. Pregnancy spacing is not widely discussed, yet it's a decision that every mother who wants more than one child will face at some point. Plus, there are a number of studies that have examined health outcomes of mothers and their children based on how much time has elapsed between pregnancies. In other words, this is not just a personal decision, but one that can affect your health and the health of your children.

For decades, doctors have observed that women who get pregnant soon after giving birth (termed "short interpregnancy interval") are more likely to have complications during pregnancy, such as intrauterine growth restriction, preterm birth, or having a child with neural tube defects, developmental delay, cerebral palsy, or autism.[116,117] In addition, maternal death, third-trimester bleeding, and anemia or more common among these women.[118]

Why might this be? No one knows for sure, but in a review of 58 studies on this topic, researchers found evidence that factors such as maternal nutritional depletion (especially folate), cervical insufficiency, incomplete healing of the uterine scar from previous cesarean delivery, transmission of infections, short duration of lactation related to breastfeeding-pregnancy overlap, and abnormal healing of endometrial blood vessels may play a role.[119] In short, pregnancy is demanding on your body and you need time to heal and rebuild nutrient stores—a challenge when your time/energy/motivation to eat well is more limited as a mother.

So, how long should you wait to get pregnant again so you can optimize your chances of an easy pregnancy and a healthy baby? And what constitutes a short interpregnancy interval?

The latest research supports pregnancy spacing of at least 18 months, meaning waiting until your infant is 18 months old to conceive your next child.[120] Not everyone wants to wait that long to get pregnant again, especially older mothers or those who want a large family. If 18 months is out of the question for you for any reason, researchers note that even waiting 12 months postpartum to get pregnant again is associated with fewer adverse outcomes, especially lower chances of developmental delays and autism in the child.[121] Another analysis found that waiting 15 months to conceive was associated with the lowest rates of fetal loss.[122] This is important to consider if you have a history of miscarriage.

Interestingly, traditional cultures encouraged pregnancy spacing. As Dr. Weston Price notes in *Nutrition and Physical Degeneration,* intentionally spacing children a minimum of 2.5 to 3 years apart was commonplace among many indigenous people. This included the Ibos of Nigeria, Indians of Peru and the Northwest Amazon, and natives of the Soloman Islands.[123] The rationale was that this time period allowed a mother to "recuperate her strength completely" and be in "thoroughly fit condition to bear another child." It was also believed to ensure the health and survival of the next child. Coincidentally, this spacing is right in line with the optimal interpregnancy intervals documented in the modern scientific literature.

If your circumstances allow, I highly encourage you to wait until your baby is around 18 months before trying to conceive again. The honest truth is that most people aren't consistently eating a nutrient-dense diet to replenish their nutrient stores. If you want to breastfeed beyond the first year, know that pregnancy can affect your milk supply (many women tandem nurse, but nursing aversions or lowered milk supply are common barriers). Connective tissues take a long time to recover and it's especially helpful for your quality of life to allow adequate time to heal, particularly if you had pelvic floor dysfunction, prolapse, or diastasis recti. Lastly, having children in quick succession brings up the obvious challenges (and exhaustion) that goes along with caring for more than one young child at once. If you want to have closely spaced children, make an extra effort to eat well, supplement well, and have extra helping hands at the ready!

Summary

Motherhood is one of the most amazing and simultaneously challenging experiences of your life. When your baby is born, life can feel like it comes to a screeching halt. Whatever had been a priority before is suddenly not (or you may simply not have the same amount of time for said priorities). Emotions run high, time is stretched thin, and getting overwhelmed is par for the course. It may sound corny, but I want to remind you that this is an intense season of life; however, it is just a season. Your baby will not always require so much focused attention or need you so frequently. You will find your new normal—and also find that what's normal is constantly shifting as your child grows and develops. Allow yourself to feel all the feels, whether it's a good day or a bad day. Taking care of yourself by having help (childcare, cooking, cleaning, etc.) and prioritizing your health (good food, mindful movement, emotional support, etc.) will go a long way in weathering this season without burning out. Here's a recap of the most important takeaways on postpartum recovery and the 4th trimester.

Tips for the 4th Trimester (short version):

- Welcome support, so you can rest, recover, and adjust to new motherhood. It's especially helpful to prearrange help for the first 4-6 weeks postpartum.
- Reframe eating well as an act of self-care, rather than a way to "get your body back." Nourishing yourself with nutrient-dense foods rebuilds your strength and boosts the nutritional value of your breast milk.
- If you are breastfeeding or plan to breastfeed, consider where you will go for professional and peer support.
- Stay on your prenatal supplements for at least the first 6 months postpartum to replenish your nutrient stores. Consult your healthcare provider about additional supplements or nutritional support.
- If you are not feeling well, talk with your healthcare provider about specific lab tests that are relevant to your symptoms.
- Embrace a slow, mindful return to exercise. Get a referral to a women's health physical therapist/pelvic floor specialist, even if you're not entirely sure you'll book the appointment.
- Be gentle with yourself and don't rush postpartum weight loss. Remember, "9 months on, 9 months off." It's OK that your body is different after having a baby.
- Explore the ways that you can support your emotional well-being and mental health. Find a tribe of like-minded mothers (online or in-person). If you have any inkling that you have postpartum depression or anxiety, seek professional help sooner rather than later.
- If you want more children, consider the amount of time you'll wait before trying to conceive again.

Well, the "short version" of this chapter is still a lot to take in. If you are reading this while you are still pregnant, I encourage you to take a quick break from planning your dream birth and consider some 4th trimester planning as well. The first bullet point is, by far, the most important.

If you are reading this with a baby in your arms, take it one day at a time. Re-read this list and see what's most feasible for you in the next week or two. Time is the most precious resource when you're caring for a baby, so tackling this huge list all at once is entirely out of the question. Think of it more as "food for thought."

I'm in no way suggesting that it's easy to do all of the above when juggling caring for an infant; however, as the months roll on, you'll find more time to care for yourself. Remember, a well-nourished and healthy mother is just as important as a healthy child. You've got this.

Recipe Appendix

BREAKFAST

Crustless Spinach Quiche
Grain-free Granola

MAIN DISHES

Grilled Lemon Pepper Salmon
Salmon Cakes
Beanless Beef Chili
Bone Broth
Chicken & Vegetable Soup
Grass-fed Beef Meatloaf
Low-Carb Shepherd's Pie
Baked Spaghetti Squash with Meatballs
Coconut Chicken Curry
Slow Cooker Carnitas

VEGETABLES

Riced Cauliflower
Roasted Brussels Sprouts
Sautéed Kale
Lemon Roasted Broccoli
Roasted Sweet Potato Fries
Roasted Curried Cauliflower
Roasted Butternut Squash

SNACKS, DESSERTS, ETC.

Spinach Dip
Nutty "Granola" Bar
Grass-fed Beef Liver Pate
Homemade Berry Sorbet
Coconut Macaroons
Maple Pots de Creme
Tart Cherry Gummies
Lily's Electrolyte Replenishment Drink

Crustless Spinach Quiche

Makes 4-6 servings

Packed with choline and protein from eggs, calcium from cheese, and folate from spinach, this quiche is a prenatal nutrition superstar. Make two and freeze one (cut into individual portions) for later.

Ingredients

- 1 tablespoon coconut oil or butter
- 1 onion, chopped
- 10 oz package frozen, chopped spinach, thawed and drained
- 6 eggs, ideally from pasture-raised chickens
- 3 cups shredded cheese (Muenster, cheddar or jack)
- ½ teaspoon salt
- ⅛ teaspoon black pepper

Directions

1. In a large skillet, cook onions in coconut oil or butter until soft.
2. Stir in spinach and allow excess moisture to evaporate.
3. In a large bowl, mix eggs, cheese, salt, and pepper.
4. Add spinach-onion mixture and stir to combine.
5. Pour into a buttered 9-inch pie dish.
6. Bake in a 350 degree oven until eggs set, about 30 minutes. Let cool for 15 minutes before serving.

NOTE: This recipe comes together quickly if you plan ahead and defrost the spinach overnight in the refrigerator. Simply poke a hole in the bag squeeze out the excess moisture, and mix it in. You may substitute any freshly cooked green for the spinach, such as kale or chard.

Grain-free Granola

Makes 10 servings (~½ cup each)

One of the biggest questions I get is "What can I have instead of cereal?" Yes, if you're following my approach, conventional breakfast cereal is off the table. My recipe for grain-free granola gives you the satisfaction of a crunchy, lightly sweet "cereal" without the refined grains.

Ingredients

- ¼ cup coconut oil or butter, melted
- 3 cups unsweetened coconut flakes
- 1 cup sliced almonds
- 1 cup chopped walnuts, pecans, hazelnuts, macadamia nuts (or combination)
- 2 tablespoons chia seeds, whole
- 2 tablespoons pure maple syrup
- 2 teaspoons ground cinnamon
- ¼ teaspoon ground nutmeg
- ½ teaspoon sea salt

Directions

1. Melt coconut oil or butter in a small saucepan.
2. Mix with remaining ingredients.
3. Spread onto a large baking sheet and bake for 25 minutes at 275 degrees until golden brown and fragrant. Be sure not to over-bake. Granola will crisp as it cools.
4. Store at room temperature in an airtight container for up to 1 month.

NOTE: You may add stevia to taste if you'd like a sweeter granola.

Grilled Lemon Pepper Salmon

Makes 2 servings

One of the best ways to get your omega-3s is wild-caught salmon. Though many are not comfortable cooking fish, it's actually quite simple. For the best quality salmon, I prefer to buy it frozen and defrost in the refrigerator overnight (virtually all "fresh" salmon at the store was flash-frozen within 24 hours of catching anyways). Good quality fish should not smell fishy, but rather like the fresh ocean air.

Ingredients

- Two 3-4 oz fillets of wild Alaskan salmon, skin on
- Juice of ½ lemon
- ¾ teaspoon of crushed lemon pepper (or less if desired)
- Sprinkle of sea salt
- Drizzle of olive oil

Directions

1. Coat salmon with spices and oil.
2. Preheat grill over medium heat. Place salmon directly on the grill, skin side down (alternatively, use a large, heavy-bottomed skillet to cook this on the stovetop). Grill for 3-5 minutes, or until edges of fish begin to turn opaque. Flip and cook an additional 1-2 minutes, or until cooked to your liking.

NOTE: You may remove the skin before serving or eat the skin (after all, it's rich in omega-3 fats and glycine). If you double or triple this recipe, you can use leftover fish to make salmon cakes.

Salmon Cakes

Makes 12-14 salmon cakes, depending on size

If you're not a big fan of fish or find salmon a little too "fishy," I encourage you to try salmon cakes. Unlike most fish cake recipes, I use a mashed potato in place of bread crumbs, making this appropriate for those who avoid grains or gluten. This is also a great way to use up leftover fish.

Ingredients

- 2 lb wild Alaskan salmon, cooked (canned salmon works well)
- 1 teaspoon salt
- ½ teaspoon black pepper
- ½ teaspoon garlic powder
- juice from ½ lemon
- 1 large russet potato, peeled, chopped
- 1 bell pepper, minced (red, orange or yellow for best color)
- 3 green onions, minced (green and white parts)
- 3-4 slices thick-cut bacon, cooked, chopped
- 2 eggs (ideally from pasture-raised hens)
- coconut oil for cooking

Directions

1. In a small pot of salted, boiling water, cook potato until easily pierced with a fork. Drain water. Mash until smooth. Let cool.
2. Once potatoes are cooled, place all ingredients in a large bowl. (If cooking fresh salmon, double check that any bones have been removed. If using canned salmon, there's no need to remove any remaining bones as they have been softened during the canning process—and are a great source of calcium.)
3. With very clean hands, thoroughly combine all ingredients. Form into patties and set aside (place in refrigerator unless cooking right away).
4. Heat 2-3 Tbsp coconut oil in a cast iron skillet over medium-high heat.
5. Fry the cakes for 1-2 minutes per side until golden brown. You may need to add additional coconut oil with each batch.

NOTE: Though salmon is nutritionally an excellent choice, other types of fish work well in this recipe. Halibut and cod are favorites in our house.

Beanless Beef Chili

Makes 6 servings

This recipe is "beanless" for the convenience of those who don't enjoy beans in their chili, prefer a low-carb chili, or have digestive issues from eating beans. If you like beans, go ahead and mix them in or serve them alongside.

Ingredients

- 1 dried chipotle pepper, stem removed
- 1 cup boiling water
- 1 ½ teaspoons coconut oil
- 1 cup chopped yellow onion
- 1 cup chopped green bell pepper
- 1 cup chopped red bell pepper
- 4 garlic cloves, minced
- 1 pound ground beef (grass-fed)
- ½ pound spicy ground pork sausage
- 3 oz beef liver, ground or finely chopped (optional)
- 1 tablespoon chili powder
- 1 tablespoon ground cumin
- 1 teaspoon dried oregano
- 1 teaspoon unsweetened cocoa powder
- 1 teaspoon Worcestershire sauce
- 1 (28 ounce) can crushed tomatoes
- 1 ½ teaspoons sea salt
- ½ teaspoon ground black pepper

Directions

1. Soak chipotle pepper in boiling water until softened, about 10 minutes. Remove pepper from water and mince.
2. Melt coconut oil in a large pot over medium heat.
3. Add onion and bell peppers to the pan. Cook until tender, 5 to 10 minutes
4. Stir garlic and minced chipotle into onion mixture and cook until fragrant, about 1 minute.
5. Add beef and sausage to the pan. Cook and stir until meat is browned and crumbly, 10 to 12 minutes.

6. Add remaining ingredients, stir to combine. Bring to a boil, reduce heat to low, and simmer until flavors are developed, 10 minutes.
7. Serve with full-fat sour cream, avocado, marinated red onions and any other low-carb toppings.

NOTE: Chili often tastes better the next day. Make a double batch and consider freezing extra for quick meals.

Bone Broth

Yields approximately 4 quarts, depending on size of your stock pot/slow cooker

This recipe is for chicken or turkey broth, however beef or pork bones may also be used. I personally like to use bones after they have been cooked, both for ease and for better flavor. For example, if I roast a whole chicken or make a batch of chicken wings, I'll save the carcass (bones, skin, and any cartilage) in the freezer for making bone broth at a later time. Ideally, I like to fill the pot about half full of bones to ensure the broth is plenty rich. This recipe can be made in a slow cooker, pressure cooker, or on the stove-top. The resulting broth will need to be seasoned (lots of salt!).

Ingredients

- 2 to 3 pounds of bones, such as necks, backs, breastbones, wings, and feet (ideally from pasture-raised chicken or turkey)
- 1 tablespoon vinegar or lemon juice
- 1 large onion, skin on, cut into quarters
- 2 carrots, whole
- 2 celery stalks, ideally with leaves
- 1 bay leaf
- 1 tablespoon kombu flakes (optional; an excellent source of iodine)
- ½ teaspoon black peppercorns (optional)
- vegetable scraps – (optionally add kale stems, parsley, garlic, ginger, etc)
- filtered water, to cover

Directions

1. Place all ingredients in a large stock pot, slow cooker, or pressure cooker. Cover with water - it should cover the contents of the pot by about an inch of water. Put the lid on your pot.
2. Stove-top or slow-cooker: Bring to a simmer and cook on low for 12-24 hours.
   Pressure cooker: cook on high pressure for 60-90 minutes.
3. The stock is done when the bones are soft. The ends of chicken or turkey bones should literally crumble, otherwise you can let it continue cooking to maximize the mineral content of the broth. (Beef or pork bones, especially knuckle bones or marrow bones, can be used for a second batch of stock.)

Real Food for Pregnancy

4. When finished, the stock should be a rich golden color (chicken and turkey make a more pale broth).
5. To strain broth, set a metal strainer over a large pot or bowl. Using a large ladle, pour broth over strainer. Discard solids. Let cool slightly before storing, however be sure to refrigerate within 2 hours, as broth is an ideal environment for bacteria to grow.
6. Store broth in the refrigerator for up to 3 days or freeze for long-term storage.

NOTE: I make big batches of stock and freeze the leftovers for later. If you're not cooking for a big crowd, consider freezing stock in ice cube trays, so you can defrost it quickly for a mug of bone broth or a small batch of soup. Don't forget to make extra in preparation for your postpartum recovery.

Chicken & Vegetable Soup

Makes 4 servings

Just about nothing compares to the flavor and comfort of grandma's chicken soup, thanks to using bone broth as a base. This recipe is easily adapted to what vegetables you have in your house. Try adding kale, cabbage, zucchini or bell peppers.

Ingredients

- 1 large onion, chopped
- 3 large carrots, peeled, chopped
- 4 stalks celery, chopped
- 2 tablespoons butter
- 1 teaspoon sea salt, or to taste
- ½ teaspoon black pepper
- ½ teaspoon dried thyme
- 6 cups chicken bone broth
- 1 lb chicken meat, picked from a roasted chicken (or pre-cooked chicken thigh meat, chopped)
- ½ cup heavy cream
- 1 tablespoon lemon juice
- 2 tablespoons fresh parsley, to garnish (optional)

Directions

1. In a large pot over high heat, sauté all vegetables in butter with salt, pepper, and thyme until lightly browned and fragrant.
2. Add chicken stock and bring to a boil.
3. Add chicken meat, heavy cream, and lemon juice. Reduce heat and simmer for 5 minutes. Adjust seasonings to taste. Serve with fresh parsley.

NOTE: Rich in gelatin and minerals, this makes an excellent soup for postpartum recovery.

Grass-fed Beef Meatloaf

Makes 8 servings

Hearty, nourishing, and packed with nutrition. This meatloaf is a an excellent source of choline, vitamin B12, iron, vitamin A, folate, zinc, and numerous other nutrients that benefit your health and your baby's health. Many meatloaf recipes call for bread crumbs or oatmeal, but I like a meatier version that uses just a bit of almond or coconut flour instead.

Ingredients

Meatloaf:

- 1 small onion, finely diced
- 8 oz mushrooms, finely diced
- 2 cloves garlic, minced
- 2 tablespoons coconut oil
- 1 small zucchini, grated
- 2 lbs grass fed ground beef
- 6 ounces grass-fed beef liver, finely chopped or ground (may substitute liver paté)
- 2 eggs, ideally from pastured chickens
- ¼ cup almond flour or coconut flour
- 2 teaspoons sea salt
- 1/2 teaspoon black pepper
- 1 teaspoon dried oregano
- 1 teaspoon dried thyme

Topping:

- 6 ounces tomato paste (1 small can)
- 1 tablespoon maple syrup or honey
- 1 packet stevia (optional, if you prefer this to be sweet, like ketchup)
- 1 teaspoon soy sauce

Directions

1. In a large skillet over medium-high heat, sauté onion, mushrooms, and garlic in coconut oil until lightly browned and all water (released from the vegetables) has evaporated from the skillet. Set aside to cool.

2. In a large mixing bowl, mix meat, cooked vegetables, and all remaining meatloaf ingredients.
3. Form into a loaf shape in a 9 x 13 inch glass baking dish.
4. Mix topping ingredients. Adjust seasonings to taste. Spoon over meatloaf.
5. Bake meatloaf in a 350 degree oven for 45-60 minutes, or until cooked through.

NOTE: This recipe is a great way to include nutrient-dense liver in your diet if you're not a fan of the taste.

Low-carb Shepherd's Pie

Makes 6-8 servings

Comfort food without all the carbs, thanks to swapping in cauliflower in place of potatoes.

Ingredients

Filling:

- 1 lb grass fed ground beef
- 3 ounces grass-fed beef liver, finely chopped (optional)
- 1 small onion, finely diced
- 3 carrots, peeled, finely diced
- 2 stalks celery, finely diced
- 2 cloves garlic, minced
- 1 tablespoon butter
- 1 teaspoon salt
- ½ teaspoon black pepper
- 2 teaspoons dried thyme

Cauliflower Topping:

- 1 large head cauliflower, chopped
- 4 tablespoons butter
- 1 teaspoon sea salt, or to taste
- ½ teaspoon black pepper

Directions

1. Steam cauliflower while preparing the filling, which takes 10-15 minutes, depending on the size of cauliflower pieces.
2. In a large skillet, cook ground beef over medium-high heat. If the pan is dry, add a bit of butter or coconut oil (grass-fed beef can be very lean).
3. With a spatula, break up meat into bite-sized pieces. Once browned, add liver and cook for 1-2 minutes.
4. Remove from heat and place in a 9x13 inch baking dish. *Do not* drain rendered fat.
5. In the same pan, add butter, onion, carrots, celery, garlic, salt, pepper, and thyme.

6. Cook for 10 minutes, being sure to scrape up browned bits.
7. Mash steamed cauliflower with butter, salt, and pepper. Spread on top of meat and vegetables.
8. Bake in a 400 degree oven for 20 minutes, until cauliflower is lightly browned.

NOTE: This recipe is a great way to include nutrient-dense liver in your diet if you're not a fan of the taste.

Twice Baked Spaghetti Squash with Meatballs

Makes 6 servings

Baking the squash twice vastly improves the flavor of spaghetti squash. Give this method a try even if you haven't liked spaghetti squash in the past.

Ingredients

Spaghetti Squash:

- 1 large spaghetti squash
- 2 tablespoons extra-virgin olive oil
- 1 teaspoon salt
- 1 jar high-quality marinara sauce (or 3-4 cups homemade marinara)
- 6 oz mozzarella cheese, shredded (from grass-fed milk, if possible)
- 6 oz Parmesan cheese, shredded (from grass-fed milk, if possible)

Meatballs:

- 1 small onion, finely diced
- 8 oz mushrooms, finely diced
- 2 cloves garlic, minced
- 2 tablespoons coconut oil
- 1 lb grass fed ground beef
- 3 ounces grass-fed beef liver, finely chopped or ground (optional)
- 1 egg, ideally from_pastured chickens
- 1 teaspoon sea salt
- 1/4 teaspoon black pepper
- 1/2 teaspoon dried oregano
- 1/8 teaspoon red pepper flakes (optional)

Directions

1. Preheat oven to 400 degrees F.
2. Slice the spaghetti squash in half lengthwise with a large, sharp knife. Scoop out the seeds (you can reserve seeds and roast separately like pumpkin seeds.)
3. Rub the inside of the squash with olive oil and sprinkle with salt. Place each squash half, cut side down, on large rimmed baking sheet, such as a lasagna pan. Add ½ cup water. Bake for 30-45 minutes,

until the squash is tender. (It's cooked when it gives slightly when you push on the outside.)

4. While squash is baking, make meatballs. In a large, cast-iron skillet over medium-high heat, sauté onion, mushrooms, and garlic in coconut oil until lightly browned and all water (released from the vegetables) has evaporated from the skillet. Set aside to cool. In a large mixing bowl, mix meat with cooked vegetables and remaining meatball ingredients. Form into 12-15 meatballs. Place meatballs on a greased baking dish, at least 1 inch apart. Bake for 15 minutes, or until cooked through.

5. Once squash is cooked, remove from oven. Fill with marinara sauce. Top with cheese. Return to oven on the top rack and bake for 20 minutes, or until cheese is melted/browned to your liking. Let sit for 10 minutes (if you can wait!) to let the juices sink in.

6. Serve by scooping the flesh of the squash with a large spoon. The squash should break apart into spaghetti-like strands while serving. Top with meatballs.

Coconut Chicken Curry

Makes 8 servings

There's something about curry that is so satisfying. The blend of spices and creamy coconut milk really make this a treat.

Ingredients

- 1 medium onion, finely diced
- 1 cup fresh green beans, trimmed, cut into 2 inch pieces
- 1 green bell pepper, thinly sliced
- 1 red bell pepper, thinly sliced
- 2 cloves garlic, minced
- 2 tablespoons freshly grated ginger
- 1 tablespoon coconut oil
- 2 tablespoons mild curry powder (such as garam masala)
- 1 teaspoon sea salt
- 15 oz can full-fat coconut milk (check ingredients to avoid preservatives and additives)
- 16 oz chicken bone broth (ideally homemade)
- 16 oz cooked, shredded chicken
- 3-4 cups fresh spinach
- juice of 2 limes
- dash of soy sauce or tamari, to taste
- chili flakes or fresh chili slices (optional)

Directions

1. In a medium pot over medium-high heat, sauté onion in coconut oil until lightly browned.
2. Add all remaining vegetables, garlic, ginger, curry powder, and salt. Cook for 5 minutes.
3. Add coconut milk, broth, and chicken.
4. Simmer for 10 minutes.
5. Add lime and tamari to taste.
6. Just before serving, add fresh spinach and stir to wilt.

NOTE: This recipe freezes extremely well. Make a double batch and freeze extra for your postpartum recovery.

Slow Cooker Carnitas

Makes 16 servings

Pulled pork is hands down one of the most delicious meals around. Turn it into carnitas by using the right blend of spices and quickly pan-frying it after cooking to crisp up the edges. Pork shoulder is an excellent source of glycine, iron, zinc, vitamin B6, and many other nutrients, so although conventional wisdom suggests it's not healthy, I beg to differ.

Ingredients

- 4-5 lb pork shoulder, ideally from a pasture-raised pig
- 1 onion, finely sliced
- 2 teaspoons sea salt
- 1 teaspoon garlic powder
- 1 teaspoon chili powder
- 1 teaspoon cumin
- 1 teaspoon oregano
- juice of 2 limes (or 2 tablespoons apple cider vinegar)
- 2 tablespoons coconut sugar or maple syrup (optional)

Directions

1. Place onions in bottom of slow cooker.
2. Mix spices and salt. Rub over pork shoulder and place in the slow cooker.
3. Add lime juice or vinegar.
4. Cook on high for 6-8 hours.
5. When finished, the pork will easily shred with a fork. Adjust cooking time as necessary.
6. Remove pork and either eat as is -or- Place drained meat in a cast iron skillet with some rendered pork fat (there'll be a layer on top of your slow cooker). Cook on high heat until pork is crisp around the edges.
7. Serve and enjoy!

NOTE: This recipe freezes extremely well. Unless I'm serving a big crowd, I'll freeze half the recipe right away in individual portions.

Riced Cauliflower

Makes ~4 servings

Cauliflower is an incredibly versatile vegetable. One of my favorite uses is turning it into "rice." At only 3g of net carbohydrates per cup (versus the 45g+ in regular rice), this is a nutritional no-brainer.

Ingredients

- 1 large head cauliflower
- 1-2 tablespoons butter or lard
- Sea salt to taste

Directions

1. Cut cauliflower into 4 large chunks.
2. With a box grater, grate cauliflower over the medium-sized or large-sized holes. Alternatively, use a food processor with the grater attachment.
3. Transfer cauliflower to a clean towel or paper towel to help absorb any excess moisture.
4. To cook, sauté cauliflower in a large skillet over medium-high heat in 1-2 tablespoons of your preferred cooking fat (I like butter or lard) and a generous pinch of salt. Cook for a total of 5-8 minutes. If the cauliflower is still a little firm for your taste, cover with a lid so the cauliflower steams and becomes more tender.
5. Use cauliflower rice in place of regular rice in all of your favorite recipes.

NOTE: Although cooking from fresh is great, you might check the freezer section at your grocery store for pre-made riced cauliflower. Thanks to the popularity of paleo and low-carb diets, more grocery stores are stocking it. Simply sauté from frozen and you have a side dish in less than 5 minutes with zero prep work and very little clean up.

Roasted Brussels Sprouts

Makes 6 servings

Brussels sprouts aren't always delicious, but when they're roasted —wow!—are they transformed. The key to yummy sprouts is to roast them cut-side down on the bottom rack of the oven, so they cook evenly and get a nice crispy, caramelized layer on the bottom.

Ingredients

- 2 pounds Brussels sprouts
- 1 onion, sliced
- a few tablespoons ghee, lard, or coconut oil
- 1 teaspoon sea salt
- ½ teaspoon black pepper
- 1 teaspoon dried thyme
- 1 teaspoon garlic powder

Directions

1. Preheat oven to 400 degrees F.
2. Prepare Brussels sprouts by trimming off the ends and peeling away discolored leaves, if any. Cut each sprout in half lengthwise (if the sprout is tiny, just leave it whole).
3. Put Brussels sprouts and onions on a large baking sheet. Add oil and seasonings, stirring to coat. Spread out in one single layer. (Tip: if they are cut-side down, they caramelize better and cook more evenly.)
4. Roast for 25-35 minutes in the bottom rack of the oven, or until soft when pierced with a fork and slightly browned. Check halfway through cooking. If they are getting too brown, move the pan to the upper rack for the remaining cooking time.

Sautéed Kale

Makes 2 servings

Packed with folate, antioxidants, and minerals, kale is most certainly a superfood. Learning how to cook it well can be a bit of an art. Using a tasty fat, like butter or bacon fat, using enough salt, and adding a bit of acidity brings out the best in kale. If that's not enough, a sprinkle of Parmesan cheese never hurts.

Ingredients

- 1 bunch fresh kale, stem removed, leaves chopped
- 1 tablespoon bacon fat or butter
- 1 clove garlic, sliced
- ¼ teaspoon salt
- Squeeze of fresh lemon juice

Directions

1. Get a large skillet with a well-fitting lid. Heat over medium-high heat. Add your cooking fat and sliced garlic. Cook until fragrant, stirring frequently.
2. Add kale, salt, 1 tablespoon of water and immediately put the lid on the pan. Allow the kale to steam for 1-2 minutes.
3. Remove lid and stir. Taste test a piece of kale. If it's too tough, continue to cook for another minute or two.
4. When done to your liking, add a squeeze of fresh lemon juice, give it a quick stir and serve.

NOTE: There are many different varieties of kale. My preference is a type called lacinato kale or black kale, since it generally has a sweeter flavor and more tender texture. Any type of kale or leafy greens can be used in this recipe. The key to making tasty sautéed greens is the combo of relatively high heat and a quick steam with the lid on. This ensures the kale stays vibrantly green, but softens. Depending on the season, you may need to adjust your cooking time. In the spring when kale is very tender, it may need less cooking time. In late summer, the opposite may be true.

Lemon Roasted Broccoli

Makes 4 servings

If you've ever steamed or boiled broccoli and shuddered at the sulfurous smell that fills your house or forced down forkfuls of limp, water-logged broccoli in the name of health, you need to give this recipe a shot.

Ingredients

- 1 lb fresh broccoli
- 1 teaspoon salt
- 1 lemon, juiced
- 1-3 large cloves garlic, minced (depends how garlicky you want it!)
- 1 small onion, sliced thin
- 2 tablespoons olive oil, coconut oil, or ghee (clarified butter)

Directions

1. Cut broccoli into individual florets. Try to cut them into similar-sized pieces so they cook evenly. (The stem can also be cut up and used in this recipe.)
2. On a large sheet pan, toss broccoli with salt, juice of 1/2 the lemon (save the other half for later use in this recipe), garlic, onion, and oil. Don't overcrowd the pan.
3. Roast at 425 degrees for 25-35 minutes, or until broccoli is tender when pierced with a fork. Turn once mid-way through cooking.
4. Remove from oven, squeeze the juice of the remaining lemon half over the top and serve.

NOTE: If they are in season, use Meyer lemons, which are sweeter and juicier than regular lemons.

Roasted Sweet Potato Fries

Makes 4-6 servings

Homemade sweet potato fries are one of my favorite comfort foods. Since they are certainly a high-carb side dish, make sure to pair them with a protein-rich meal or snack. Thanks to their high vitamin B6 and potassium content, sweet potato fries are a good option if you're feeling nauseous.

Ingredients

- 2 large sweet potatoes
- 3 tablespoons lard, ghee, or coconut oil
- 1 teaspoon sea salt
- ½ teaspoon garlic powder
- ½ teaspoon fresh pepper

Directions

1. Preheat oven to 400 degrees. Wash and dry sweet potatoes (leave unpeeled).
2. Cut into sticks, roughly 1 cm thick.
3. Place on a large baking sheet and toss with remaining ingredients. Lay out in a single layer.
4. Roast for 25 minutes on the bottom rack. Flip. Roast for another 10-15 minutes, or until easily pierced with a fork and lightly browned.

Roasted Curried Cauliflower

Makes 6 servings

Don't let the long list of ingredients dissuade you from making this dish. It's one of the most requested vegetable dishes in my family. The coconut milk and spices combine to create a rich sauce (I won't tell if you lick your plate).

Ingredients

- 1 large head cauliflower (about 2 lbs) cut into small florets
- 1 onion, sliced
- 1 bell pepper, sliced
- 1-2 inch piece of fresh ginger, finely grated OR 1 teaspoon ground dried ginger
- 2-3 heaping tablespoons mild curry powder
- 2 cloves garlic, minced OR 1 teaspoon garlic powder
- 2 teaspoons sea salt
- ½ teaspoon freshly ground pepper
- 16 oz can coconut milk (full-fat)
- 1-2 tablespoons coconut oil or ghee
- 1 tablespoons balsamic vinegar or pomegranate molasses

Directions

1. Cut up all vegetables (into similarly-sized pieces) and place in a large baking pan, such as a lasagne dish. You want a single layer, so if it's piled up, split it into 2 pans. The smaller the pieces, the faster it will cook.
2. Add all remaining ingredients and toss to combine.
3. Bake in preheated 425 degree oven for 30 min or until cauliflower is lightly browned and tender when pierced with a fork. Serve hot or cold.

NOTE: The addition of balsamic vinegar or pomegranate molasses probably sounds weird, but the flavor is drab without it. Pomegranate molasses is found in Middle Eastern markets. Feel free to add additional vegetables to this dish or, for a little protein, consider adding cooked garbanzo beans, chicken, or roasted cashews.

Real Food for Pregnancy

Roasted Butternut Squash

Makes 6-8 servings

Winter squash is a great side dish, rich in magnesium and vitamin B6. This makes it a great choice in early pregnancy if you're feeling nauseous. Though it's naturally sweet, it has about half the carbs of sweet potato.

Ingredients

- 1 large butternut squash
- 2 tablespoons softened butter
- 1 teaspoon sea salt (or about ½ teaspoon per pound of squash)
- ½ teaspoon pepper

Directions

1. Preheat oven to 425 degrees F.
2. With a large knife, carefully cut butternut squash in half, lengthwise.
3. Coat inside with softened butter and sprinkle with salt and pepper.
4. Roast cut-side down on a large baking pan for 35 minutes, or until squash is easily pierced with a fork.
5. Serve by scooping out the cooked squash with a large spoon. Top with additional butter.

Spinach Dip

Makes 6 servings

Spinach dip is a great way to sneak extra greens into your diet. This recipe was developed during the winter when I couldn't get my hands on good quality greens, hence the use of frozen spinach. I like to serve it with fresh, cut-up vegetables. Remember, fat helps you absorb the nutrients and antioxidants in vegetables, so don't feel guilty about using a whole block of cream cheese.

Ingredients

- 10 oz frozen spinach, defrosted
- 8 oz cream cheese, full fat
- 1 garlic clove, minced
- 1 teaspoon olive oil
- ½ cup shredded Parmesan cheese
- Sea salt and pepper, to taste

Directions

1. Poke a hole in the bag of defrosted spinach and squeeze over the sink to remove extra liquid.
2. In a small saucepan set over medium heat, sautéed garlic in olive oil until slightly softened and fragrant.
3. Add spinach and cream cheese, stirring occasionally with a wooden spoon as cream cheese softens.
4. Once heated through and fully combined, mix in Parmesan cheese.
5. Taste and add a little salt & pepper if desired.
6. Serve warm or cold with sliced carrots, celery, bell peppers, or any other fresh produce.

NOTE: Spinach dip keeps well in the refrigerator for up to a week.

Real Food for Pregnancy

Nutty "Granola" Bars

Makes ~24 bars

Most granola bars pack in a lot of sugar and not much protein. Thanks to nuts, seeds, egg, and (optional) collagen protein, these bars are packed with protein and micronutrients.

Ingredients

- 4 tablespoons ground flaxseeds or chia seeds
- ½ cup raw honey
- 2 heaping tablespoons collagen protein (optional)
- 1 egg, ideally from pasture-raised chicken
- 1 teaspoon sea salt
- 1 cup raw almonds pieces
- 1 cup raw walnuts pieces (or other nuts)
- 1 cup unsweetened large coconut flakes
- 1 cup unsweetened fine coconut flakes

Directions

1. In a large bowl, mix the ground flaxseeds or chia seeds, honey, and collagen protein (optional). Add remaining ingredients and mix thoroughly to combine.
2. Line a sheet tray with parchment paper and scoop mixture onto paper.
3. Lay another piece of parchment paper on top of the mixture and with your hands spread it evenly on tray so that it extends all the way to the sides.
4. Press the mixture down firmly with a flat surface, such as the bottom of a small pot.
5. Remove top layer of parchment paper and place in 350 degree oven.
6. Bake for 24 minutes, rotating the tray at 12 minutes.
7. Let cool and cut into 24 bars.

NOTE: For long-term storage, wrap individually in parchment or wax paper and store in an airtight container in the fridge.

Grass-fed Beef Liver Pate

Makes 8 servings

I'll be honest. Taste-wise, liver is *not* my favorite food. But on a nutritional scale of 1-10, it gets an 11. And since nutritionally there are literally no foods that can take its place, liver is something I've learned to incorporate into my diet – and I think you should, too.

Ingredients

- 1 lb grass-fed beef liver (or pasture-raised chicken liver)
- 1 tablespoon arrowroot powder (or organic corn starch)
- 4 tablespoon (½ stick) butter (from grass-fed cows)
- 1 medium onion, sliced
- ½ teaspoon salt
- ½ teaspoon dried thyme
- pinch of black pepper
- ½ cup heavy whipping cream (ideally from grass-fed cows)

Directions

1. With a paper towel, pat any excess moisture off the liver. Sprinkle with salt, thyme, pepper, then the arrowroot powder (arrowroot is a gluten-free alternative to flour).
2. Heat a large cast iron skillet over medium heat. Add butter.
3. Cook liver until lightly browned on both sides. Transfer to the food processor.
4. Meanwhile, add onions to the skillet. Cook until lightly browned and soft.
5. Add heavy cream to deglaze the pan (scraping up any caramelized bits with a metal spatula).
6. Transfer contents of pan to the food processor.
7. Process/pulse until you have a nice, thick pate. Taste test and add additional salt if needed.
8. Transfer to small mason jars, ensuring no air bubbles are present. Use within 1 week or freeze jars for later use.

NOTE: If eating straight-up pate with crackers or vegetables isn't your thing, you can mix liver pate into any recipe that uses ground meat. I often make a large batch of pate and freeze it in small containers (4-8 oz jars or even ice cube trays) specifically for this purpose. Then, the next time I go to make meatloaf, meatballs, chili, or shepherd's pie, I can simply defrost a small amount and mix it right in.

Homemade Berry Sorbet

Makes 2 servings

Ready in less than a minute and deeply satisfying, homemade berry sorbet is a recipe you'll make again and again.

Ingredients

- 1 cup frozen berries (blueberries, raspberries, cherries, or blackberries)
- ½ cup heavy whipping cream, ideally from grass-fed cows
- 1 tablespoon collagen protein (optional)
- 1 packet stevia sweetener or 5-10 drops liquid stevia extract (optional)

Directions

1. Puree all ingredients using a blender, immersion blender, or food processor.
2. Serve immediately.

NOTE: There are several brands of collagen and gelatin powder made from grass-fed beef. Great Lakes is one of them. I prefer collagen protein because it dissolves completely, even in cold liquids. This provides a nourishing source of protein and glycine to this recipe, but is not required. Stevia is also optional for those who like a sweeter sorbet.

Coconut Macaroons

Makes 36 cookies

These cookies are packed with healthy fat and fiber from coconut and protein from egg whites, making them a filling option for dessert. For a real treat, dip the baked cookies in a little melted dark chocolate.

Ingredients

- 5 egg whites*
- ¼ teaspoon sea salt
- ⅓ cup honey
- 1 tablespoon vanilla extract (or almond extract)
- 3 cups shredded coconut, unsweetened

Directions

1. In a large bowl, whisk egg whites and salt until stiff.
2. Fold in remaining ingredients.
3. With a spoon, scoop out 1 tablespoon portions and drop onto a parchment-lined baking sheet.
4. Bake at 350 degrees for 10-15 minutes, until lightly browned.

* Save the egg yolks for maple pots de creme, scrambled eggs, mixing into meatloaf/meatballs, or another recipe. They are too good to throw away!

Maple Pots de Creme

Makes 4 servings

Pots de creme are like the bottom of creme brulee – delicious little baked custards minus the burnt sugar crust. These "pots of cream" or "pots of custard" originate from France. They are a decadent dessert, but low in sugar and full of important nutrients for baby (choline, vitamin B12, vitamin A, DHA, just to name a few). One serving provides more than 60% of your daily choline needs.

Ingredients

- 1 ½ cups heavy cream, ideally from grass-fed cows
- ¼ cup maple syrup
- ¼ teaspoon sea salt
- 4 egg yolks, ideally from pasture-raised hens*
- ½ teaspoon vanilla extract
- ¼ teaspoon maple extract (optional)

Directions

1. Preheat the oven to 300 degrees. Place 4 ramekins in a rimmed baking dish, such as a brownie pan.
2. Combine the cream, maple syrup, and salt in a small saucepan. Heat until it comes to a simmer. Turn off heat.
3. In a medium bowl, whisk together the egg yolks and vanilla extract (and, if using, the maple extract).
4. Temper the egg yolks - Using a small ladle, add some hot cream to the egg yolks a few tablespoons at a time while stirring the eggs (this prevents the egg yolks from scrambling). Once you've added ~1 cup of cream, pour the rest of the cream into the bowl and whisk to combine.
5. Strain the mixture through a fine sieve.
6. Using a ladle, pour the mixture into ramekins (8 oz wide mouth Mason jars work well if you don't have ramekins).
7. Carefully pour enough hot water into the rimmed baking dish to come halfway up the sides of the ramekins.
8. Bake the custards until the edges are set but the center jiggles slightly, 45-50 minutes.
9. Remove the ramekins from the water bath and cool to room temperature.

10. You can either eat at room temperature or refrigerate until cold. (I prefer them cold.)

*Save the egg whites for use in other recipes, such as frittatas, scrambles, or coconut macaroons

NOTE: Extra pots de creme keep well in the refrigerator for up to a week.

Tart Cherry Gummies

Makes ~20 gummies

If you ever encountered "Jello Jigglers" as a child, these are my health-ified version. Though traditional jello is a far cry from a health food, with refined sugar and food dyes, homemade versions using high-quality gelatin and fruit juice are a great way to get additional gelatin (and the amino acid glycine) into your diet. Tart cherry gummies have a naturally sweet-tart flavor from unsweetened tart cherry juice. If you find yourself craving sour candies or gummy candies when you're nauseous, these make a great alternative. Some research supports the use of tart cherry juice as a mild sleep aid, which may prove helpful in later pregnancy and early postpartum.

Ingredients

- 1 ½ cups organic tart cherry juice*
- 4 tablespoons gelatin, ideally from grass-fed cows
- A few drops of stevia extract or a tablespoon of honey (optional, if you prefer it sweeter)

Directions

1. Mix ingredients in a small saucepan. Let gelatin sit for a few minutes (this helps it dissolve).
2. Heat saucepan on the stove set at medium-low heat.
3. Stir with a metal spoon while the mixture heats, so the gelatin completely dissolves.
4. Once you no longer see gelatin granules, remove from heat and pour into a glass dish, such as a pie plate.
5. Place in the refrigerator to chill for 30 min, or until gelatin sets.
6. Cut into bite-sized pieces with a knife (or make fun shapes with cookie cutters) and store in an airtight container in the refrigerator.

NOTE: *Some don't find tart cherry juice sweet enough, so if that's you, feel free to swap in a sweeter fruit juice, add some stevia extract, or add a little honey. You may use any juice you'd like with the exception of pineapple (because it contains the protein-digesting enzyme bromelain, so the gelatin won't gel!).

Lily's Electrolyte Replenishment Drink

Makes 4 servings

This beverage is a good choice if you are dehydrated or have been vomiting (it's also helpful for labor!). It's essential to replenish lost fluids and electrolytes quickly when pregnant. Though many people rely on sports drinks, the artificial colors, flavors, and preservatives are not ideal. Try my homemade version instead.

Ingredients

- 1 quart coconut water (unsweetened)
- ¼ teaspoon sea salt (such as Himalayan pink salt)
- ½ cup fruit juice (such as 100% pineapple, orange, cherry or apple juice)
- Juice of 1 lemon
- 10 drops trace mineral concentrate (optional)

Directions

1. Mix all ingredients in a large pitcher and enjoy. Store leftovers in the refrigerator.

NOTE: Trace Mineral Drops are an excellent addition to boost the mineral content of the drink, but they are not an essential ingredient. I prefer ConcenTrace® Trace Mineral Drops from the company Trace Minerals Research, which are available online or at most health food stores.

References

Introduction

[1] Holder, Tara, et al. "A low disposition index in adolescent offspring of mothers with gestational diabetes: a risk marker for the development of impaired glucose tolerance in youth." *Diabetologia* 57.11 (2014): 2413-2420.

[2] Dabelea, Dana, et al. "Prevalence of type 1 and type 2 diabetes among children and adolescents from 2001 to 2009." *JAMA* 311.17 (2014): 1778-1786.

Chapter 1

[1] Godfrey, Keith M., and David JP Barker. "Fetal programming and adult health." *Public Health Nutrition* 4.2b (2001): 611-624.

[2] Ladipo, Oladapo A. "Nutrition in pregnancy: mineral and vitamin supplements." *The American Journal of Clinical Nutrition* 72.1 (2000): 280s-290s.

[3] Price, Weston A. *Nutrition and Physical Degeneration A Comparison of Primitive and Modern Diets and Their Effects.* New York: Hoeber. 1939. Print.

[4] Loche, Elena, and Susan E. Ozanne. "Early nutrition, epigenetics, and cardiovascular disease." *Current Opinion in Lipidology* 27.5 (2016): 449-458.

[5] Denham, Joshua. "Exercise and epigenetic inheritance of disease risk." *Acta Physiologica* (2017).

[6] Hoffman, Jessie B., Michael C. Petriello, and Bernhard Hennig. "Impact of nutrition on pollutant toxicity: an update with new insights into epigenetic regulation." *Reviews on Environmental Health* 32.1-2 (2017): 65-72.

[7] Denhardt, David. "Effect of Stress on Human Biology: Epigenetics, Adaptation, Inheritance and Social Significance." *Journal of Cellular Physiology* (2017).

[8] D'Vaz, Nina, and Rae-Chi Huang. "Nutrition, Epigenetics and the Early Life Origins of Disease: Evidence from Human Studies." *Nutrition, Epigenetics and Health.* 2017. 25-40.

[9] Geraghty, Aisling A., et al. "Nutrition during pregnancy impacts offspring's epigenetic status—Evidence from human and animal studies." *Nutrition and Metabolic Insights* 8.Suppl 1 (2015): 41.

Chapter 2

[1] Adams, Kelly M., Martin Kohlmeier, and Steven H. Zeisel. "Nutrition education in US medical schools: latest update of a national survey." *Academic medicine: journal of the Association of American Medical Colleges* 85.9 (2010): 1537.

[2] Dufour, Darna L., and Michelle L. Sauther. "Comparative and evolutionary dimensions of the energetics of human pregnancy and lactation." *American Journal of Human Biology* 14.5 (2002): 584-602.

[3] Dufour, Darna L., and Michelle L. Sauther. "Comparative and evolutionary dimensions of the energetics of human pregnancy and lactation." *American Journal of Human Biology* 14.5 (2002): 584-602.

[4] Ladipo, Oladapo A. "Nutrition in pregnancy: mineral and vitamin supplements." *The American journal of clinical nutrition* 72.1 (2000): 280s-290s.

[5] Priest, James R et al. "Maternal Mid-Pregnancy Glucose Levels and Risk of Congenital Heart Disease in Offspring." *JAMA pediatrics* 169.12 (2015): 1112–1116.

[6] Hendricks, Kate A., et al. "Effects of hyperinsulinemia and obesity on risk of neural tube defects among Mexican Americans." *Epidemiology* 12.6 (2001): 630-635.

[7] Menke, Andy, et al. "Prevalence of and trends in diabetes among adults in the United States, 1988-2012." *JAMA* 314.10 (2015): 1021-1029.

[8] Clapp JF: Maternal carbohydrate intake and pregnancy outcome. Proc Nutr Soc. (2002): 61 (1): 45-50.

[9] Moses RG, Luebcke M, Davis WS, Coleman KJ, Tapsell LC, Petocz P, Brand-Miller JC: Effect of a low-glycemic-index diet during pregnancy on obstetric outcomes. Am J Clin Nutr. 2006, 84 (4): 807-12.

[10] Clapp III, James F. "Maternal carbohydrate intake and pregnancy outcome." *Proceedings of the Nutrition Society* 61.01 (2002): 45-50.

[11] Chen, Ling-Wei, et al. "Associations of maternal macronutrient intake during pregnancy with infant BMI peak characteristics and childhood BMI." *The American Journal of Clinical Nutrition* 105.3 (2017): 705-713.

[12] Chen, Ling-Wei, et al. "Associations of maternal macronutrient intake during pregnancy with infant BMI peak characteristics and childhood BMI." *The American Journal of Clinical Nutrition* 105.3 (2017): 705-713.

[13] Wong, Alan C., and Cynthia W. Ko. "Carbohydrate Intake as a Risk Factor for Biliary Sludge and Stones during Pregnancy." *Journal of clinical gastroenterology* 47.8 (2013): 700–705.

[14] Regnault, T. R., Gentili, S., Sarr, O., Toop, C. R. and Sloboda, D. M. (2013), "Fructose, pregnancy and later life impacts." Clin Exp Pharmacol Physiol, 40: 824–837.

[15] Clausen, Torun et al. "High intake of energy, sucrose, and polyunsaturated fatty acids is associated with increased risk of preeclampsia. American Journal of Obstetrics & Gynecology. (2001) Vol 185, Issue 2, 451-458

[16] Ferolla FM¹, Hijano DR, Acosta PL, et al. "Macronutrients during pregnancy and life-threatening respiratory syncytial virus infections in children." Am J Respir Crit Care Med. (2013); 187(9):983-90.

[17] Goletzke, Janina, et al. "Dietary micronutrient intake during pregnancy is a function of carbohydrate quality." *The American Journal of Clinical Nutrition* 102.3 (2015): 626-632.

[18] Procter, Sandra B., and Christina G. Campbell. "Position of the Academy of Nutrition and Dietetics: nutrition and lifestyle for a healthy pregnancy outcome." *Journal of the Academy of Nutrition and Dietetics* 114.7 (2014): 1099-1103.

[19] Chen, Ling-Wei, et al. "Associations of maternal macronutrient intake during pregnancy with infant BMI peak characteristics and childhood BMI." *The American Journal of Clinical Nutrition* 105.3 (2017): 705-713.

[20] Ströhle, Alexander, and Andreas Hahn. "Diets of modern hunter-gatherers vary substantially in their carbohydrate content depending on ecoenvironments: results from an ethnographic analysis." *Nutrition Research* 31.6 (2011): 429-435.

[21] Ströhle, Alexander, and Andreas Hahn. "Diets of modern hunter-gatherers vary substantially in their carbohydrate content depending on ecoenvironments: results from an ethnographic analysis." *Nutrition Research* 31.6 (2011): 429-435.

[22] Spreadbury, Ian. "Comparison with ancestral diets suggests dense acellular carbohydrates promote an inflammatory microbiota, and may be the primary dietary cause of leptin resistance and obesity." *Diabetes, metabolic syndrome and obesity: targets and therapy* 5 (2012): 175.

[23] Brawley, L., et al. "Glycine rectifies vascular dysfunction induced by dietary protein imbalance during pregnancy." *The Journal of physiology* 554.2 (2004): 497-504.

[24] Brawley, Lee, et al. "Dietary protein restriction in pregnancy induces hypertension and vascular defects in rat male offspring." *Pediatric Research* 54.1 (2003): 83-90.

[25] Kalhan, Satish C. "One-carbon metabolism, fetal growth and long-term consequences." *Maternal and Child Nutrition: The First 1,000 Days*. Vol. 74. Karger Publishers, 2013. 127-138.

[26] Cuco, G., et al. "Association of maternal protein intake before conception and throughout pregnancy with birth weight." *Acta obstetricia et gynecologica Scandinavica* 85.4 (2006): 413-421.

[27] Moore, Vivienne M., and Michael J. Davies. "Diet during pregnancy, neonatal outcomes and later health." *Reproduction, Fertility and Development* 17.3 (2005): 341-348.

[28] Godfrey, Keith, et al. "Maternal nutrition in early and late pregnancy in relation to placental and fetal growth." *Bmj* 312.7028 (1996): 410.

[29] Moore, Vivienne M., and Michael J. Davies. "Diet during pregnancy, neonatal outcomes and later health." *Reproduction, Fertility and Development* 17.3 (2005): 341-348.

[30] Thone-Reineke, Christa, et al. "High-protein nutrition during pregnancy and lactation programs blood pressure, food efficiency, and body weight of the offspring in a sex-dependent manner." *American Journal of Physiology-Regulatory, Integrative and Comparative Physiology* 291.4 (2006): R1025-R1030.

[31] Institute of Medicine Food and Nutrition Board. Dietary reference intakes: energy, carbohydrates, fiber, fat, fatty acids, cholesterol, protein, and amino acids. Washington, DC: The National Academy Press; 2005.

[32] Stephens, Trina V., et al. "Protein requirements of healthy pregnant women during early and late gestation are higher than current recommendations." *The Journal of Nutrition* 145.1 (2015): 73-78.

[33] Stephens, Trina V., et al. "Healthy pregnant women in Canada are consuming more dietary protein at 16-and 36-week gestation than currently recommended by the Dietary Reference Intakes, primarily from dairy food sources." *Nutrition Research* 34.7 (2014): 569-576.

[34] C.A. Daley, et al. "A review of fatty acid profiles and antioxidant content in grass-fed and grain-fed beef." Nutrition Journal 2010, 9:10.

[35] Mathews Jr, Kenneth H., and Rachel J. Johnson. "Alternative beef production systems: issues and implications." *US Department of Agriculture, Economic Research Service, LDPM-218-01* (2013).

[36] Wallace, Taylor C., and Victor L. Fulgoni III. "Assessment of total choline intakes in the United States." *Journal of the American College of Nutrition* 35.2 (2016): 108-112.

[37] Strobel, Manuela, Jana Tinz, and Hans-Konrad Biesalski. "The importance of β-carotene as a source of vitamin A with special regard to pregnant and breastfeeding women." *European journal of nutrition* 46.9 (2007): 1-20.

[38] Van den Berg, H., K. F. A. M. Hulshof, and J. P. Deslypere. "Evaluation of the effect of the use of vitamin supplements on vitamin A intake among (potentially) pregnant women in relation to the consumption of liver and liver products." *European Journal of Obstetrics & Gynecology and Reproductive Biology* 66.1 (1996): 17-21.

Real Food for Pregnancy

[39] Zeisel, Steven H. "The fetal origins of memory: the role of dietary choline in optimal brain development." *The Journal of pediatrics* 149.5 (2006): S131-S136.

[40] Shaw, Gary M., et al. "Choline and risk of neural tube defects in a folate-fortified population." *Epidemiology* 20.5 (2009): 714-719.

[41] Strobel, Manuela, Jana Tinz, and Hans-Konrad Biesalski. "The importance of β-carotene as a source of vitamin A with special regard to pregnant and breastfeeding women." *European Journal of Nutrition* 46.9 (2007): 1-20.

[42] DeLany JP, Windhauser MM, Champagne CM, Bray GA. Differential oxidation of individual dietary fatty acids in human. Am J Clin Nutr 2000; 72: 905–911.

[43] Gimpfl, Martina, et al. "Modification of the fatty acid composition of an obesogenic diet improves the maternal and placental metabolic environment in obese pregnant mice." *Biochimica et Biophysica Acta (BBA)-Molecular Basis of Disease* 1863.6 (2017): 1605-1614.

[44] Chang, Chia-Yu, Der-Shin Ke, and Jen-Yin Chen. "Essential fatty acids and human brain." *Acta Neurol Taiwan* 18.4 (2009): 231-41.

[45] Chang, Chia-Yu, Der-Shin Ke, and Jen-Yin Chen. "Essential fatty acids and human brain." *Acta Neurol Taiwan* 18.4 (2009): 231-41.

[46] Herrera, Emilio. "Lipid metabolism in pregnancy and its consequences in the fetus and newborn." *Endocrine* 19.1 (2002): 43-55.

[47] Al, M. D., et al. "Fat intake of women during normal pregnancy: relationship with maternal and neonatal essential fatty acid status." *Journal of the American College of Nutrition* 15.1 (1996): 49-55.

[48] Sakayori, Nobuyuki, et al. "Maternal dietary imbalance between omega-6 and omega-3 polyunsaturated fatty acids impairs neocortical development via epoxy metabolites." *Stem Cells* 34.2 (2016): 470-482.

[49] Herrera, Emilio. "Lipid metabolism in pregnancy and its consequences in the fetus and newborn." *Endocrine* 19.1 (2002): 43-55.

[50] Kim, Hyejin, et al. "Association between maternal intake of n-6 to n-3 fatty acid ratio during pregnancy and infant neurodevelopment at 6 months of age: results of the MOCEH cohort study." *Nutrition journal* 16.1 (2017): 23.

[51] Candela, C. Gómez, LMa Bermejo López, and V. Loria Kohen. "Importance of a balanced omega 6/omega 3 ratio for the maintenance of health. Nutritional recommendations." *Nutricion hospitalaria* 26.2 (2011): 323-329.

[52] Price, Weston A. *Nutrition and Physical Degeneration A Comparison of Primitive and Modern Diets and Their Effects.* New York: Hoeber. 1939. Print.

[53] Daley, Cynthia A., et al. "A review of fatty acid profiles and antioxidant content in grass-fed and grain-fed beef." *Nutrition journal* 9.1 (2010): 10.

[54] Chavarro, J. E., et al. "A prospective study of dairy foods intake and anovulatory infertility." *Human Reproduction* 22.5 (2007): 1340-1347.

[55] Afeiche, M. C., et al. "Dairy intake in relation to in vitro fertilization outcomes among women from a fertility clinic." *Human Reproduction* 31.3 (2016): 563-571.

[56] Siri-Tarino, Patty W., et al. "Meta-analysis of prospective cohort studies evaluating the association of saturated fat with cardiovascular disease." *The American journal of clinical nutrition* (2010): ajcn-27725.

[57] Malhotra, Aseem, Rita F. Redberg, and Pascal Meier. "Saturated fat does not clog the arteries: coronary heart disease is a chronic inflammatory condition, the risk of which can be effectively reduced from healthy lifestyle interventions." (2017): bjsports-2016.

[58] Veerman, J. Lennert. "Dietary fats: a new look at old data challenges established wisdom." *The BMJ* 353 (2016).

[59] Hamley, Steven. "The effect of replacing saturated fat with mostly n-6 polyunsaturated fat on coronary heart disease: a meta-analysis of randomised controlled trials." *Nutrition journal* 16.1 (2017): 30.

[60] Brown, Melody J., et al. "Carotenoid bioavailability is higher from salads ingested with full-fat than with fat-reduced salad dressings as measured with electrochemical detection." *The American journal of clinical nutrition* 80.2 (2004): 396-403.

[61] Cooke, L., and A. Fildes. "The impact of flavour exposure in utero and during milk feeding on food acceptance at weaning and beyond." *Appetite* 57.3 (2011): 808-811.

[62] Montgomery, Kristen S. "Nutrition column an update on water needs during pregnancy and beyond." *The Journal of perinatal education* 11.3 (2002): 40.

[63] Popkin, Barry M., Kristen E. D'anci, and Irwin H. Rosenberg. "Water, hydration, and health." *Nutrition reviews* 68.8 (2010): 439-458.

[64] Scaife, Paula Juliet, and Markus Georg Mohaupt. "Salt, aldosterone and extrarenal Na+-sensitive responses in pregnancy." *Placenta* (2017).

[65] Ingram, M, and AG Kitchell. "Salt as a preservative for foods." *International Journal of Food Science & Technology* 2.1 (1967): 1-15.

[66] Gildea, John J et al. "A linear relationship between the ex-vivo sodium mediated expression of two sodium regulatory pathways as a surrogate marker of salt sensitivity of blood pressure in exfoliated human renal proximal tubule cells: the virtual renal biopsy." *Clinica Chimica Acta* 421 (2013): 236-242.

[67] Schoenaker, Danielle AJM, Sabita S. Soedamah-Muthu, and Gita D. Mishra. "The association between dietary factors and gestational hypertension and preeclampsia: a systematic review and meta-analysis of observational studies." *BMC medicine* 12.1 (2014): 157.

References

68 Sakuyama, Hiroe, et al. "Influence of gestational salt restriction in fetal growth and in development of diseases in adulthood." *Journal of biomedical science* 23.1 (2016): 12.

69 Guan J, Mao C, Feng X, Zhang H, Xu F, Geng C, et al. Fetal development of regulatory mechanisms for body fluid homeostasis. Brazil J Med Biol Res. 2008;41:446–54.

70 Iwaoka, T., et al. "The effect of low and high NaCl diets on oral glucose tolerance." *Journal of Molecular Medicine* 66.16 (1988): 724-728.

71 Klein, Alice Victoria, and Hosen Kiat. "The mechanisms underlying fructose-induced hypertension: a review." *Journal of hypertension* 33.5 (2015): 912-920.

72 Liebman, Michael. "When and why carbohydrate restriction can be a viable option." *Nutrition* 30.7 (2014): 748-754.

73 Hutchinson, A. D., et al. "Understanding maternal dietary choices during pregnancy: The role of social norms and mindful eating." *Appetite* 112 (2017): 227-234.

Chapter 3

1 Shaw, Gary M et al. "Periconceptional dietary intake of choline and betaine and neural tube defects in offspring." *American Journal of Epidemiology* 160.2 (2004): 102-109.

2 Jiang, Xinyin et al. "Maternal choline intake alters the epigenetic state of fetal cortisol-regulating genes in humans." *The FASEB Journal* 26.8 (2012): 3563-3574.

3 Zeisel, Steven H. "Nutritional importance of choline for brain development." *Journal of the American College of Nutrition* 23.sup6 (2004): 621S-626S.

4 Wallace, Taylor C., and Victor L. Fulgoni III. "Assessment of total choline intakes in the United States." *Journal of the American College of Nutrition* 35.2 (2016): 108-112.

5 Cohen, Joshua T., et al. "A quantitative analysis of prenatal intake of n-3 polyunsaturated fatty acids and cognitive development." *American Journal of Preventive Medicine* 29.4 (2005): 366-366.

6 West, Allyson A et al. "Choline intake influences phosphatidylcholine DHA enrichment in nonpregnant women but not in pregnant women in the third trimester." *The American Journal of Clinical Nutrition* 97.4 (2013): 718-727.

7 Thomas Rajarethnem, Huban, et al. "Combined Supplementation of Choline and Docosahexaenoic Acid during Pregnancy Enhances Neurodevelopment of Fetal Hippocampus." *Neurology research international* (2017).

8 Karsten, HD et al. "Vitamins A, E and fatty acid composition of the eggs of caged hens and pastured hens." *Renewable Agriculture and Food Systems* 25.01 (2010): 45-54.

9 Ratliff, Joseph et al. "Consuming eggs for breakfast influences plasma glucose and ghrelin, while reducing energy intake during the next 24 hours in adult men." *Nutrition Research* 30.2 (2010): 96-103.

10 Lemos, Bruno S., et al. "Consumption of up to Three Eggs per Day Increases Dietary Cholesterol and Choline while Plasma LDL Cholesterol and Trimethylamine N-oxide Concentrations Are Not Increased in a Young, Healthy Population." *The FASEB Journal* 31.1 Supplement (2017): 447-3.

11 Geiker, Nina Rica Wium, et al. "Egg consumption, cardiovascular diseases and type 2 diabetes." *European journal of clinical nutrition* (2017).

12 Kishimoto, Yoshimi, et al. "Additional consumption of one egg per day increases serum lutein plus zeaxanthin concentration and lowers oxidized low-density lipoprotein in moderately hypercholesterolemic males." *Food Research International* (2017).

13 Fernandez, Maria Luz, and Mariana Calle. "Revisiting dietary cholesterol recommendations: does the evidence support a limit of 300 mg/d?." *Current Atherosclerosis Reports* 12.6 (2010): 377-383.

14 Volek, Jeff S et al. "Carbohydrate restriction has a more favorable impact on the metabolic syndrome than a low fat diet." *Lipids* 44.4 (2009): 297-309.

15 Centers for Disease Control and Prevention (CDC). Surveillance for Foodborne Disease Outbreaks, United States, 2012, Annual Report. Atlanta, Georgia: US Department of Health and Human Services, CDC, 2014.

16 Painter, John A., et al. "Attribution of foodborne illnesses, hospitalizations, and deaths to food commodities by using outbreak data, United States, 1998–2008." *Emerging infectious diseases* 19.3 (2013): 407.

17 Alali, Walid Q et al. "Prevalence and distribution of Salmonella in organic and conventional broiler poultry farms." *Foodborne pathogens and disease* 7.11 (2010): 1363-1371.

18 Ebel, Eric, and Wayne Schlosser. "Estimating the annual fraction of eggs contaminated with Salmonella enteritidis in the United States." *International journal of food microbiology* 61.1 (2000): 51-62.

19 Wallace, Taylor C., and Victor L. Fulgoni. "Usual Choline Intakes Are Associated with Egg and Protein Food Consumption in the United States." *Nutrients* 9.8 (2017): 839.

20 Breymann, Christian. "Iron deficiency anemia in pregnancy." *Seminars in hematology*. Vol. 52. No. 4. WB Saunders, 2015.

21 Perez, Eva M., et al. "Mother-infant interactions and infant development are altered by maternal iron deficiency anemia." *The Journal of nutrition* 135.4 (2005): 850-855.

22 Greenberg, James A., and Stacey J. Bell. "Multivitamin supplementation during pregnancy: emphasis on folic acid and l-methylfolate." *Reviews in Obstetrics and Gynecology* 4.3-4 (2011): 126.

23 Molloy, Anne M et al. "Effects of folate and vitamin B12 deficiencies during pregnancy on fetal, infant, and child development." *Food & Nutrition Bulletin* 29.Supplement 1 (2008): 101-111.

[24] Rogne, Tormod, et al. "Associations of Maternal Vitamin B12 Concentration in Pregnancy With the Risks of Preterm Birth and Low Birth Weight: A Systematic Review and Meta-Analysis of Individual Participant Data." *American journal of epidemiology* (2017).

[25] Bae, Sajin, et al. "Vitamin B-12 status differs among pregnant, lactating, and control women with equivalent nutrient intakes." *The Journal of Nutrition* 145.7 (2015): 1507-1514.

[26] Masterjohn, Christopher. "Vitamin D toxicity redefined: vitamin K and the molecular mechanism." *Medical Hypotheses* 68.5 (2007): 1026-1034.

[27] Buss, NE et al. "The teratogenic metabolites of vitamin A in women following supplements and liver." *Human & Experimental Toxicology* 13.1 (1994): 33-43.

[28] Strobel, Manuela, Jana Tinz, and Hans-Konrad Biesalski. "The importance of β-carotene as a source of vitamin A with special regard to pregnant and breastfeeding women." *European Journal of Nutrition* 46.9 (2007): 1-20.

[29] National Institutes of Health. "Vitamin A — Health Professional Fact Sheet." (2016) https://ods.od.nih.gov/factsheets/VitaminA-HealthProfessional/. Accessed 6 Oct. 2017.

[30] Van den Berg, H., K. F. A. M. Hulshof, and J. P. Deslypere. "Evaluation of the effect of the use of vitamin supplements on vitamin A intake among (potentially) pregnant women in relation to the consumption of liver and liver products." *European Journal of Obstetrics & Gynecology and Reproductive Biology* 66.1 (1996): 17-21.

[31] Strobel, Manuela, Jana Tinz, and Hans-Konrad Biesalski. "The importance of β-carotene as a source of vitamin A with special regard to pregnant and breastfeeding women." *European Journal of Nutrition* 46.9 (2007): 1-20.

[32] Harrison, Earl H. "Mechanisms involved in the intestinal absorption of dietary vitamin A and provitamin A carotenoids." *Biochimica et Biophysica Acta (BBA)-Molecular and Cell Biology of Lipids* 1821.1 (2012): 70-77.

[33] Tang, Guangwen. "Bioconversion of dietary provitamin A carotenoids to vitamin A in humans." *The American Journal of Clinical Nutrition* 91.5 (2010): 1468S-1473S.

[34] Novotny, Janet A et al. "β-Carotene conversion to vitamin A decreases as the dietary dose increases in humans." *The Journal of Nutrition* 140.5 (2010): 915-918.

[35] van Stuijvenberg, Martha E., et al. "Serum retinol in 1–6-year-old children from a low socio-economic South African community with a high intake of liver: implications for blanket vitamin A supplementation." *Public health nutrition* 15.4 (2012): 716-724.

[36] Rodahl, K., and T. Moore. "The vitamin A content and toxicity of bear and seal liver." *Biochemical Journal* 37.2 (1943): 166.

[37] Hoffman, Jay R., and Michael J. Falvo. "Protein-Which is best." *Journal of Sports Science and Medicine* 3.3 (2004): 118-130.

[38] Foster, Meika, et al. "Zinc status of vegetarians during pregnancy: a systematic review of observational studies and meta-analysis of zinc intake." *Nutrients* 7.6 (2015): 4512-4525.

[39] Hunt, Janet R. "Bioavailability of iron, zinc, and other trace minerals from vegetarian diets." *The American Journal of Clinical Nutrition* 78.3 (2003): 633S-639S.

[40] Wang, Hua, et al. "Maternal zinc deficiency during pregnancy elevates the risks of fetal growth restriction: a population-based birth cohort study." *Scientific reports* 5 (2015).

[41] Morris, M.S.; Picciano, M.F.; Jacques, P.F.; Selhub, J. Plasma pyridoxal 5'-phosphate in the US population: The National Health and Nutrition Examination Survey, 2003–2004. Am. J. Clin. Nutr. 2008, 87, 1446–1454.

[42] Ho, Chia-ling, et al. "Prevalence and Predictors of Low Vitamin B6 Status in Healthy Young Adult Women in Metro Vancouver." *Nutrients* 8.9 (2016): 538.

[43] Godfrey, Keith, et al. "Maternal nutrition in early and late pregnancy in relation to placental and fetal growth." *Bmj* 312.7028 (1996): 410.

[44] Rees, William D, Fiona A Wilson, and Christopher A Maloney. "Sulfur amino acid metabolism in pregnancy: the impact of methionine in the maternal diet." *The Journal of Nutrition* 136.6 (2006): 1701S-1705S.

[45] Persaud, Chandarika et al. "The excretion of 5-oxoproline in urine, as an index of glycine status, during normal pregnancy." *BJOG: An International Journal of Obstetrics & Gynaecology* 96.4 (1989): 440-444.

[46] Morrione, Thomas G, and Sam Seifter. "Alteration in the collagen content of the human uterus during pregnancy and postpartum involution." *The Journal of Experimental Medicine* 115.2 (1962): 357-365.

[47] Aziz, Jazli, et al. "Molecular mechanisms of stress-responsive changes in collagen and elastin networks in skin." *Skin Pharmacology and Physiology* 29.4 (2016): 190-203.

[48] Dasarathy, Jaividhya et al. "Methionine metabolism in human pregnancy." *The American Journal of Clinical Nutrition* 91.2 (2010): 357-365.

[49] Rees, William D, Fiona A Wilson, and Christopher A Maloney. "Sulfur amino acid metabolism in pregnancy: the impact of methionine in the maternal diet." *The Journal of Nutrition* 136.6 (2006): 1701S-1705S.

[50] Jackson, Alan A., Michael C. Marchand, and Simon C. Langley-Evans. "Increased systolic blood pressure in rats induced by a maternal low-protein diet is reversed by dietary supplementation with glycine." *Clinical Science* 103.6 (2002): 633-639.

[51] Rees, William D. "Manipulating the sulfur amino acid content of the early diet and its implications for long-term health." *Proceedings of the Nutrition Society* 61.01 (2002): 71-77.

References

[52] El Hafidi, Mohammed, Israel Perez, and Guadalupe Banos. "Is glycine effective against elevated blood pressure?." (2006): 26-31.

[53] Austdal, Marie, et al. "Metabolomic biomarkers in serum and urine in women with preeclampsia." *PloS one* 9.3 (2014): e91923.

[54] Friesen, Russell W et al. "Relationship of dimethylglycine, choline, and betaine with oxoproline in plasma of pregnant women and their newborn infants." *The Journal of Nutrition* 137.12 (2007): 2641-2646.

[55] Kalhan, Satish C. "One-carbon metabolism, fetal growth and long-term consequences." *Maternal and Child Nutrition: The First 1,000 Days.* Vol. 74. Karger Publishers, 2013. 127-138.

[56] Leite, Isabel Cristina Gonçalves, Francisco José Roma Paumgartten, and Sérgio Koifman. "Chemical exposure during pregnancy and oral clefts in newborns." *Cadernos de saude publica* 18.1 (2002): 17-31.

[57] Brown, Melody J et al. "Carotenoid bioavailability is higher from salads ingested with full-fat than with fat-reduced salad dressings as measured with electrochemical detection." *The American Journal of Clinical Nutrition* 80.2 (2004): 396-403.

[58] Fabbri, Adriana DT, and Guy A. Crosby. "A review of the impact of preparation and cooking on the nutritional quality of vegetables and legumes." *International Journal of Gastronomy and Food Science* 3 (2016): 2-11.

[59] Baker, Brian P., et al. "Pesticide residues in conventional, integrated pest management (IPM)-grown and organic foods: insights from three US data sets." *Food Additives & Contaminants* 19.5 (2002): 427-446.

[60] Ralston, Nicholas VC, and Laura J Raymond. "Dietary selenium's protective effects against methylmercury toxicity." *Toxicology* 278.1 (2010): 112-123.

[61] Hibbeln, Joseph R., et al. "Maternal seafood consumption in pregnancy and neurodevelopmental outcomes in childhood (ALSPAC study): an observational cohort study." *The Lancet* 369.9561 (2007): 578-585.

[62] Burger, Joanna, and Michael Gochfeld. "Mercury and selenium levels in 19 species of saltwater fish from New Jersey as a function of species, size, and season." *Science of the Total Environment* 409.8 (2011): 1418-1429.

[63] Bodnar, Lisa M et al. "High prevalence of vitamin D insufficiency in black and white pregnant women residing in the northern United States and their neonates." *The Journal of Nutrition* 137.2 (2007): 447-452.

[64] Zimmermann, Michael B. "The effects of iodine deficiency in pregnancy and infancy." *Paediatric and Perinatal Epidemiology* 26.s1 (2012): 108-117.

[65] Stagnaro-Green, Alex, Scott Sullivan, and Elizabeth N Pearce. "Iodine supplementation during pregnancy and lactation." *JAMA* 308.23 (2012): 2463-2464.

[66] Mozaffarian, Dariush, and Eric B Rimm. "Fish intake, contaminants, and human health: evaluating the risks and the benefits." *JAMA* 296.15 (2006): 1885-1899.

[67] Cabello, Felipe C., et al. "Aquaculture as yet another environmental gateway to the development and globalisation of antimicrobial resistance." *The Lancet Infectious Diseases* 16.7 (2016): e127-e133.

[68] Conti, Gea Oliveri, et al. "Determination of illegal antimicrobials in aquaculture feed and fish: an ELISA study." *Food Control* 50 (2015): 937-941.

[69] Hossain, M. A. "Fish as source of n-3 polyunsaturated fatty acids (PUFAs), which one is better-farmed or wild?." *Advance Journal of Food Science and Technology* 3.6 (2011): 455-466.

[70] Tsuchie, Hiroyuki et al. "Amelioration of pregnancy-associated osteoporosis after treatment with vitamin K2: a report of four patients." *Upsala Journal of Medical Sciences* 117.3 (2012): 336-341.

[71] Choi, Hyung Jin et al. "Vitamin K2 supplementation improves insulin sensitivity via osteocalcin metabolism: a placebo-controlled trial." *Diabetes Care* 34.9 (2011): e147-e147.

[72] "Iodine — Health Professional Fact Sheet - Office of Dietary Supplements." National Institutes of Health. 24 Jun. 2011, https://ods.od.nih.gov/factsheets/Iodine-HealthProfessional/. Accessed 13 Jun. 2017.

[73] Bertelsen, Randi J et al. "Probiotic milk consumption in pregnancy and infancy and subsequent childhood allergic diseases." *Journal of Allergy and Clinical Immunology* 133.1 (2014): 165-171. e8.

[74] Myhre, Ronny et al. "Intake of probiotic food and risk of spontaneous preterm delivery." *The American Journal of Clinical Nutrition* 93.1 (2011): 151-157.

[75] Cordain, Loren, et al. "Plant-animal subsistence ratios and macronutrient energy estimations in worldwide hunter-gatherer diets." *The American journal of clinical nutrition* 71.3 (2000): 682-692.

[76] Price, Weston A. *Nutrition and Physical Degeneration A Comparison of Primitive and Modern Diets and Their Effects.* New York: Hoeber. 1939. Print.

[77] Chmurzynska, Agata. "Fetal programming: link between early nutrition, DNA methylation, and complex diseases." *Nutrition Reviews* 68.2 (2010): 87-98.

[78] Molloy, Anne M et al. "Effects of folate and vitamin B12 deficiencies during pregnancy on fetal, infant, and child development." *Food & Nutrition Bulletin* 29.Supplement 1 (2008): 101-111.

[79] Rogne, Tormod, et al. "Associations of Maternal Vitamin B12 Concentration in Pregnancy With the Risks of Preterm Birth and Low Birth Weight: A Systematic Review and Meta-Analysis of Individual Participant Data." *American Journal of Epidemiology* (2017).

[80] Pawlak, Roman, et al. "How prevalent is vitamin B12 deficiency among vegetarians?." *Nutrition reviews* 71.2 (2013): 110-117.

[81] Koebnick, Corinna, et al. "Long-term ovo-lacto vegetarian diet impairs vitamin B-12 status in pregnant women." *The Journal of nutrition* 134.12 (2004): 3319-3326.

Real Food for Pregnancy

[82] Smulders, Y. M., et al. "Cellular folate vitamer distribution during and after correction of vitamin B12 deficiency: a case for the methylfolate trap." *British journal of haematology* 132.5 (2006): 623-629.

[83] Bae, Sajin, et al. "Vitamin B-12 status differs among pregnant, lactating, and control women with equivalent nutrient intakes." *The Journal of Nutrition* 145.7 (2015): 1507-1514.

[84] Black, Maureen M. "Effects of vitamin B12 and folate deficiency on brain development in children." *Food and nutrition bulletin* 29.2_suppl1 (2008): S126-S131.

[85] "The ethical case for eating oysters and mussels | Diana Fleischman." 20 May. 2013, https://sentientist.org/2013/05/20/the-ethical-case-for-eating-oysters-and-mussels/. Accessed 31 Jul. 2017.

[86] Zeisel SH. Nutrition in pregnancy: the argument for including a source of choline. *Int J Womens Health.* 2013;5:193-199.

[87] Wallace, Taylor C., and Victor L. Fulgoni. "Usual Choline Intakes Are Associated with Egg and Protein Food Consumption in the United States." *Nutrients* 9.8 (2017): 839.

[88] Davenport, Crystal, et al. "Choline intakes exceeding recommendations during human lactation improve breast milk choline content by increasing PEMT pathway metabolites." *The Journal of nutritional biochemistry* 26.9 (2015): 903-911.

[89] Jiang, Xinyin, et al. "Maternal choline intake alters the epigenetic state of fetal cortisol-regulating genes in humans." *The FASEB Journal* 26.8 (2012): 3563-3574.

[90] Jiang, Xinyin, et al. "A higher maternal choline intake among third-trimester pregnant women lowers placental and circulating concentrations of the antiangiogenic factor fms-like tyrosine kinase-1 (sFLT1)." *The FASEB Journal* 27.3 (2013): 1245-1253.

[91] Caudill, Marie A., et al. "Maternal choline supplementation during the third trimester of pregnancy improves infant information processing speed: a randomized, double-blind, controlled feeding study." *The FASEB Journal* (2017): fj-201700692RR.

[92] Ganz, Ariel B., et al. "Genetic impairments in folate enzymes increase dependence on dietary choline for phosphatidylcholine production at the expense of betaine synthesis." *The FASEB Journal* 30.10 (2016): 3321-3333.

[93] Meléndez-Hevia, Enrique, et al. "A weak link in metabolism: the metabolic capacity for glycine biosynthesis does not satisfy the need for collagen synthesis." *Journal of biosciences* 34.6 (2009): 853-872.

[94] Lewis, Rohan M., et al. "Low serine hydroxymethyltransferase activity in the human placenta has important implications for fetal glycine supply." *The Journal of Clinical Endocrinology & Metabolism* 90.3 (2005): 1594-1598.

[95] Lewis, Rohan M., et al. "Low serine hydroxymethyltransferase activity in the human placenta has important implications for fetal glycine supply." *The Journal of Clinical Endocrinology & Metabolism* 90.3 (2005): 1594-1598.

[96] Meléndez-Hevia, Enrique, et al. "A weak link in metabolism: the metabolic capacity for glycine biosynthesis does not satisfy the need for collagen synthesis." *Journal of biosciences* 34.6 (2009): 853-872.

[97] Meléndez-Hevia, Enrique, et al. "A weak link in metabolism: the metabolic capacity for glycine biosynthesis does not satisfy the need for collagen synthesis." *Journal of biosciences* 34.6 (2009): 853-872.

[98] Solomons NW. Vitamin A and carotenoids. In: Bowman BA, Russell RM, eds. *Present Knowledge in Nutrition.* Washington, D.C.: ILSI Press; 2001:127-145.

[99] Ross AC. Vitamin A and retinoids. In: Shils ME, Olson JA, Shike M, Ross AC, eds. *Modern Nutrition in Health and Disease.* Baltimore: Lippincott Williams & Wilkins; 1999:305-327.

[100] Novotny, Janet A et al. "β-Carotene conversion to vitamin A decreases as the dietary dose increases in humans." *The Journal of Nutrition* 140.5 (2010): 915-918.

[101] Elder, Sonya J., et al. "Vitamin K contents of meat, dairy, and fast food in the US diet." *Journal of agricultural and food chemistry* 54.2 (2006): 463-467.

[102] Maresz, Katarzyna. "Proper calcium use: vitamin K2 as a promoter of bone and cardiovascular health." *Integrative Medicine: A Clinician's Journal* 14.1 (2015): 34.

[103] Innis, Sheila M. "Dietary (n-3) fatty acids and brain development." *The Journal of Nutrition* 137.4 (2007): 855-859.

[104] Singh, Meharban. "Essential fatty acids, DHA and human brain." *The Indian Journal of Pediatrics* 72.3 (2005): 239-242.

[105] Gerster, H. "Can adults adequately convert alpha-linolenic acid (18: 3n-3) to eicosapentaenoic acid (20: 5n-3) and docosahexaenoic acid (22: 6n-3)?." *International Journal for Vitamin and Nutrition Research.* 68.3 (1997): 159-173.

[106] Creighton, C. "Vegetarian diets in pregnancy: RD resources for consumers." *Vegetarian Nutrition DPG of the Academy of Nutrition and Dietetics* (2010). Available at: https://vegetariannutrition.net/docs/Pregnancy-Vegetarian-Nutrition.pdf

[107] Kim, Hyejin, et al. "Association between maternal intake of n-6 to n-3 fatty acid ratio during pregnancy and infant neurodevelopment at 6 months of age: results of the MOCEH cohort study." *Nutrition journal* 16.1 (2017): 23.

[108] Sakayori, Nobuyuki, et al. "Maternal dietary imbalance between omega-6 and omega-3 polyunsaturated fatty acids impairs neocortical development via epoxy metabolites." *Stem Cells* 34.2 (2016): 470-482.

[109] Sanders, T. A., Frey R. Ellis, and J. W. Dickerson. "Studies of vegans: the fatty acid composition of plasma choline phosphoglycerides, erythrocytes, adipose tissue, and breast milk, and some indicators of susceptibility to ischemic heart disease in vegans and omnivore controls." *The American journal of clinical nutrition* 31.5 (1978): 805-813.

[110] Sanders, Thomas AB. "DHA status of vegetarians." *Prostaglandins, Leukotrienes and Essential Fatty Acids* 81.2 (2009): 137-141.

[111] dos Santos Vaz, Juliana, et al. "Dietary patterns, n-3 fatty acids intake from seafood and high levels of anxiety symptoms during pregnancy: findings from the Avon Longitudinal Study of Parents and Children." *PLoS One* 8.7 (2013): e67671.

[112] da Rocha, Camilla MM, and Gilberto Kac. "High dietary ratio of omega-6 to omega-3 polyunsaturated acids during pregnancy and prevalence of postpartum depression." *Maternal & child nutrition* 8.1 (2012): 36-48.

[113] Marangoni, Franca, et al. "Maternal Diet and Nutrient Requirements in Pregnancy and Breastfeeding. An Italian Consensus Document." *Nutrients* 8.10 (2016): 629.

[114] Hurrell, Richard F., et al. "Degradation of phytic acid in cereal porridges improves iron absorption by human subjects." *The American Journal of Clinical Nutrition* 77.5 (2003): 1213-1219.

[115] Haddad, Ella H., et al. "Dietary intake and biochemical, hematologic, and immune status of vegans compared with nonvegetarians." *The American journal of clinical nutrition* 70.3 (1999): 586s-593s.

[116] Hunt, Janet R. "Bioavailability of iron, zinc, and other trace minerals from vegetarian diets." *The American Journal of Clinical Nutrition* 78.3 (2003): 633S-639S.

[117] Breymann, Christian. "Iron deficiency anemia in pregnancy." *Seminars in hematology*. Vol. 52. No. 4. WB Saunders, 2015.

[118] Breymann, Christian. "Iron deficiency anemia in pregnancy." *Seminars in hematology*. Vol. 52. No. 4. WB Saunders, 2015.

[119] Hunt, Janet R. "Bioavailability of iron, zinc, and other trace minerals from vegetarian diets." *The American Journal of Clinical Nutrition* 78.3 (2003): 633S-639S.

[120] Schüpbach, R., et al. "Micronutrient status and intake in omnivores, vegetarians and vegans in Switzerland." *European journal of nutrition* 56.1 (2017): 283-293.

[121] Wang, Hua, et al. "Maternal zinc deficiency during pregnancy elevates the risks of fetal growth restriction: a population-based birth cohort study." *Scientific reports* 5 (2015).

[122] Uriu-Adams, Janet Y., and Carl L. Keen. "Zinc and reproduction: effects of zinc deficiency on prenatal and early postnatal development." *Birth Defects Research Part B: Developmental and Reproductive Toxicology* 89.4 (2010): 313-325.

[123] Hunt, Janet R. "Bioavailability of iron, zinc, and other trace minerals from vegetarian diets." *The American Journal of Clinical Nutrition* 78.3 (2003): 633S-639S.

[124] Gibson, Rosalind S., Leah Perlas, and Christine Hotz. "Improving the bioavailability of nutrients in plant foods at the household level." *Proceedings of the Nutrition Society* 65.2 (2006): 160-168.

[125] Gilani, G. Sarwar, Kevin A. Cockell, and Estatira Sepehr. "Effects of antinutritional factors on protein digestibility and amino acid availability in foods." *Journal of AOAC International* 88.3 (2005): 967-987.

[126] Janelle, K. Christina, and Susan I. Barr. "Nutrient intakes and eating behavior see of vegetarian and nonvegetarian women." *Journal of the American Dietetic Association* 95.2 (1995): 180-189.

[127] Haddad, Ella H., and Jay S. Tanzman. "What do vegetarians in the United States eat?." *The American journal of clinical nutrition* 78.3 (2003): 626S-632S.

[128] "The ethical case for eating oysters and mussels | Diana Fleischman." 20 May. 2013, https://sentientist.org/2013/05/20/the-ethical-case-for-eating-oysters-and-mussels/. Accessed 31 Jul. 2017.

[129] Lopez, Hubert W., et al. "Making bread with sourdough improves mineral bioavailability from reconstituted whole wheat flour in rats." *Nutrition* 19.6 (2003): 524-530.

[130] Hurrell, Richard F., et al. "Degradation of phytic acid in cereal porridges improves iron absorption by human subjects." *The American Journal of Clinical Nutrition* 77.5 (2003): 1213-1219.

Chapter 4

[1] Janakiraman, Vanitha. "Listeriosis in pregnancy: diagnosis, treatment, and prevention." *Rev Obstet Gynecol* 1.4 (2008): 179-85.

[2] Pezdirc, Kristine B., et al. "Listeria monocytogenes and diet during pregnancy; balancing nutrient intake adequacy v. adverse pregnancy outcomes." *Public health nutrition* 15.12 (2012): 2202-2209.

[3] Einarson, Adrienne, et al. "Food-borne illnesses during pregnancy." *Canadian Family Physician* 56.9 (2010): 869-870.

[4] Tam, Carolyn, Aida Erebara, and Adrienne Einarson. "Food-borne illnesses during pregnancy Prevention and treatment." *Canadian Family Physician* 56.4 (2010): 341-343.

[5] Ebel, Eric, and Wayne Schlosser. "Estimating the annual fraction of eggs contaminated with Salmonella enteritidis in the United States." *International journal of food microbiology* 61.1 (2000): 51-62.

[6] Alali, Walid Q et al. "Prevalence and distribution of Salmonella in organic and conventional broiler poultry farms." *Foodborne pathogens and disease* 7.11 (2010): 1363-1371.

Real Food for Pregnancy

[7] Bloomingdale, Arienne, et al. "A qualitative study of fish consumption during pregnancy." *The American Journal of Clinical Nutrition* 92.5 (2010): 1234-1240.

[8] Bloomingdale, Arienne, et al. "A qualitative study of fish consumption during pregnancy." *The American Journal of Clinical Nutrition* 92.5 (2010): 1234-1240.

[9] Ito, Misae, and Nancy C. Sharts-Hopko. "Japanese women's experience of childbirth in the United States." *Health care for women International* 23.6-7 (2002): 666-677.

[10] "Is it safe to eat sushi during pregnancy? - Health questions - NHS ...." http://www.nhs.uk/chq/Pages/is-it-safe-to-eat-sushi-during-pregnancy.aspx. Accessed 11 Feb. 2017.

[11] Tam, Carolyn, Aida Erebara, and Adrienne Einarson. "Food-borne illnesses during pregnancy Prevention and treatment." *Canadian Family Physician* 56.4 (2010): 341-343.

[12] Laird, Brian D., and Hing Man Chan. "Bioaccessibility of metals in fish, shellfish, wild game, and seaweed harvested in British Columbia, Canada." *Food and chemical toxicology* 58 (2013): 381-387.

[13] Costa, Sara, et al. "Fatty acids, mercury, and methylmercury bioaccessibility in salmon (Salmo salar) using an in vitro model: effect of culinary treatment." *Food chemistry* 185 (2015): 268-276.

[14] Harrison, Michael, et al. "Nature and availability of iodine in fish." *The American journal of clinical nutrition* 17.2 (1965): 73-77.

[15] Conti, Gea Oliveri, et al. "Determination of illegal antimicrobials in aquaculture feed and fish: an ELISA study." *Food Control* 50 (2015): 937-941.

[16] Iwamoto, Martha, et al. "Epidemiology of seafood-associated infections in the United States." *Clinical Microbiology Reviews* 23.2 (2010): 399-411.

[17] Centers for Disease Control and Prevention (CDC. "Vital signs: Listeria illnesses, deaths, and outbreaks--United States, 2009-2011." *MMWR. Morbidity and mortality weekly report* 62.22 (2013): 448.

[18] "Outbreaks Involving Salmonella | CDC." 28 Nov. 2016, http://www.cdc.gov/salmonella/outbreaks.html.

[19] D'amico, D. J., and C. W. Donnelly. "Microbiological quality of raw milk used for small-scale artisan cheese production in Vermont: effect of farm characteristics and practices." *Journal of dairy science* 93.1 (2010): 134-147.

[20] Painter, John A., et al. "Attribution of foodborne illnesses, hospitalizations, and deaths to food commodities by using outbreak data, United States, 1998–2008." *Emerging infectious diseases* 19.3 (2013): 407.

[21] Painter, John A., et al. "Attribution of foodborne illnesses, hospitalizations, and deaths to food commodities by using outbreak data, United States, 1998–2008." *Emerging infectious diseases* 19.3 (2013): 407.

[22] Sivapalasingam, Sumathi, et al. "Fresh produce: a growing cause of outbreaks of foodborne illness in the United States, 1973 through 1997." *Journal of food protection* 67.10 (2004): 2342-2353.

[23] Tam, Carolyn, Aida Erebara, and Adrienne Einarson. "Food-borne illnesses during pregnancy Prevention and treatment." *Canadian Family Physician* 56.4 (2010): 341-343.

[24] Harris, L. J., et al. "Outbreaks associated with fresh produce: incidence, growth, and survival of pathogens in fresh and fresh-cut produce." *Comprehensive reviews in food science and food safety* 2.s1 (2003): 78-141.

[25] Centers for Disease Control and Prevention (CDC). Surveillance for Foodborne Disease Outbreaks, United States, 2012, Annual Report. Atlanta, Georgia: US Department of Health and Human Services, CDC, 2014.

[26] Schley, P. D., and C. J. Field. "The immune-enhancing effects of dietary fibres and prebiotics." *British Journal of Nutrition* 87.S2 (2002): S221-S230.

[27] Sanchez, Albert, et al. "Role of sugars in human neutrophilic phagocytosis." *The American journal of clinical nutrition* 26.11 (1973): 1180-1184.

[28] Alali, Walid Q et al. "Prevalence and distribution of Salmonella in organic and conventional broiler poultry farms." *Foodborne pathogens and disease* 7.11 (2010): 1363-1371.

[29] Berge, Anna C., et al. "Geographic, farm, and animal factors associated with multiple antimicrobial resistance in fecal Escherichia coli isolates from cattle in the western United States." *Journal of the American Veterinary Medical Association* 236.12 (2010): 1338-1344.

[30] D'amico, D. J., and C. W. Donnelly. "Microbiological quality of raw milk used for small-scale artisan cheese production in Vermont: effect of farm characteristics and practices." *Journal of dairy science* 93.1 (2010): 134-147.

[31] Wilhoit, Lauren F., David A. Scott, and Brooke A. Simecka. "Fetal Alcohol Spectrum Disorders: Characteristics, Complications, and Treatment." *Community Mental Health Journal* (2017): 1-8.

[32] Sood, Beena, et al. "Prenatal alcohol exposure and childhood behavior at age 6 to 7 years: I. dose-response effect." *Pediatrics* 108.2 (2001): e34-e34.

[33] Flak, Audrey L., et al. "The association of mild, moderate, and binge prenatal alcohol exposure and child neuropsychological outcomes: a meta-analysis." *Alcoholism: Clinical and Experimental Research* 38.1 (2014): 214-226.

[34] Robinson, Marc, et al. "Low–moderate prenatal alcohol exposure and risk to child behavioural development: a prospective cohort study." *BJOG: An International Journal of Obstetrics & Gynaecology* 117.9 (2010): 1139-1152.

[35] O'Callaghan, Frances V., et al. "Prenatal alcohol exposure and attention, learning and intellectual ability at 14 years: a prospective longitudinal study." *Early human development* 83.2 (2007): 115-123.

36 O'Keeffe, Linda M., Richard A. Greene, and Patricia M. Kearney. "The effect of moderate gestational alcohol consumption during pregnancy on speech and language outcomes in children: a systematic review." *Systematic reviews* 3.1 (2014): 1.

37 O'Keeffe, Linda M., Richard A. Greene, and Patricia M. Kearney. "The effect of moderate gestational alcohol consumption during pregnancy on speech and language outcomes in children: a systematic review." *Systematic Reviews* 3.1 (2014): 1.

38 Uriu-Adams, Janet Y., and Carl L. Keen. "Zinc and reproduction: effects of zinc deficiency on prenatal and early postnatal development." *Birth Defects Research Part B: Developmental and Reproductive Toxicology* 89.4 (2010): 313-325.

39 Zeisel, Steven H. "What choline metabolism can tell us about the underlying mechanisms of fetal alcohol spectrum disorders." *Molecular neurobiology* 44.2 (2011): 185-191.

40 Dudley, Robert. "Ethanol, fruit ripening, and the historical origins of human alcoholism in primate frugivory." *Integrative and Comparative Biology* 44.4 (2004): 315-323.

41 Chen, Ling-Wei, et al. "Maternal caffeine intake during pregnancy is associated with risk of low birth weight: a systematic review and dose-response meta-analysis." *BMC medicine* 12.1 (2014): 174.

42 Chen, Ling-Wei, et al. "Maternal caffeine intake during pregnancy is associated with risk of low birth weight: a systematic review and dose-response meta-analysis." *BMC medicine* 12.1 (2014): 174.

43 American College of Obstetricians and Gynecologists. "Moderate caffeine consumption during pregnancy. ACOG Committee Opinion No. 462." *Obstetrics and Gynecology* 116.2 (2010): 467-468.

44 Greenwood, Darren C., et al. "Caffeine intake during pregnancy and adverse birth outcomes: a systematic review and dose–response meta-analysis." *European Journal of Epidemiology* 29.10 (2014): 725-734.

45 Chen, Lei, et al. "Exploring Maternal Patterns Of Dietary Caffeine Consumption Before Conception And During Pregnancy." *Maternal & Child Health Journal* 18.10 (2014): 2446-2455. *CINAHL Plus with Full Text.* Web. 26 Jan. 2017.

46 Goletzke, Janina, et al. "Dietary micronutrient intake during pregnancy is a function of carbohydrate quality." *The American Journal of Clinical Nutrition* 102.3 (2015): 626-632.

47 Cordain, Loren, et al. "Origins and evolution of the Western diet: health implications for the 21st century." *The American Journal of Clinical Nutrition* 81.2 (2005): 341-354.

48 Cordain, Loren, et al. "Origins and evolution of the Western diet: health implications for the 21st century." *The American Journal of Clinical Nutrition* 81.2 (2005): 341-354.

49 Korem, Tal, et al. "Bread Affects Clinical Parameters and Induces Gut Microbiome-Associated Personal Glycemic Responses." *Cell Metabolism* 25.6 (2017): 1243-1253.

50 Czaja-Bulsa, Grażyna. "Non coeliac gluten sensitivity–A new disease with gluten intolerance." *Clinical Nutrition* 34.2 (2015): 189-194.

51 Quero, JC Salazar, et al. "Nutritional assessment of gluten-free diet. Is gluten-free diet deficient in some nutrient?." *Anales de Pediatría (English Edition)* 83.1 (2015): 33-39.

52 Clapp III, James F. "Maternal carbohydrate intake and pregnancy outcome." *Proceedings of the Nutrition Society* 61.01 (2002): 45-50.

53 Zhang, Cuilin, and Yi Ning. "Effect of dietary and lifestyle factors on the risk of gestational diabetes: review of epidemiologic evidence." *The American journal of clinical nutrition* 94.6 Suppl (2011): 1975S-1979S.

54 Bédard, Annabelle, et al. "Maternal intake of sugar during pregnancy and childhood respiratory and atopic outcomes." *European Respiratory Journal* 50.1 (2017): 1700073.

55 Wiss, David A., et al. "Preclinical evidence for the addiction potential of highly palatable foods: Current developments related to maternal influence." *Appetite* 115 (2017): 19-27.

56 Choi, Chang Soon, et al. "High sucrose consumption during pregnancy induced ADHD-like behavioral phenotypes in mice offspring." *The Journal of nutritional biochemistry* 26.12 (2015): 1520-1526.

57 Yang, Qing. "Gain weight by "going diet?" Artificial sweeteners and the neurobiology of sugar cravings: Neuroscience 2010." *The Yale Journal of Biology and Medicine* 83.2 (2010): 101.

58 Suez, Jotham et al. "Artificial sweeteners induce glucose intolerance by altering the gut microbiota." *Nature* 514.7521 (2014): 181-186.

59 Abou-Donia, Mohamed B et al. "Splenda alters gut microflora and increases intestinal p-glycoprotein and cytochrome p-450 in male rats." *Journal of Toxicology and Environmental Health, Part A* 71.21 (2008): 1415-1429.

60 Pałkowska-Goździk, Ewelina, Anna Bigos, and Danuta Rosołowska-Huszcz. "Type of sweet flavour carrier affects thyroid axis activity in male rats." *European journal of nutrition* (2016): 1-10.

61 Zhu, Yeyi, et al. "Maternal consumption of artificially sweetened beverages during pregnancy, and offspring growth through 7 years of age: a prospective cohort study." *International Journal of Epidemiology* (2017).

62 Zhu, Yeyi, et al. "Maternal consumption of artificially sweetened beverages during pregnancy, and offspring growth through 7 years of age: a prospective cohort study." *International Journal of Epidemiology* (2017).

63 Mohd-Radzman, Nabilatul Hani, et al. "Potential roles of Stevia rebaudiana Bertoni in abrogating insulin resistance and diabetes: a review." *Evidence-Based Complementary and Alternative Medicine* 2013 (2013).

Real Food for Pregnancy

[64] Simopoulos, A. P., and J. J. DiNicolantonio. "The importance of a balanced ω-6 to ω-3 ratio in the prevention and management of obesity." *Open Heart* 3.2 (2016): e000385.

[65] Al-Gubory, K. H., P. A. Fowler, and C. Garrel. "The roles of cellular reactive oxygen species, oxidative stress and antioxidants in pregnancy outcomes." *The international journal of biochemistry & cell biology* 42.10 (2010): 1634-1650.

[66] Donahue, S. M. A., et al. "Associations of maternal prenatal dietary intake of n-3 and n-6 fatty acids with maternal and umbilical cord blood levels." *Prostaglandins, Leukotrienes and Essential Fatty Acids* 80.5 (2009): 289-296.

[67] Candela, C. Gómez, LMa Bermejo López, and V. Loria Kohen. "Importance of a balanced omega 6/omega 3 ratio for the maintenance of health. Nutritional recommendations." *Nutricion hospitalaria* 26.2 (2011): 323-329.

[68] Simopoulos, A. P. "Evolutionary aspects of diet, the omega-6/omega-3 ratio and genetic variation: nutritional implications for chronic diseases." *Biomedicine & pharmacotherapy* 60.9 (2006): 502-507.

[69] Coletta, Jaclyn M., Stacey J. Bell, and Ashley S. Roman. "Omega-3 fatty acids and pregnancy." *Reviews in Obstetrics and Gynecology* 3.4 (2010): 163.

[70] Strain, J. J., et al. "Associations of maternal long-chain polyunsaturated fatty acids, methyl mercury, and infant development in the Seychelles Child Development Nutrition Study." *Neurotoxicology* 29.5 (2008): 776-782.

[71] Kim, Hyejin, et al. "Association between maternal intake of n-6 to n-3 fatty acid ratio during pregnancy and infant neurodevelopment at 6 months of age: results of the MOCEH cohort study." *Nutrition journal* 16.1 (2017): 23.

[72] Moon, R. J., et al. "Maternal plasma polyunsaturated fatty acid status in late pregnancy is associated with offspring body composition in childhood." *The Journal of Clinical Endocrinology & Metabolism* 98.1 (2012): 299-307.

[73] Muhlhausler, Beverly S., and Gérard P. Ailhaud. "Omega-6 polyunsaturated fatty acids and the early origins of obesity." *Current Opinion in Endocrinology, Diabetes and Obesity* 20.1 (2013): 56-61.

[74] Innis, Sheila M. "Trans fatty intakes during pregnancy, infancy and early childhood." *Atherosclerosis Supplements* 7.2 (2006): 17-20.

[75] Micha, Renata, and Dariush Mozaffarian. "Trans fatty acids: effects on metabolic syndrome, heart disease and diabetes." *Nature Reviews Endocrinology* 5.6 (2009): 335-344.

[76] Grootendorst-van Mil, Nina H., et al. "Maternal Midpregnancy Plasma trans 18: 1 Fatty Acid Concentrations Are Positively Associated with Risk of Maternal Vascular Complications and Child Low Birth Weight." *The Journal of Nutrition* 147.3 (2017): 398-403.

[77] Morrison, John A, Charles J Glueck, and Ping Wang. "Dietary trans fatty acid intake is associated with increased fetal loss." *Fertility and Sterility* 90.2 (2008): 385-390.

[78] Carlson, Susan E., et al. "trans Fatty acids: infant and fetal development." *The American journal of clinical nutrition* 66.3 (1997): 717S-736S.

[79] Ferlay, Anne, et al. "Production of trans and conjugated fatty acids in dairy ruminants and their putative effects on human health: A review." *Biochimie* (2017).

[80] Daley, Cynthia A., et al. "A review of fatty acid profiles and antioxidant content in grass-fed and grain-fed beef." *Nutrition journal* 9.1 (2010): 10.

[81] Lopez, H. Walter, et al. "Minerals and phytic acid interactions: is it a real problem for human nutrition?." *International Journal of Food Science & Technology* 37.7 (2002): 727-739.

[82] Egounlety, M., and O. C. Aworh. "Effect of soaking, dehulling, cooking and fermentation with Rhizopus oligosporus on the oligosaccharides, trypsin inhibitor, phytic acid and tannins of soybean (Glycine max Merr.), cowpea (Vigna unguiculata L. Walp) and groundbean (Macrotyloma geocarpa Harms)." *Journal of Food Engineering* 56.2 (2003): 249-254.

[83] Anderson, Robert L., and Walter J. Wolf. "Compositional changes in trypsin inhibitors, phytic acid, sa." *The Journal of nutrition* 125.3 (1995): S581.

[84] Pearce, Elizabeth N. "Iodine in Pregnancy: Is Salt Iodization Enough?." *J Clin Endocrinol Metab* 93.7 (2008): 2466-2468.

[85] Korevaar, Tim IM, et al. "Association of maternal thyroid function during early pregnancy with offspring IQ and brain morphology in childhood: a population-based prospective cohort study." *The Lancet Diabetes & Endocrinology* 4.1 (2016): 35-43.

[86] Pearce, Elizabeth N. "Iodine in Pregnancy: Is Salt Iodization Enough?." *J Clin Endocrinol Metab* 93.7 (2008): 2466-2468.

[87] Caldwell KL, Makhmudov A, Ely E, Jones RL, Wang RY. Iodine status of the U.S. population, National Health and Nutrition Examination Survey, 2005-2006 and 2007-2008. *Thyroid* 21 (2011): 419–427.

[88] Pearce, Elizabeth N. "Iodine in Pregnancy: Is Salt Iodization Enough?." *J Clin Endocrinol Metab* 93.7 (2008): 2466-2468.

[89] Korevaar, Tim IM, et al. "Association of maternal thyroid function during early pregnancy with offspring IQ and brain morphology in childhood: a population-based prospective cohort study." *The Lancet Diabetes & Endocrinology* 4.1 (2016): 35-43.

[90] Cederroth, Christopher Robin, Céline Zimmermann, and Serge Nef. "Soy, phytoestrogens and their impact on reproductive health." *Molecular and cellular endocrinology* 355.2 (2012): 192-200.

[91] Jacobsen, Bjarne K., et al. "Soy isoflavone intake and the likelihood of ever becoming a mother: the Adventist Health Study-2." *International journal of women's health* 6 (2014): 377.

[92] "eCFR — Code of Federal Regulations - acamedia.info." 2 Sep. 2016, http://www.acamedia.info/sciences/sciliterature/globalw/reference/glyphosate/US_eCFR.pdf. Accessed 24 Feb. 2017.

[93] Bøhn, Thomas, et al. "Compositional differences in soybeans on the market: glyphosate accumulates in Roundup Ready GM soybeans." *Food Chemistry* 153 (2014): 207-215.

[94] Benachour, Nora, et al. "Time-and dose-dependent effects of roundup on human embryonic and placental cells." *Archives of Environmental Contamination and Toxicology* 53.1 (2007): 126-133.

[95] Paganelli, Alejandra, et al. "Glyphosate-based herbicides produce teratogenic effects on vertebrates by impairing retinoic acid signaling." *Chemical research in toxicology* 23.10 (2010): 1586-1595.

[96] Romano, Marco Aurelio, et al. "Glyphosate impairs male offspring reproductive development by disrupting gonadotropin expression." *Archives of toxicology* 86.4 (2012): 663-673.

[97] Saldana, Tina M., et al. "Pesticide exposure and self-reported gestational diabetes mellitus in the Agricultural Health Study." *Diabetes Care* 30.3 (2007): 529-534.

[98] Krüger, Monika, et al. "Detection of glyphosate in malformed piglets." *J Environ Anal Toxicol* 4.230 (2014): 2161-0525.

[99] Richard, Sophie, et al. "Differential effects of glyphosate and roundup on human placental cells and aromatase." *Environmental Health Perspectives* (2005): 716-720.

[100] Nayak, Prasunpriya. "Aluminum: impacts and disease." *Environmental research* 89.2 (2002): 101-115.

[101] Agostoni, Carlo, et al. "Soy protein infant formulae and follow-on formulae: a commentary by the ESPGHAN Committee on Nutrition." *Journal of pediatric gastroenterology and nutrition* 42.4 (2006): 352-361.

[102] Karimour, A., et al. "Toxicity Effects of Aluminum Chloride on Uterus and Placenta of Pregnant Mice." *JBUMS*, (2005): 22-27.

[103] Abu-Taweel, Gasem M., Jamaan S. Ajarem, and Mohammad Ahmad. "Neurobehavioral toxic effects of perinatal oral exposure to aluminum on the developmental motor reflexes, learning, memory and brain neurotransmitters of mice offspring." *Pharmacology Biochemistry and Behavior* 101.1 (2012): 49-56.

[104] Fanni, Daniela, et al. "Aluminum exposure and toxicity in neonates: a practical guide to halt aluminum overload in the prenatal and perinatal periods." *World J Pediatr* 10.2 (2014): 101-107.

[105] Seneff, Stephanie, Nancy Swanson, and Chen Li. "Aluminum and glyphosate can synergistically induce pineal gland pathology: connection to gut dysbiosis and neurological disease." *Agricultural Sciences* 6.1 (2015): 42.

Chapter 6

[1] Giddens, Jacqueline Borah, et al. "Pregnant adolescent and adult women have similarly low intakes of selected nutrients." *Journal of the American Dietetic Association* 100.11 (2000): 1334-1340.

[2] Ladipo, Oladapo A. "Nutrition in pregnancy: mineral and vitamin supplements." *The American Journal of Clinical Nutrition* 72.1 (2000): 280s-290s.

[3] Bae, Sajin, et al. "Vitamin B-12 status differs among pregnant, lactating, and control women with equivalent nutrient intakes." *The Journal of Nutrition* 145.7 (2015): 1507-1514.

[4] Kim, Denise, et al. "Maternal intake of vitamin B6 and maternal and cord plasma levels of pyridoxal 5'phosphate in a cohort of Canadian pregnant women and newborn infants." *The FASEB Journal* 29.1 Supplement (2015): 919-4.

[5] Greenberg, James A, and Stacey J Bell. "Multivitamin supplementation during pregnancy: emphasis on folic acid and L-methylfolate." *Reviews in Obstetrics and Gynecology* 4.3-4 (2011): 126.

[6] Schmid, Alexandra, and Barbara Walther. "Natural vitamin D content in animal products." *Advances in Nutrition: An International Review Journal* 4.4 (2013): 453-462.

[7] Bodnar, Lisa M et al. "High prevalence of vitamin D insufficiency in black and white pregnant women residing in the northern United States and their neonates." *The Journal of Nutrition* 137.2 (2007): 447-452.

[8] Dawodu, Adekunle, and Reginald C Tsang. "Maternal vitamin D status: effect on milk vitamin D content and vitamin D status of breastfeeding infants." *Advances in Nutrition: An International Review Journal* 3.3 (2012): 353-361.

[9] Lee, Joyce M et al. "Vitamin D deficiency in a healthy group of mothers and newborn infants." *Clinical Pediatrics* 46.1 (2007): 42-44.

[10] Viljakainen, HT et al. "Maternal vitamin D status determines bone variables in the newborn." *The Journal of Clinical Endocrinology & Metabolism* 95.4 (2010): 1749-1757.

[11] Wei, Shu-Qin et al. "Maternal vitamin D status and adverse pregnancy outcomes: a systematic review and meta-analysis." *The Journal of Maternal-Fetal & Neonatal Medicine* 26.9 (2013): 889-899.

[12] Aghajafari, Fariba et al. "Association between maternal serum 25-hydroxyvitamin D level and pregnancy and neonatal outcomes: systematic review and meta-analysis of observational studies." *BMJ: British Medical Journal* 346 (2013).

[13] Nozza, Josephine M, and Christine P Rodda. "Vitamin D deficiency in mothers of infants with rickets." *The Medical Journal of Australia* 175.5 (2001): 253-255.

[14] Javaid, MK et al. "Maternal vitamin D status during pregnancy and childhood bone mass at age 9 years: a longitudinal study." *The Lancet* 367.9504 (2006): 36-43.

[15] Litonjua, Augusto A. "Childhood asthma may be a consequence of vitamin D deficiency." *Current Opinion in Allergy and Clinical Immunology* 9.3 (2009): 202.

[16] Brehm, John M et al. "Serum vitamin D levels and markers of severity of childhood asthma in Costa Rica." *American Journal of Respiratory and Critical Care Medicine* 179.9 (2009): 765-771.

[17] Whitehouse, Andrew JO et al. "Maternal serum vitamin D levels during pregnancy and offspring neurocognitive development." *Pediatrics* 129.3 (2012): 485-493.

[18] Kinney, Dennis K et al. "Relation of schizophrenia prevalence to latitude, climate, fish consumption, infant mortality, and skin color: a role for prenatal vitamin d deficiency and infections?." *Schizophrenia Bulletin* (2009): sbp023.

[19] Stene, LC et al. "Use of cod liver oil during pregnancy associated with lower risk of Type I diabetes in the offspring." *Diabetologia* 43.9 (2000): 1093-1098.

[20] Salzer, Jonatan, Anders Svenningsson, and Peter Sundström. "Season of birth and multiple sclerosis in Sweden." *Acta Neurologica Scandinavica* 121.1 (2010): 20-23.

[21] Hollis, Bruce W et al. "Vitamin D supplementation during pregnancy: Double-blind, randomized clinical trial of safety and effectiveness." *Journal of Bone and Mineral Research* 26.10 (2011): 2341-2357.

[22] ACOG Committee on Obstetric Practice. "ACOG Committee Opinion No. 495: Vitamin D: Screening and supplementation during pregnancy." *Obstetrics and Gynecology* 118.1 (2011): 197.

[23] Veugelers, Paul J., and John Paul Ekwaru. "A statistical error in the estimation of the recommended dietary allowance for vitamin D." *Nutrients* 6.10 (2014): 4472-4475.

[24] Papadimitriou, Dimitrios T. "The big Vitamin D mistake." *Journal of Preventive Medicine and Public Health* (2017).

[25] Heaney, Robert P., et al. "Vitamin D3 is more potent than vitamin D2 in humans." *The Journal of Clinical Endocrinology & Metabolism* 96.3 (2011): E447-E452.

[26] Masterjohn, Christopher. "Vitamin D toxicity redefined: vitamin K and the molecular mechanism." *Medical Hypotheses* 68.5 (2007): 1026-1034.

[27] Innis, Sheila M. "Dietary (n-3) fatty acids and brain development." *The Journal of Nutrition* 137.4 (2007): 855-859.

[28] Candela, C. Gómez, LMa Bermejo López, and V. Loria Kohen. "Importance of a balanced omega 6/omega 3 ratio for the maintenance of health. Nutritional recommendations." *Nutricion hospitalaria* 26.2 (2011): 323-329.

[29] Dunstan, J. A., et al. "Cognitive assessment of children at age 2½ years after maternal fish oil supplementation in pregnancy: a randomised controlled trial." *Archives of Disease in Childhood-Fetal and Neonatal Edition* 93.1 (2008): F45-F50.

[30] Helland, Ingrid B., et al. "Maternal supplementation with very-long-chain n-3 fatty acids during pregnancy and lactation augments children's IQ at 4 years of age." *Pediatrics* 111.1 (2003): e39-e44.

[31] Greenberg, James A., Stacey J. Bell, and Wendy Van Ausdal. "Omega-3 fatty acid supplementation during pregnancy." *Reviews in obstetrics and Gynecology* 1.4 (2008): 162.

[32] Dunlop, Anne L., et al. "The maternal microbiome and pregnancy outcomes that impact infant health: A review." *Advances in neonatal care: official journal of the National Association of Neonatal Nurses* 15.6 (2015): 377.

[33] Brantsæter, Anne Lise, et al. "Intake of probiotic food and risk of preeclampsia in primiparous women: the Norwegian Mother and Child Cohort Study." *American journal of epidemiology* 174.7 (2011): 807-815.

[34] Luoto, Raakel et al. "Impact of maternal probiotic-supplemented dietary counselling on pregnancy outcome and prenatal and postnatal growth: a double-blind, placebo-controlled study." *British Journal of Nutrition* 103.12 (2010): 1792-1799.

[35] Luoto, Raakel et al. "Impact of maternal probiotic-supplemented dietary counselling on pregnancy outcome and prenatal and postnatal growth: a double-blind, placebo-controlled study." *British Journal of Nutrition* 103.12 (2010): 1792-1799.

[36] Aagaard, Kjersti et al. "The placenta harbors a unique microbiome." *Science Translational Medicine* 6.237 (2014): 237ra65-237ra65.

[37] Mueller, Noel T et al. "Prenatal exposure to antibiotics, cesarean section and risk of childhood obesity." *International Journal of Obesity* (2014).

[38] "Jędrychowski, Wiesław, et al. "The prenatal use of antibiotics and the development of allergic disease in one year old infants. A preliminary study." *International journal of occupational medicine and environmental health* 19.1 (2006): 70-76.

[39] Timm, Signe, et al. "Prenatal antibiotics and atopic dermatitis among 18-month-old children in the Danish National Birth Cohort." *Clinical & Experimental Allergy* (2017).

[40] Gray, Lawrence EK, et al. "The Maternal Diet, Gut Bacteria, and Bacterial Metabolites during Pregnancy influence Offspring Asthma." *Frontiers in Immunology* 8 (2017).

[41] Rautava, Samuli, Marko Kalliomäki, and Erika Isolauri. "Probiotics during pregnancy and breast-feeding might confer immunomodulatory protection against atopic disease in the infant." *Journal of Allergy and Clinical Immunology* 109.1 (2002): 119-121.

[42] Baldassarre, Maria Elisabetta, et al. "Administration of a multi-strain probiotic product to women in the perinatal period differentially affects the breast milk cytokine profile and may have beneficial effects on neonatal gastrointestinal functional symptoms. A randomized clinical trial." *Nutrients* 8.11 (2016): 677.

[43] Yoon, Kyung Young, Edward E. Woodams, and Yong D. Hang. "Production of probiotic cabbage juice by lactic acid bacteria." *Bioresource technology* 97.12 (2006): 1427-1430.

[44] Timar, A. V. "Comparative study of kefir lactic microflora." *Analele Universității din Oradea, Fascicula: Ecotoxicologie, Zootehnie și Tehnologii de Industrie Alimentară* (2010): 847-858.

[45] Bird, A., et al. "Resistant starch, large bowel fermentation and a broader perspective of prebiotics and probiotics." *Beneficial Microbes* 1.4 (2010): 423-431.

46 Thoma, Marie E et al. "Bacterial vaginosis is associated with variation in dietary indices." *The Journal of Nutrition* 141.9 (2011): 1698-1704.

47 De Gregorio, P. R., et al. "Preventive effect of Lactobacillus reuteri CRL1324 on Group B Streptococcus vaginal colonization in an experimental mouse model." *Journal of Applied Microbiology* 118.4 (2015): 1034-1047.

48 Martinez, Rafael CR, et al. "Improved cure of bacterial vaginosis with single dose of tinidazole (2 g), Lactobacillus rhamnosus GR-1, and Lactobacillus reuteri RC-14: a randomized, double-blind, placebo-controlled trial." *Canadian Journal of Microbiology* 55.2 (2009): 133-138.

49 Ho, Ming, et al. "Oral Lactobacillus rhamnosus GR-1 and Lactobacillus reuteri RC-14 to reduce Group B Streptococcus colonization in pregnant women: a randomized controlled trial." *Taiwanese Journal of Obstetrics and Gynecology* 55.4 (2016): 515-518.

50 Bailey, Regan L et al. "Estimation of total usual calcium and vitamin D intakes in the United States." *The Journal of Nutrition* 140.4 (2010): 817-822.

51 Kovacs, Christopher S. "Maternal mineral and bone metabolism during pregnancy, lactation, and post-weaning recovery." *Physiological reviews* 96.2 (2016): 449-547.

52 Rosanoff, Andrea, Connie M Weaver, and Robert K Rude. "Suboptimal magnesium status in the United States: are the health consequences underestimated?." *Nutrition Reviews* 70.3 (2012): 153-164.

53 Bardicef, Mordechai et al. "Extracellular and intracellular magnesium depletion in pregnancy and gestational diabetes." *American Journal of Obstetrics and Gynecology* 172.3 (1995): 1009-1013.

54 Dahle, Lars O., et al. "The effect of oral magnesium substitution on pregnancy-induced leg cramps." *American Journal of Obstetrics and Gynecology* 173.1 (1995): 175-180.

55 Rylander, Ragnar, and Maria Bullarbo. "[304-POS]: Use of oral magnesium to prevent gestational hypertension." *Pregnancy Hypertension: An International Journal of Women's Cardiovascular Health* 5.1 (2015): 150.

56 Guo, Wanli, et al. "Magnesium deficiency in plants: An urgent problem." *The crop journal* 4.2 (2016): 83-91.

57 Mäder, Paul et al. "Soil fertility and biodiversity in organic farming." *Science* 296.5573 (2002): 1694-1697.

58 Chandrasekaran, Navin Chandrakanth, et al. "Permeation of topically applied Magnesium ions through human skin is facilitated by hair follicles." *Magnesium Research* 29.2 (2016): 35-42.

59 Edwards, Marshall J. "Hyperthermia and fever during pregnancy." *Birth Defects Research Part A: Clinical and Molecular Teratology* 76.7 (2006): 507-516.

60 Aggett PJ. Iron. In: Erdman JW, Macdonald IA, Zeisel SH, eds. Present Knowledge in Nutrition. 10th ed. Washington, DC: Wiley-Blackwell; 2012: 506-20.

61 Breymann, Christian. "Iron deficiency anemia in pregnancy." *Seminars in Hematology.* Vol. 52. No. 4. WB Saunders, 2015.

62 Zimmermann, Michael B., Hans Burgi, and Richard F. Hurrell. "Iron deficiency predicts poor maternal thyroid status during pregnancy." *The Journal of Clinical Endocrinology & Metabolism* 92.9 (2007): 3436-3440.

63 Hyder, SM Ziauddin, et al. "Do side-effects reduce compliance to iron supplementation? A study of daily- and weekly-dose regimens in pregnancy." *Journal of Health, Population and Nutrition* (2002): 175-179.

64 Melamed, Nir, et al. "Iron supplementation in pregnancy—does the preparation matter?." *Archives of Gynecology and Obstetrics* 276.6 (2007): 601-604.

65 Hurrell R, Egli I. Iron bioavailability and dietary reference values. *Am J Clin Nutr* 2010;91:1461S-7S.

66 Moore CV. Iron nutrition and requirements. In "Iron Metabolism," *Series Haematologica, Scandinavia J. Hematol.* 1965. Vol 6: 1-14.

67 Melamed, Nir, et al. "Iron supplementation in pregnancy—does the preparation matter?." *Archives of Gynecology and Obstetrics* 276.6 (2007): 601-604.

68 Tompkins, Winslow T. "The clinical significance of nutritional deficiencies in pregnancy." *Bulletin of the New York Academy of Medicine* 24.6 (1948): 376.

69 Niang, Khadim, et al. "Spirulina Supplementation in Pregnant Women in the Dakar Region (Senegal)." *Open Journal of Obstetrics and Gynecology* 7.01 (2016): 147.

70 Rees, William D, Fiona A Wilson, and Christopher A Maloney. "Sulfur amino acid metabolism in pregnancy: the impact of methionine in the maternal diet." *The Journal of Nutrition* 136.6 (2006): 1701S-1705S.

71 Dante, Giulia, et al. "Herbal therapies in pregnancy: what works?." *Current Opinion in Obstetrics and Gynecology* 26.2 (2014): 83-91.

72 Holst, Lone, Svein Haavik, and Hedvig Nordeng. "Raspberry leaf–Should it be recommended to pregnant women?." *Complementary therapies in clinical practice* 15.4 (2009): 204-208.

73 Burn JH, Withell ER. A principle in raspberry leaves which relaxes uterine muscle. *Lancet.* 1941; 241:6149–6151.

74 Pavlović, Aleksandra V., et al. "Phenolics composition of leaf extracts of raspberry and blackberry cultivars grown in Serbia." *Industrial Crops and Products* 87 (2016): 304-314.

75 Holst, Lone, Svein Haavik, and Hedvig Nordeng. "Raspberry leaf–Should it be recommended to pregnant women?." *Complementary therapies in clinical practice* 15.4 (2009): 204-208.

76 Holst, Lone, Svein Haavik, and Hedvig Nordeng. "Raspberry leaf–Should it be recommended to pregnant women?." *Complementary therapies in clinical practice* 15.4 (2009): 204-208.

[77] Dante, G., et al. "Herb remedies during pregnancy: a systematic review of controlled clinical trials." *The Journal of Maternal-Fetal & Neonatal Medicine* 26.3 (2013): 306-312.

[78] Vutyavanich, Teraporn, Theerajana Kraisarin, and Rung-aroon Ruangsri. "Ginger for nausea and vomiting in pregnancy: randomized, double-masked, placebo-controlled trial." *Obstetrics & Gynecology* 97.4 (2001): 577-582.

[79] Niebyl, Jennifer R. "Nausea and vomiting in pregnancy." *New England Journal of Medicine* 363.16 (2010): 1544-1550.

[80] Anderson, F. W. J., and C. T. Johnson. "Complementary and alternative medicine in obstetrics." *International Journal of Gynecology & Obstetrics* 91.2 (2005): 116-124.

[81] Gholami, Fereshte, et al. "Onset of Labor in Post-Term Pregnancy by Chamomile." *Iranian Red Crescent Medical Journal* 18.11 (2016).

[82] Srivastava, Janmejai K., Eswar Shankar, and Sanjay Gupta. "Chamomile: a herbal medicine of the past with a bright future." *Molecular medicine reports* 3.6 (2010): 895-901.

[83] Silva, Fernando V., et al. "Chamomile reveals to be a potent galactogogue: the unexpected effect." *The Journal of Maternal-Fetal & Neonatal Medicine* (2017): 1-3.

[84] Chang, Shao-Min, and Chung-Hey Chen. "Effects of an intervention with drinking chamomile tea on sleep quality and depression in sleep disturbed postnatal women: a randomized controlled trial." *Journal of advanced nursing* 72.2 (2016): 306-315.

[85] Dante, Giulia, et al. "Herbal therapies in pregnancy: what works?." *Current Opinion in Obstetrics and Gynecology* 26.2 (2014): 83-91.

[86] Prabu, P. C., and S. Panchapakesan. "Prenatal developmental toxicity evaluation of Withania somnifera root extract in Wistar rats." *Drug and chemical toxicology* 38.1 (2015): 50-56.

[87] Dar, Nawab John, Abid Hamid, and Muzamil Ahmad. "Pharmacologic overview of Withania somnifera, the Indian Ginseng." *Cellular and molecular life sciences* 72.23 (2015): 4445-4460.

[88] Jafarzadeh, Lobat, et al. "Antioxidant activity and teratogenicity evaluation of Lawsonia Inermis in BALB/c mice." *Journal of clinical and diagnostic research: JCDR* 9.5 (2015): FF01.

[89] Domaracký, M., et al. "Effects of selected plant essential oils on the growth and development of mouse preimplantation embryos in vivo." *Physiological Research* 56.1 (2007): 97.

[90] Marcus, Donald M., and Arthur P. Grollman. "Botanical medicines--the need for new regulations." *The New England Journal of Medicine* 347.25 (2002): 2073.

[91] American Herbal Products Association's Botanical Safety Handbook, 2nd ed. (CRC Press, 2013).

Chapter 7

[1] Niebyl, Jennifer R. "Nausea and vomiting in pregnancy." *New England Journal of Medicine* 363.16 (2010): 1544-1550.

[2] Ghani, Rania Mahmoud Abdel, and Adlia Tawfik Ahmed Ibrahim. "The effect of aromatherapy inhalation on nausea and vomiting in early pregnancy: a pilot randomized controlled trial." *J Nat Sci Res* 3.6 (2013): 10-22.

[3] Niebyl, Jennifer R. "Nausea and vomiting in pregnancy." *New England Journal of Medicine* 363.16 (2010): 1544-1550.

[4] Vutyavanich, Teraporn, Theerajana Kraisarin, and Rung-aroon Ruangsri. "Ginger for nausea and vomiting in pregnancy: randomized, double-masked, placebo-controlled trial." *Obstetrics & Gynecology* 97.4 (2001): 577-582.

[5] Niebyl, Jennifer R. "Nausea and vomiting in pregnancy." *New England Journal of Medicine* 363.16 (2010): 1544-1550.

[6] O'brien, Beverley, M. Joyce Relyea, and Terry Taerum. "Efficacy of P6 acupressure in the treatment of nausea and vomiting during pregnancy." *American Journal of Obstetrics and Gynecology* 174.2 (1996): 708-715.

[7] Forbes, Scott. "Pregnancy sickness and parent-offspring conflict over thyroid function." *Journal of Theoretical Biology* 355 (2014): 61-67.

[8] Forbes, Scott. "Pregnancy sickness and embryo quality." *Trends in Ecology & Evolution* 17.3 (2002): 115-120.

[9] Orloff, Natalia C., and Julia M. Hormes. "Pickles and ice cream! Food cravings in pregnancy: hypotheses, preliminary evidence, and directions for future research." *Food Cravings* (2015): 66.

[10] Sorenson, R. L., and T. C. Brelje. "Adaptation of islets of Langerhans to pregnancy: β-cell growth, enhanced insulin secretion and the role of lactogenic hormones." *Hormone and metabolic research* 29.06 (1997): 301-307.

[11] Barbour, Linda A., et al. "Cellular mechanisms for insulin resistance in normal pregnancy and gestational diabetes." *Diabetes care* 30.Supplement 2 (2007): S112-S119.

[12] Young, Sera L. "Pica in pregnancy: new ideas about an old condition." *Annual review of nutrition* 30 (2010): 403-422.

[13] Costa, Sara, et al. "Fatty acids, mercury, and methylmercury bioaccessibility in salmon (Salmo salar) using an in vitro model: effect of culinary treatment." *Food chemistry* 185 (2015): 268-276.

[14] Harrison, Michael, et al. "Nature and availability of iodine in fish." *The American journal of clinical nutrition* 17.2 (1965): 73-77.

[15] Laird, Brian D., and Hing Man Chan. "Bioaccessibility of metals in fish, shellfish, wild game, and seaweed harvested in British Columbia, Canada." *Food and chemical toxicology* 58 (2013): 381-387.

[16] Pearce, Elizabeth N., et al. "Sources of dietary iodine: bread, cows' milk, and infant formula in the Boston area." *The Journal of Clinical Endocrinology & Metabolism* 89.7 (2004): 3421-3424.

[17] Scaife, Paula Juliet, and Markus Georg Mohaupt. "Salt, aldosterone and extrarenal Na+-sensitive responses in pregnancy." *Placenta* (2017).

[18] Flaxman, S. M., and Sherman, P. W. (2000). Morning sickness: a mechanism for protecting mother and embryo. Q. Rev. Biol. 75, 113–148.

[19] Orloff, Natalia C., and Julia M. Hormes. "Pickles and ice cream! Food cravings in pregnancy: hypotheses, preliminary evidence, and directions for future research." *Food Cravings* (2015): 66.

[20] Leonti, Marco. "The co-evolutionary perspective of the food-medicine continuum and wild gathered and cultivated vegetables." *Genetic Resources and Crop Evolution* 59.7 (2012): 1295-1302.

[21] Fessler, D. M. T. (2002). Reproductive immunosuppression and diet: an evolutionary perspective on pregnancy sickness and meat consumption. Curr. Anthropol. 43, 19–61.

[22] Fessler, D. M. T. (2002). Reproductive immunosuppression and diet: an evolutionary perspective on pregnancy sickness and meat consumption. Curr. Anthropol. 43, 19–61.

[23] Rasmussen, K. M., and Yaktine, A. L. (eds). (2009). *Weight Gain During Pregnancy: Reexamining the Guidelines*. Washington, DC: The National Academies Press.

[24] Nordin, S., Broman, D. A., Olofsson, J. K., and Wulff, M. (2004). A longitudinal descriptive study of self-reported abnormal smell and taste perception in pregnant women. *Chem. Senses* 29, 391–402.

[25] Nordin, S., Broman, D. A., Olofsson, J. K., and Wulff, M. (2004). A longitudinal descriptive study of self-reported abnormal smell and taste perception in pregnant women. *Chem. Senses* 29, 391–402.

[26] Orloff, Natalia C., and Julia M. Hormes. "Pickles and ice cream! Food cravings in pregnancy: hypotheses, preliminary evidence, and directions for future research." *Food Cravings* (2015): 66.

[27] Wideman, C. H., G. R. Nadzam, and H. M. Murphy. "Implications of an animal model of sugar addiction, withdrawal and relapse for human health." *Nutritional neuroscience* 8.5-6 (2005): 269-276.

[28] Avena, Nicole M., Pedro Rada, and Bartley G. Hoebel. "Evidence for sugar addiction: behavioral and neurochemical effects of intermittent, excessive sugar intake." *Neuroscience & Biobehavioral Reviews* 32.1 (2008): 20-39.

[29] Fuhrman, Joel, et al. "Changing perceptions of hunger on a high nutrient density diet." *Nutrition journal* 9.1 (2010): 51.

[30] Chang, Kevin T., et al. "Low glycemic load experimental diet more satiating than high glycemic load diet." *Nutrition and cancer* 64.5 (2012): 666-673.

[31] Chandler-Laney, Paula C., et al. "Return of hunger following a relatively high carbohydrate breakfast is associated with earlier recorded glucose peak and nadir." *Appetite* 80 (2014): 236-241.

[32] Fallaize, Rosalind, et al. "Variation in the effects of three different breakfast meals on subjective satiety and subsequent intake of energy at lunch and evening meal." *European journal of nutrition* 52.4 (2013): 1353-1359.

[33] Orloff, Natalia C., and Julia M. Hormes. "Pickles and ice cream! Food cravings in pregnancy: hypotheses, preliminary evidence, and directions for future research." *Food Cravings* (2015): 66.

[34] Bailey, L. (2001). Gender shows: first-time mothers and embodied selves. Gend. Soc. 15, 110–129.

[35] Orloff, Natalia C., and Julia M. Hormes. "Pickles and ice cream! Food cravings in pregnancy: hypotheses, preliminary evidence, and directions for future research." *Food Cravings* (2015): 66.

[36] Katterman, Shawn N., et al. "Mindfulness meditation as an intervention for binge eating, emotional eating, and weight loss: a systematic review." *Eating behaviors* 15.2 (2014): 197-204.

[37] Phupong, Vorapong, and Tharangrut Hanprasertpong. "Interventions for heartburn in pregnancy." *The Cochrane Library* (2015).

[38] Tan, Eng Kien, and Eng Loy Tan. "Alterations in physiology and anatomy during pregnancy." *Best Practice & Research Clinical Obstetrics & Gynaecology* 27.6 (2013): 791-802.

[39] Reinke, Claudia M., Jörg Breitkreutz, and Hans Leuenberger. "Aluminium in over-the-counter drugs." *Drug Safety* 26.14 (2003): 1011-1025.

[40] Wu, Keng-Liang, et al. "Effect of liquid meals with different volumes on gastroesophageal reflux disease." *Journal of Gastroenterology and Hepatology* 29.3 (2014): 469-473.

[41] Zhang, Qing, et al. "Effect of hyperglycemia on triggering of transient lower esophageal sphincter relaxations." *American Journal of Physiology-Gastrointestinal and Liver Physiology* 286.5 (2004): G797-G803.

[42] Austin, Gregory L., et al. "A very low-carbohydrate diet improves gastroesophageal reflux and its symptoms." *Digestive Diseases and Sciences* 51.8 (2006): 1307-1312.

[43] Altomare, Annamaria, et al. "Gastroesophageal reflux disease: Update on inflammation and symptom perception." *World J Gastroenterol* 19.39 (2013): 6523-8.

[44] Zou, Duowu, et al. "Inhibition of transient lower esophageal sphincter relaxations by electrical acupoint stimulation." *American Journal of Physiology-Gastrointestinal and Liver Physiology* 289.2 (2005): G197-G201.

[45] Longo, Sherri A., et al. "Gastrointestinal conditions during pregnancy." *Clinics in colon and rectal surgery* 23.02 (2010): 080-089.

[46] Longo, Sherri A., et al. "Gastrointestinal conditions during pregnancy." *Clinics in colon and rectal surgery* 23.02 (2010): 080-089.

[47] Avsar, A. F., and H. L. Keskin. "Haemorrhoids during pregnancy." *Journal of Obstetrics and Gynaecology* 30.3 (2010): 231-237.

Real Food for Pregnancy

[48] Wong, Banny S., et al. "Effects of A3309, an ileal bile acid transporter inhibitor, on colonic transit and symptoms in females with functional constipation." *The American Journal of Gastroenterology* 106.12 (2011): 2154.

[49] Sikirov, Dov. "Comparison of straining during defecation in three positions: results and implications for human health." *Digestive diseases and sciences* 48.7 (2003): 1201-1205.

[50] Dimmer, Christine, et al. "Squatting for the Prevention of Haemorrhoids?." *Townsend Letter for Doctors and Patients* (1996): 66-71.

[51] de Milliano, Inge, et al. "Is a multispecies probiotic mixture effective in constipation during pregnancy?'A pilot study'." *Nutrition Journal* 11.1 (2012): 80.

[52] Bradley, Catherine S., et al. "Constipation in pregnancy: prevalence, symptoms, and risk factors." *Obstetrics & Gynecology* 110.6 (2007): 1351-1357.

[53] Talley, Nicholas J., et al. "Risk factors for chronic constipation based on a general practice sample." *The American Journal of Gastroenterology* 98.5 (2003): 1107.

[54] Shulman, Rachel, and Melissa Kottke. "Impact of maternal knowledge of recommended weight gain in pregnancy on gestational weight gain." *American journal of obstetrics and gynecology* 214.6 (2016): 754-e1.

[55] Siega-Riz, Anna Maria, et al. "A systematic review of outcomes of maternal weight gain according to the Institute of Medicine recommendations: birthweight, fetal growth, and postpartum weight retention." *AJOG.* 201.4 (2009): 339-e1.

[56] National Research Council and Institute of Medicine. (2007). *Influence of Pregnancy Weight on Maternal and Child Health (Workshop Report).* Washington, DC: The National Academies Press.

[57] Shapiro, A. L. B., et al. "Maternal diet quality in pregnancy and neonatal adiposity: The healthy start study." *International Journal of Obesity* 40.7 (2016): 1056-1062.

[58] Centers for Disease Control and Prevention (CDC. "Trends in intake of energy and macronutrients--United States, 1971-2000." *MMWR. Morbidity and mortality weekly report* 53.4 (2004): 80.

[59] Clapp III, James F. "Maternal carbohydrate intake and pregnancy outcome." *Proceedings of the Nutrition Society* 61.01 (2002): 45-50.

[60] Bello, Jennifer K., et al. "Pregnancy Weight Gain, Postpartum Weight Retention, and Obesity." *Current Cardiovascular Risk Reports* 10.1 (2016): 1-12.

[61] Alavi, N., et al. "Comparison of national gestational weight gain guidelines and energy intake recommendations." *Obesity Reviews* 14.1 (2013): 68-85.

[62] Lain, Kristine Y., and Patrick M. Catalano. "Metabolic changes in pregnancy." *Clinical Obstetrics and Gynecology* 50.4 (2007): 938-948.

[63] Flegal KM, Carroll MD, Ogden CL, Curtin LR. Prevalence and trends in obesity among US adults, 1999-2008. JAMA 2010; 303: 235–241.

[64] Kiel, Deborah W., et al. "Gestational weight gain and pregnancy outcomes in obese women: how much is enough?." *Obstetrics & Gynecology* 110.4 (2007): 752-758.

[65] Shapiro, A. L. B., et al. "Maternal diet quality in pregnancy and neonatal adiposity: The healthy start study." *International Journal of Obesity* 40.7 (2016): 1056-1062.

[66] Report of the American College of Obstetricians and Gynecologists' Task Force on Hypertension in Pregnancy. *ObstetGynecol.* 2013;122(5):1122-1131.

[67] Villar J, Repke J, Markush L, Calvert W, Rhoads G. The measuring of blood pressure during pregnancy. American Journal of Obstetrics and Gynecology 1989;161:1019-24.

[68] Aune, Dagfinn, et al. "Physical activity and the risk of preeclampsia: a systematic review and meta-analysis." *Epidemiology* 25.3 (2014): 331-343.

[69] Gildea, John J et al. "A linear relationship between the ex-vivo sodium mediated expression of two sodium regulatory pathways as a surrogate marker of salt sensitivity of blood pressure in exfoliated human renal proximal tubule cells: the virtual renal biopsy." *Clinica Chimica Acta* 421 (2013): 236-242.

[70] Schoenaker, Danielle AJM, Sabita S. Soedamah-Muthu, and Gita D. Mishra. "The association between dietary factors and gestational hypertension and pre-eclampsia: a systematic review and meta-analysis of observational studies." *BMC medicine* 12.1 (2014): 157.

[71] "Nabeshima, K. "Effect of salt restriction on preeclampsia." Nihon Jinzo Gakkai Shi 36.3 (1994): 227-232.

[72] Iwaoka, Taisuke, et al. "Dietary NaCl restriction deteriorates oral glucose tolerance in hypertensive patients with impairment of glucose tolerance." *American journal of hypertension* 7.5 (1994): 460-463.

[73] Sakuyama, Hiroe, et al. "Influence of gestational salt restriction in fetal growth and in development of diseases in adulthood." *Journal of biomedical science* 23.1 (2016): 12.

[74] Guan J, Mao C, Feng X, Zhang H, Xu F, Geng C, et al. Fetal development of regulatory mechanisms for body fluid homeostasis. Brazil J Med Biol Res. 2008;41:446–54.

[75] Duley, L., and D. Henderson-Smart. "Reduced salt intake compared to normal dietary salt, or high intake, in pregnancy." *The Cochrane database of systematic reviews* 2 (2000): CD001687.

[76] Robinson, Margaret. "Salt in pregnancy." *The Lancet* 271.7013 (1958): 178-181.

[77] Gennari, Carine, et al. "Normotensive blood pressure in pregnancy–the role of salt and aldosterone." *Hypertension* 63.2 (2014): 362-368.

[78] Scaife, Paula Juliet, and Markus Georg Mohaupt. "Salt, aldosterone and extrarenal Na+-sensitive responses in pregnancy." *Placenta* (2017).

[79] Rakova, Natalia, et al. "Novel ideas about salt, blood pressure, and pregnancy." *Journal of reproductive immunology* 101 (2014): 135-139.

[80] Klein, Alice Victoria, and Hosen Kiat. "The mechanisms underlying fructose-induced hypertension: a review." *Journal of hypertension* 33.5 (2015): 912-920.

[81] Borgen, I., et al. "Maternal sugar consumption and risk of preeclampsia in nulliparous Norwegian women." *European journal of clinical nutrition* 66.8 (2012): 920-925.

[82] Bodnar, Lisa M., et al. "Inflammation and triglycerides partially mediate the effect of prepregnancy body mass index on the risk of preeclampsia." *American journal of epidemiology* 162.12 (2005): 1198-1206.

[83] Bahado-Singh, Ray O., et al. "Metabolomic determination of pathogenesis of late-onset preeclampsia." *The Journal of Maternal-Fetal & Neonatal Medicine* 30.6 (2017): 658-664.

[84] Bryson, Chris L., et al. "Association between gestational diabetes and pregnancy-induced hypertension." *American journal of epidemiology* 158.12 (2003): 1148-1153.

[85] Liebman, Michael. "When and why carbohydrate restriction can be a viable option." *Nutrition* 30.7 (2014): 748-754.

[86] Mehendale, Savita, et al. "Fatty acids, antioxidants, and oxidative stress in pre-eclampsia." *International Journal of Gynecology & Obstetrics* 100.3 (2008): 234-238.

[87] Grootendorst-van Mil, Nina H., et al. "Maternal Midpregnancy Plasma trans 18: 1 Fatty Acid Concentrations Are Positively Associated with Risk of Maternal Vascular Complications and Child Low Birth Weight." *The Journal of Nutrition* 147.3 (2017): 398-403.

[88] Bej, Punyatoya, et al. "Role of nutrition in pre-eclampsia and eclampsia cases, a case control study." *Indian Journal of Community Health* 26.6 (2014): 233-236.

[89] El Hafidi, Mohammed, Israel Perez, and Guadalupe Banos. "Is glycine effective against elevated blood pressure?" (2006): 26-31.

[90] Austdal, Marie, et al. "Metabolomic biomarkers in serum and urine in women with preeclampsia." *PloS one* 9.3 (2014): e91923.

[91] Kwan, Sze Ting Cecilia, et al. "Maternal choline supplementation during pregnancy improves placental vascularization and modulates placental nutrient supply in a sexually dimorphic manner." *Placenta* 45 (2016): 130.

[92] Zhang, Min, et al. "77 Choline supplementation during pregnancy protects against lipopolysaccharide-induced preeclampsia symptoms: Immune and inflammatory mechanisms." *Pregnancy Hypertension: An International Journal of Women's Cardiovascular Health* 6.3 (2016): 175.

[93] Kwan, Sze Ting Cecilia, et al. "Maternal choline supplementation during murine pregnancy modulates placental markers of inflammation, apoptosis and vascularization in a fetal sex-dependent manner." *Placenta* (2017).

[94] Jiang, Xinyin, et al. "Choline inadequacy impairs trophoblast function and vascularization in cultured human placental trophoblasts." *Journal of cellular physiology* 229.8 (2014): 1016-1027.

[95] Jiang, Xinyin, et al. "A higher maternal choline intake among third-trimester pregnant women lowers placental and circulating concentrations of the antiangiogenic factor fms-like tyrosine kinase-1 (sFLT1)." *The FASEB Journal* 27.3 (2013): 1245-1253.

[96] Galleano, Monica, Olga Pechanova, and Cesar G Fraga. "Hypertension, nitric oxide, oxidants, and dietary plant polyphenols." *Current pharmaceutical biotechnology* 11.8 (2010): 837-848.

[97] Rumbold, Alice R., et al. "Vitamins C and E and the risks of preeclampsia and perinatal complications." *New England Journal of Medicine* 354.17 (2006): 1796-1806.

[98] Bodnar, Lisa M., et al. "Maternal vitamin D deficiency increases the risk of preeclampsia." *The Journal of Clinical Endocrinology & Metabolism* 92.9 (2007): 3517-3522.

[99] Hyppönen, Elina, et al. "Vitamin D and pre-eclampsia: original data, systematic review and meta-analysis." *Annals of Nutrition and Metabolism* 63.4 (2013): 331-340.

[100] Schoenaker, Danielle AJM, Sabita S. Soedamah-Muthu, and Gita D. Mishra. "The association between dietary factors and gestational hypertension and pre-eclampsia: a systematic review and meta-analysis of observational studies." *BMC medicine* 12.1 (2014): 157.

[101] Rylander, Ragnar, and Maria Bullarbo. "[304-POS]: Use of oral magnesium to prevent gestational hypertension." *Pregnancy Hypertension: An International Journal of Women's Cardiovascular Health* 5.1 (2015): 150.

[102] Hofmeyr, G. J. "Prevention of pre-eclampsia: calcium supplementation and other strategies: review." *Obstetrics and Gynaecology Forum.* Vol. 26. No. 3. In House Publications, 2016.

[103] Asemi, Zatollah, and Ahmad Esmaillzadeh. "The effect of multi mineral-vitamin D supplementation on pregnancy outcomes in pregnant women at risk for pre-eclampsia." *International journal of preventive medicine* 6 (2015).

[104] Gulaboglu, Mine, Bunyamin Borekci, and Ilhan Delibas. "Urine iodine levels in preeclamptic and normal pregnant women." *Biological trace element research* 136.3 (2010): 249-257.

[105] Borekci, Bunyamin, Mine Gulaboglu, and Mustafa Gul. "Iodine and magnesium levels in maternal and umbilical cord blood of preeclamptic and normal pregnant women." *Biological trace element research* 129.1-3 (2009): 1.

[106] Dempsey, F. C., F. L. Butler, and F. A. Williams. "No need for a pregnant pause: physical activity may reduce the occurrence of gestational diabetes mellitus and preeclampsia." *Exercise and sport sciences reviews* 33.3 (2005): 141-149.

[107] Barakat, Ruben, et al. "Exercise during pregnancy protects against hypertension and macrosomia: randomized clinical trial." *American journal of obstetrics and gynecology* 214.5 (2016): 649-e1.

[108] Vianna, Priscila, et al. "Distress conditions during pregnancy may lead to pre-eclampsia by increasing cortisol levels and altering lymphocyte sensitivity to glucocorticoids." *Medical hypotheses* 77.2 (2011): 188-191.

[109] Shirazi, Marzieh Amohammadi. "Investigating the effectiveness of mindfulness training in the first trimester of pregnancy on improvement of pregnancy outcomes and stress reduction in pregnant women referred to Moheb Yas General Women Hospital." *International Journal of Humanities and Cultural Studies (IJHCS) ISSN 2356-5926* (2016): 2291-2301.

[110] Barbour, Linda A., et al. "Cellular mechanisms for insulin resistance in normal pregnancy and gestational diabetes." *Diabetes care* 30.Supplement 2 (2007): S112-S119.

[111] Hernandez, Teri L., et al. "Patterns of glycemia in normal pregnancy." *Diabetes Care* 34.7 (2011): 1660-1668.

[112] Hughes, Ruth CE, et al. "An early pregnancy HbA1c≥ 5.9%(41 mmol/mol) is optimal for detecting diabetes and identifies women at increased risk of adverse pregnancy outcomes." *Diabetes Care* 37.11 (2014): 2953-2959.

[113] Coustan, Donald R., et al. "The Hyperglycemia and Adverse Pregnancy Outcome (HAPO) study: paving the way for new diagnostic criteria for gestational diabetes mellitus." *American journal of obstetrics and gynecology* 202.6 (2010): 654-e1.

[114] Ma, Ronald CW, et al. "Maternal diabetes, gestational diabetes and the role of epigenetics in their long term effects on offspring." *Progress in biophysics and molecular biology* 118.1 (2015): 55-68.

[115] Holder, Tara, et al. "A low disposition index in adolescent offspring of mothers with gestational diabetes: a risk marker for the development of impaired glucose tolerance in youth." *Diabetologia* 57.11 (2014): 2413-2420.

[116] Oken, Emily, and Matthew W. Gillman. "Fetal origins of obesity." *Obesity* 11.4 (2003): 496-506.

[117] HAPO Study Cooperative Research Group, Metzger BE, Lowe LP et al (2008) Hyperglycemia and adverse pregnancy outcomes. N Engl J Med 358:1991–2002

[118] Priest, James R., et al. "Maternal Midpregnancy Glucose Levels and Risk of Congenital Heart Disease in Offspring." *JAMA pediatrics* 169.12 (2015): 1112-1116.

[119] Kremer, Carrie J., and Patrick Duff. "Glyburide for the treatment of gestational diabetes." *American journal of obstetrics and gynecology* 190.5 (2004): 1438-1439.

[120] Moses, Robert G., et al. "Can a low–glycemic index diet reduce the need for insulin in gestational diabetes mellitus? A randomized trial." *Diabetes care* 32.6 (2009): 996-1000.

[121] Kizirian, Nathalie V., et al. "Lower glycemic load meals reduce diurnal glycemic oscillations in women with risk factors for gestational diabetes." *BMJ Open Diabetes Research and Care* 5.1 (2017): e000351.

[122] Kokic SI, Ivanisevic M, Biolo G, Simunic B, Kokic T, Pisot R. P-68 The impact of structured aerobic and resistance exercise on the course and outcomes of gestational diabetes mellitus: a randomised controlled trial. Poster Presentations. *Br J Sports Med* 2016;50:A69

[123] Kim, Hail, et al. "Serotonin regulates pancreatic beta cell mass during pregnancy." *Nature medicine* 16.7 (2010): 804-808.

[124] Ruiz-Gracia, Teresa, et al. "Lifestyle patterns in early pregnancy linked to gestational diabetes mellitus diagnoses when using IADPSG criteria. The St Carlos gestational study." *Clinical Nutrition* 35.3 (2016): 699-705.

[125] Huang, Wu-Qing, et al. "Excessive fruit consumption during the second trimester is associated with increased likelihood of gestational diabetes mellitus: a prospective study." *Scientific Reports* 7 (2017).

[126] Clapp III, James F. "Maternal carbohydrate intake and pregnancy outcome." *Proceedings of the Nutrition Society* 61.01 (2002): 45-50.

[127] Dempsey, Jennifer C., et al. "A case-control study of maternal recreational physical activity and risk of gestational diabetes mellitus." *Diabetes research and clinical practice* 66.2 (2004): 203-215.

[128] Wei, Shu-Qin et al. "Maternal vitamin D status and adverse pregnancy outcomes: a systematic review and meta-analysis." *The Journal of Maternal-Fetal & Neonatal Medicine* 26.9 (2013): 889-899.

[129] Mostafavi, Ebrahim, et al. "Abdominal obesity and gestational diabetes: the interactive role of magnesium." *Magnesium Research* 28.4 (2015): 116-125.

[130] Asemi, Zatollah, et al. "Magnesium supplementation affects metabolic status and pregnancy outcomes in gestational diabetes: a randomized, double-blind, placebo-controlled trial." *The American journal of clinical nutrition* 102.1 (2015): 222-229.

Chapter 8

[1] Downs, Danielle Symons, and Jan S Ulbrecht. "Understanding exercise beliefs and behaviors in women with gestational diabetes mellitus." *Diabetes Care* 29.2 (2006): 236-240.

[2] Evenson, Kelly R, A Savitz, and Sara L Huston. "Leisure-time physical activity among pregnant women in the US." *Paediatric and Perinatal Epidemiology* 18.6 (2004): 400-407.

[3] Garland, Meghan. "Physical Activity During Pregnancy: A Prescription for Improved Perinatal Outcomes." *The Journal for Nurse Practitioners* 13.1 (2017): 54-58.

[4] Artal, Raul. "Exercise in Pregnancy: Guidelines." *Clinical Obstetrics and Gynecology* 59.3 (2016): 639-644.

[5] Jovanovic-Peterson, Lois, Eric P Durak, and Charles M Peterson. "Randomized trial of diet versus diet plus cardiovascular conditioning on glucose levels in gestational diabetes." *American Journal of Obstetrics and Gynecology* 161.2 (1989): 415-419.

[6] "Brzęk, Anna, et al. "Physical activity in pregnancy and its impact on duration of labor and postpartum period." *Annales Academiae Medicae Silesiensis*. Vol. 70. 2016.

[7] Zhang, Cuilin, et al. "A prospective study of pregravid physical activity and sedentary behaviors in relation to the risk for gestational diabetes mellitus." *Archives of internal medicine* 166.5 (2006): 543-548.

[8] Barakat, Ruben, et al. "Exercise during pregnancy protects against hypertension and macrosomia: randomized clinical trial." *American journal of obstetrics and gynecology* 214.5 (2016): 649-e1.

[9] Collings, CA, LB Curet, and JP Mullin. "Maternal and fetal responses to a maternal aerobic exercise program." *American Journal of Obstetrics and Gynecology* 145.6 (1983): 702-707.

[10] Lassen, Kait, "Does Aerobic Exercise During Pregnancy Prevent Cesarean Sections?" (2016). *PCOM Physician Assistant Studies Student Scholarship*. 276.

[11] Babbar, Shilpa, and Jaye Shyken. "Yoga in Pregnancy." *Clinical obstetrics and gynecology* 59.3 (2016): 600-612.

[12] Lotgering, Frederik K. "30+ Years of Exercise in Pregnancy." *Advances in Fetal and Neonatal Physiology*. Springer New York, 2014. 109-116.

[13] May LE, Glaros A, Yeh HW, Clapp JF 3rd, Gustafson KM. Aerobic exercise during pregnancy influences fetal cardiac autonomic control of heart rate and heart rate variability. Early Hum Dev (2010) 86: 213–217.

[14] Labonte-Lemoyne, Elise, Daniel Curnier, and Dave Ellemberg. "Exercise during pregnancy enhances cerebral maturation in the newborn: A randomized controlled trial." *Journal of Clinical and Experimental Neuropsychology* 39.4 (2017): 347-354.

[15] Hillman, Charles H, Kirk I Erickson, and Arthur F Kramer. "Be smart, exercise your heart: exercise effects on brain and cognition." *Nature Reviews Neuroscience* 9.1 (2008): 58-65.

[16] Dempsey, Jennifer C et al. "A case-control study of maternal recreational physical activity and risk of gestational diabetes mellitus." *Diabetes Research and Clinical Practice* 66.2 (2004): 203-215.

[17] Moyer, Carmen, Olga Roldan Reoyo, and Linda May. "The Influence of Prenatal Exercise on Offspring Health: A Review." *Clinical medicine insights. Women's health* 9 (2016): 37.

[18] Perales, Maria, et al. "Benefits of aerobic or resistance training during pregnancy on maternal health and perinatal outcomes: A systematic review." *Early human development* 94 (2016): 43-48.

[19] Hammer, Roger L, Jan Perkins, and Richard Parr. "Exercise during the childbearing year." *The Journal of Perinatal Education* 9.1 (2000): 1.

[20] Brenner, IK et al. "Physical conditioning effects on fetal heart rate responses to graded maternal exercise." *Medicine and Science in Sports and Exercise* 31.6 (1999): 792-799.

[21] Zumwalt, Mimi. "Prevention and management of common musculoskeletal injuries incurred through exercise during pregnancy." *The Active Female*. Humana Press, 2008. 183-197.

[22] Belogolovsky, Inna, et al. "The Effectiveness of Exercise in Treatment of Pregnancy-Related Lumbar and Pelvic Girdle Pain: A Meta-Analysis and Evidence-Based Review." *Journal of Women's Health Physical Therapy* 39.2 (2015): 53-64.

[23] Sangsawang, Bussara, and Nucharee Sangsawang. "Is a 6-week supervised pelvic floor muscle exercise program effective in preventing stress urinary incontinence in late pregnancy in primigravid women?: a randomized controlled trial." *European Journal of Obstetrics & Gynecology and Reproductive Biology* 197 (2016): 103-110.

[24] Elenskaia, Ksena, et al. "The effect of pregnancy and childbirth on pelvic floor muscle function." *International urogynecology journal* 22.11 (2011): 1421.

[25] Benjamin, D. R., A. T. M. Van de Water, and C. L. Peiris. "Effects of exercise on diastasis of the rectus abdominis muscle in the antenatal and postnatal periods: a systematic review." *Physiotherapy* 100.1 (2014): 1-8.

[26] Candido, G., T. Lo, and P. A. Janssen. "Risk factors for diastasis of the recti abdominis." *Journal - Association of Chartered Physiotherapists in Women's Health*. (2005): 49.

[27] Chiarello, Cynthia M., et al. "The effects of an exercise program on diastasis recti abdominis in pregnant women." *Journal of Women's Health Physical Therapy* 29.1 (2005): 11-16.

[28] Benjamin, D. R., A. T. M. Van de Water, and C. L. Peiris. "Effects of exercise on diastasis of the rectus abdominis muscle in the antenatal and postnatal periods: a systematic review." *Physiotherapy* 100.1 . W(2014): 1-8.

[29] Kluge, Judith, et al. "Specific exercises to treat pregnancy-related low back pain in a South African population." *International Journal of Gynecology & Obstetrics* 113.3 (2011): 187-191.

[30] Richardson, Carolyn A., et al. "The relation between the transversus abdominis muscles, sacroiliac joint mechanics, and low back pain." *Spine* 27.4 (2002): 399-405.

[31] Chan, Justin, Aniket Natekar, and Gideon Koren. "Hot yoga and pregnancy." *Canadian Family Physician* 60.1 (2014): 41-42.

[32] Bacchi, Elisabetta, et al. "Physical Activity Patterns in Normal-Weight and Overweight/Obese Pregnant Women." *PloS one* 11.11 (2016): e0166254.

[33] Ward-Ritacco, Christie, Mélanie S. Poudevigne, and Patrick J. O'Connor. "Muscle strengthening exercises during pregnancy are associated with increased energy and reduced fatigue." *Journal of Psychosomatic Obstetrics & Gynecology* 37.2 (2016): 68-72.

Real Food for Pregnancy

Chapter 9

[1] Bodnar, Lisa M et al. "High prevalence of vitamin D insufficiency in black and white pregnant women residing in the northern United States and their neonates." *The Journal of Nutrition* 137.2 (2007): 447-452.

[2] Wei, Shu-Qin et al. "Maternal vitamin D status and adverse pregnancy outcomes: a systematic review and meta-analysis." *The Journal of Maternal-Fetal & Neonatal Medicine* 26.9 (2013): 889-899.

[3] Aghajafari, Fariba et al. "Association between maternal serum 25-hydroxyvitamin D level and pregnancy and neonatal outcomes: systematic review and meta-analysis of observational studies." *BMJ: British Medical Journal* 346 (2013).

[4] Javaid, MK et al. "Maternal vitamin D status during pregnancy and childhood bone mass at age 9 years: a longitudinal study." *The Lancet* 367.9504 (2006): 36-43.

[5] Elsori, Deena H., and Majeda S. Hammoud. "Vitamin D deficiency in mothers, neonates and children." *The Journal of Steroid Biochemistry and Molecular Biology* (2017).

[6] Hollis, Bruce W et al. "Vitamin D supplementation during pregnancy: Double-blind, randomized clinical trial of safety and effectiveness." *Journal of Bone and Mineral Research* 26.10 (2011): 2341-2357.

[7] "Vitamin D Council | Testing for vitamin D." https://www.vitamindcouncil.org/about-vitamin-d/testing-for-vitamin-d/. Accessed 8 May. 2017.

[8] Luxwolda, Martine F., et al. "Traditionally living populations in East Africa have a mean serum 25-hydroxyvitamin D concentration of 115 nmol/l." *British Journal of Nutrition* 108.09 (2012): 1557-1561.

[9] Dawodu, Adekunle, and Reginald C. Tsang. "Maternal vitamin D status: effect on milk vitamin D content and vitamin D status of breastfeeding infants." *Advances in Nutrition: An International Review Journal* 3.3 (2012): 353-361.

[10] Brunner C, Wuillemin WA. [Iron deficiency and iron deficiency anemia—symptoms and therapy]. Ther Umsch. 2010;67(5):219–23.

[11] Scholl TO, Hediger ML, Fischer RL, et al. Anemia vs iron deficiency— Increased risk of preterm delivery in a prospective study. Am J Clin Nutr. 1992;55:985-988.

[12] Zimmermann, Michael B., Hans Burgi, and Richard F. Hurrell. "Iron deficiency predicts poor maternal thyroid status during pregnancy." *The Journal of Clinical Endocrinology & Metabolism* 92.9 (2007): 3436-3440.

[13] Walsh, Thomas, et al. "Laboratory assessment of iron status in pregnancy." *Clinical chemistry and laboratory medicine* 49.7 (2011): 1225-1230.

[14] Vandevijvere, Stefanie, et al. "Iron status and its determinants in a nationally representative sample of pregnant women." *Journal of the Academy of Nutrition and Dietetics* 113.5 (2013): 659-666.

[15] "Moog, Nora K., et al. "Influence of maternal thyroid hormones during gestation on fetal brain development." *Neuroscience* 342 (2017): 68-100.

[16] Moog, Nora K., et al. "Influence of maternal thyroid hormones during gestation on fetal brain development." *Neuroscience* 342 (2017): 68-100.

[17] Johns, Lauren E., et al. "Longitudinal Profiles of Thyroid Hormone Parameters in Pregnancy and Associations with Preterm Birth." *PloS one* 12.1 (2017): e0169542.

[18] Almomin AM, Mansour AA, Sharief M. Trimester-Specific Reference Intervals of Thyroid Function Testing in Pregnant Women from Basrah, Iraq Using Electrochemiluminescent Immunoassay. Diseases. (2016) Apr 26;4(2):20.

[19] Abalovich, M., et al. "Overt and subclinical hypothyroidism complicating pregnancy." *Thyroid* 12.1 (2002): 63-68.

[20] Moog, Nora K., et al. "Influence of maternal thyroid hormones during gestation on fetal brain development." *Neuroscience* 342 (2017): 68-100.

[21] Alexander, Erik K., et al. "2017 Guidelines of the American Thyroid Association for the diagnosis and management of thyroid disease during pregnancy and the postpartum." *Thyroid* 27.3 (2017): 315-389.

[22] Stricker, R. T., et al. "Evaluation of maternal thyroid function during pregnancy: the importance of using gestational age-specific reference intervals." *European Journal of Endocrinology* 157.4 (2007): 509-514.

[23] Alexander, Erik K., et al. "2017 Guidelines of the American Thyroid Association for the diagnosis and management of thyroid disease during pregnancy and the postpartum." *Thyroid* 27.3 (2017): 315-389.

[24] Alexander, Erik K., et al. "2017 Guidelines of the American Thyroid Association for the diagnosis and management of thyroid disease during pregnancy and the postpartum." *Thyroid* 27.3 (2017): 315-389.

[25] Practice Committee of the American Society for Reproductive Medicine. "Subclinical hypothyroidism in the infertile female population: a guideline." *Fertility and sterility* 104.3 (2015): 545-553.

[26] Forbes, Scott. "Pregnancy sickness and parent-offspring conflict over thyroid function." *Journal of theoretical biology* 355 (2014): 61-67.

[27] Caldwell KL, Makhmudov A, Ely E, Jones RL, Wang RY. Iodine status of the U.S. population, National Health and Nutrition Examination Survey, 2005-2006 and 2007-2008. *Thyroid* 21 (2011): 419–427.

[28] Dunn, John T. "Iodine should be routinely added to complementary foods." *The Journal of nutrition* 133.9 (2003): 3008S-3010S.

[29] Zava, Theodore T., and David T. Zava. "Assessment of Japanese iodine intake based on seaweed consumption in Japan: A literature-based analysis." *Thyroid research* 4.1 (2011): 14.

[30] Fuse, Yozen, et al. "Iodine status of pregnant and postpartum Japanese women: effect of iodine intake on maternal and neonatal thyroid function in an iodine-sufficient area." *The Journal of Clinical Endocrinology & Metabolism* 96.12 (2011): 3846-3854.

[31] Leung, Angela M., Elizabeth N. Pearce, and Lewis E. Braverman. "Iodine content of prenatal multivitamins in the United States." *New England Journal of Medicine* 360.9 (2009): 939-940.

[32] "Iodine — Health Professional Fact Sheet - Office of Dietary Supplements." 24 Jun. 2011, https://ods.od.nih.gov/factsheets/Iodine-HealthProfessional/. Accessed 13 Jun. 2017.

[33] Fordyce, F. M. "Database of the iodine content of food and diets populated with data from published literature." (2003). Nottingham, UK, British Geological Survey.

[34] Diosady, L. L., et al. "Stability of iodine in iodized salt used for correction of iodine-deficiency disorders. II." *Food and Nutrition Bulletin* 19.3 (1998): 240-250.

[35] BaJaJ, Jagminder K., Poonam Salwan, and Shalini Salwan. "Various possible toxicants involved in thyroid dysfunction: A Review." *Journal of clinical and diagnostic research: JCDR* 10.1 (2016): FE01.

[36] Veltri, Flora, et al. "Prevalence of thyroid autoimmunity and dysfunction in women with iron deficiency during early pregnancy: is it altered?." *European Journal of Endocrinology* 175.3 (2016): 191-199.

[37] Mahmoodianfard, Salma, et al. "Effects of zinc and selenium supplementation on thyroid function in overweight and obese hypothyroid female patients: a randomized double-blind controlled trial." *Journal of the American College of Nutrition* 34.5 (2015): 391-399.

[38] Negro, Roberto, et al. "The influence of selenium supplementation on postpartum thyroid status in pregnant women with thyroid peroxidase autoantibodies." *The Journal of Clinical Endocrinology & Metabolism* 92.4 (2007): 1263-1268.

[39] "Wang, Jiying, et al. "Meta-analysis of the association between vitamin D and autoimmune thyroid disease." *Nutrients* 7.4 (2015): 2485-2498.

[40] Lundin, Knut EA, and Cisca Wijmenga. "Coeliac disease and autoimmune disease [mdash] genetic overlap and screening." *Nature Reviews Gastroenterology & Hepatology* 12.9 (2015): 507-515.

[41] Leung, Angela M., et al. "Exposure to thyroid-disrupting chemicals: a transatlantic call for action." (2016): 479-480.

[42] Fong, Alex, et al. "Use of hemoglobin A1c as an early predictor of gestational diabetes mellitus." *American journal of obstetrics and gynecology* 211.6 (2014): 641-e1.

[43] Hughes, Ruth CE, et al. "An early pregnancy HbA1c≥ 5.9%(41 mmol/mol) is optimal for detecting diabetes and identifies women at increased risk of adverse pregnancy outcomes." *Diabetes Care* 37.11 (2014): 2953-2959.

[44] Ahmeda, Sheikh Salahuddin, and Tarafdar Runa Lailaa. "Hemoglobin A1c and Fructosamine in Diabetes: Clinical Use and Limitations."

[45] Shang, M., and L. Lin. "IADPSG criteria for diagnosing gestational diabetes mellitus and predicting adverse pregnancy outcomes." *Journal of Perinatology* 34.2 (2014): 100-104.

[46] Lamar, Michael E., et al. "Jelly beans as an alternative to a fifty-gram glucose beverage for gestational diabetes screening." *American journal of obstetrics and gynecology* 181.5 (1999): 1154-1157.

[47] Damayanti, Sophi, Benny Permana, and Choong Chie Weng. "Determination of Sugar Content in Fruit Juices Using High Performance Liquid Chromatography." *Acta Pharmaceutica Indonesia* 37.4 (2017): 131-139.

[48] Kuwa, Katsuhiko, et al. "Relationships of glucose concentrations in capillary whole blood, venous whole blood and venous plasma." *Clinica Chimica Acta* 307.1 (2001): 187-192.

[49] Hoffman, R. M., et al. "Glucose clearance in grazing mares is affected by diet, pregnancy, and lactation." *Journal of animal science* 81.7 (2003): 1764-1771.

[50] Wilkerson, Hugh LC, et al. "Diagnostic evaluation of oral glucose tolerance tests in nondiabetic subjects after various levels of carbohydrate intake." *New England Journal of Medicine* 262.21 (1960): 1047-1053.

[51] Tajima, Ryoko, et al. "Carbohydrate intake during early pregnancy is inversely associated with abnormal glucose challenge test results in Japanese pregnant women." *Diabetes/Metabolism Research and Reviews* (2017).

[52] Agarwal, Mukesh M. "Gestational diabetes mellitus: Screening with fasting plasma glucose." *World Journal of Diabetes* 7.14 (2016): 279.

[53] Agarwal, Mukesh M. "Gestational diabetes mellitus: Screening with fasting plasma glucose." *World Journal of Diabetes* 7.14 (2016): 279.

[54] Rudland, Victoria L., et al. "Gestational Diabetes: Seeing Both the Forest and the Trees." *Current Obstetrics and Gynecology Reports* 1.4 (2012): 198-206.

[55] Hernandez, Teri L., et al. "Patterns of glycemia in normal pregnancy." *Diabetes Care* 34.7 (2011): 1660-1668.

[56] Greenberg, James A, and Stacey J Bell. "Multivitamin supplementation during pregnancy: emphasis on folic acid and L-methylfolate." *Reviews in Obstetrics and Gynecology* 4.3-4 (2011): 126.

[57] Liu, Laura X., and Zolt Arany. "Maternal cardiac metabolism in pregnancy." *Cardiovascular research* 101.4 (2014): 545-553.

[58] Rizzo, Thomas A et al. "Prenatal and perinatal influences on long-term psychomotor development in offspring of diabetic mothers." American Journal of Obstetrics and Gynecology 173.6 (1995): 1753-1758.

[59] Liu, Laura X., and Zolt Arany. "Maternal cardiac metabolism in pregnancy." *Cardiovascular research* 101.4 (2014): 545-553.

[60] Felig, Philip, and Vincent Lynch. "Starvation in human pregnancy: hypoglycemia, hypoinsulinemia, and hyperketonemia." Science 170.3961 (1970): 990-992.

[61] Institute of Medicine (US). Panel on Macronutrients, and Institute of Medicine (US). Standing Committee on the Scientific Evaluation of Dietary Reference Intakes. Dietary Reference Intakes for energy,

Real Food for Pregnancy

carbohydrate, fiber, fat, fatty acids, cholesterol, protein, and amino acids. Natl Academy Pr, 2005. pg 275-277.

[62] Coetzee, EJ, WPU Jackson, and PA Berman. "Ketonuria in pregnancy—with special reference to calorie-restricted food intake in obese diabetics." Diabetes 29.3 (1980): 177-181.

[63] Institute of Medicine (US). Panel on Macronutrients, and Institute of Medicine (US). Standing Committee on the Scientific Evaluation of Dietary Reference Intakes. Dietary Reference Intakes for energy, carbohydrate, fiber, fat, fatty acids, cholesterol, protein, and amino acids. Natl Academy Pr, 2005. pg 275-277.

[64] Bon, C et al. "[Feto-maternal metabolism in human normal pregnancies: study of 73 cases]." Annales de Biologie Clinique Dec. 2006: 609-619.

[65] Muneta, Tetsuo, et al. "Ketone body elevation in placenta, umbilical cord, newborn and mother in normal delivery." Glycative Stress Research 3 (2016): 133-140.

Chapter 10

[1] Sultan, Charles, et al. "Environmental xenoestrogens, antiandrogens and disorders of male sexual differentiation." Molecular and cellular endocrinology 178.1 (2001): 99-105.

[2] Nagel, S. C., vom Saal, F. S., Thayer, K. A., Dhar, M. G., Boechler, M., & Welshons, W. V. (1997). Relative binding affinity-serum modified access (RBA-SMA) assay predicts the relative in vivo bioactivity of the xenoestrogens bisphenol A and octylphenol. Environmental health perspectives, 105(1), 70.

[3] Kass, Laura, et al. "Perinatal exposure to xenoestrogens impairs mammary gland differentiation and modifies milk composition in Wistar rats." Reproductive Toxicology 33.3 (2012): 390-400.

[4] Nadal, Angel, et al. "The pancreatic β-cell as a target of estrogens and xenoestrogens: Implications for blood glucose homeostasis and diabetes." Molecular and cellular endocrinology 304.1 (2009): 63-68.

[5] Alonso-Magdalena, Paloma, et al. "Bisphenol A exposure during pregnancy disrupts glucose homeostasis in mothers and adult male offspring." Environmental health perspectives 118.9 (2010): 1243.

[6] Rochester, Johanna R. "Bisphenol A and human health: a review of the literature." Reproductive toxicology 42 (2013): 132-155.

[7] Evans, Sarah F., et al. "Prenatal bisphenol A exposure and maternally reported behavior in boys and girls." Neurotoxicology 45 (2014): 91-99.

[8] Harley KG, et al. (2013) Prenatal and early childhood bisphenol A concentrations and behavior in school-aged children. Environ Res 126:43–50

[9] Kinch, Cassandra D., et al. "Low-dose exposure to bisphenol A and replacement bisphenol S induces precocious hypothalamic neurogenesis in embryonic zebrafish." Proceedings of the National Academy of Sciences 112.5 (2015): 1475-1480.

[10] Vandenberg, Laura N., et al. "Human exposure to bisphenol A (BPA)." Reproductive toxicology 24.2 (2007): 139-177.

[11] Ikezuki, Yumiko, et al. "Determination of bisphenol A concentrations in human biological fluids reveals significant early prenatal exposure." Human reproduction 17.11 (2002): 2839-2841.

[12] Rudel RA, Gray JM, Engel CL, et al. Food packaging and bisphenol A and bis(2-ethyhexyl) phthalate exposure: findings from a dietary intervention. Environ Health Perspect. 2011;119:914–920.

[13] Vandenberg, Laura N., et al. "Human exposure to bisphenol A (BPA)." Reproductive toxicology 24.2 (2007): 139-177.

[14] Qiu, Wenhui, et al. "Actions of bisphenol A and bisphenol S on the reproductive neuroendocrine system during early development in zebrafish." Endocrinology 157.2 (2016): 636-647.

[15] Kinch, Cassandra D., et al. "Low-dose exposure to bisphenol A and replacement bisphenol S induces precocious hypothalamic neurogenesis in embryonic zebrafish." Proceedings of the National Academy of Sciences 112.5 (2015): 1475-1480.

[16] Hormann, Annette M., et al. "Holding thermal receipt paper and eating food after using hand sanitizer results in high serum bioactive and urine total levels of bisphenol A (BPA)." PloS one 9.10 (2014): e110509.

[17] SCCNFP. 2002. Opinion of the Scientific Committee on Cosmetic Products and Non-Food Products Intended for Consumers. Concerning Diethyl Phthalate. Available: http://ec.europa.eu/health/archive/ph_risk/committees/sccp/documents/out168_en.pdf Accessed 22 May. 2017.

[18] Adibi, Jennifer J., et al. "Prenatal exposures to phthalates among women in New York City and Krakow, Poland." Environmental Health Perspectives 111.14 (2003): 1719.

[19] Adibi, Jennifer J., et al. "Prenatal exposures to phthalates among women in New York City and Krakow, Poland." Environmental Health Perspectives 111.14 (2003): 1719.

[20] Albert, O.; Jegou, B. (2013). "A critical assessment of the endocrine susceptibility of the human testis to phthalates from fetal life to adulthood". Human Reproduction Update. 20 (2): 231–49.

[21] Barrett, Julia R. "Phthalates and baby boys: potential disruption of human genital development." Environmental health perspectives 113.8 (2005): A542.

[22] Tilson HA (June 2008). "EHP Papers of the Year, 2008". Environ. Health Perspect. 116 (6): A234.

[23] Swan SH; Liu F; Hines M; et al. (April 2010). "Prenatal phthalate exposure and reduced masculine play in boys". International Journal of Andrology. 33: 259–269.

[24] Factor-Litvak, P; Insel, B; Calafat, A. M.; Liu, X; Perera, F; Rauh, V. A.; Whyatt, R. M. (2014). "Persistent Associations between Maternal Prenatal Exposure to Phthalates on Child IQ at Age 7 Years". *PLoS ONE.* **9** (12): e114003.

[25] Ferguson, Kelly K.; McElrath, Thomas F.; Meeker, John D. (2014-01-01). "Environmental phthalate exposure and preterm birth". *JAMA pediatrics.* 168 (1): 61–67.

[26] Geer, Laura A., et al. "Association of birth outcomes with fetal exposure to parabens, triclosan and triclocarban in an immigrant population in Brooklyn, New York." *Journal of hazardous materials* 323 (2017): 177-183.

[27] Vo, Thuy TB, and Eui-Bae Jeung. "An evaluation of estrogenic activity of parabens using uterine calbindin-D9k gene in an immature rat model." *Toxicological sciences* 112.1 (2009): 68-77.

[28] "European Commission - PRESS RELEASES - Press ... - Europa.eu." 26 Sep. 2014, http://europa.eu/rapid/press-release_IP-14-1051_en.htm. Accessed 25 May. 2017.

[29] Braun, Joe M., et al. "Personal care product use and urinary phthalate metabolite and paraben concentrations during pregnancy among women from a fertility clinic." *Journal of Exposure Science and Environmental Epidemiology* 24.5 (2014): 459-466.

[30] Fisher, Mandy, et al. "Paraben Concentrations in Maternal Urine and Breast Milk and Its Association with Personal Care Product Use." *Environmental Science & Technology* 51.7 (2017): 4009-4017.

[31] Philippat, Claire, et al. "Prenatal exposure to environmental phenols: concentrations in amniotic fluid and variability in urinary concentrations during pregnancy." *Environmental Health Perspectives (Online)* 121.10 (2013): 1225.

[32] Geer, Laura A., et al. "Association of birth outcomes with fetal exposure to parabens, triclosan and triclocarban in an immigrant population in Brooklyn, New York." *Journal of hazardous materials* 323 (2017): 177-183.

[33] Aker, Amira M., et al. "Phenols and parabens in relation to reproductive and thyroid hormones in pregnant women." *Environmental Research* 151 (2016): 30-37.

[34] Philippat, Claire, et al. "Prenatal exposure to phenols and growth in boys." *Epidemiology (Cambridge, Mass.)* 25.5 (2014): 625.

[35] Harley, Kim G., et al. "Reducing phthalate, paraben, and phenol exposure from personal care products in adolescent girls: findings from the HERMOSA Intervention Study." *Environmental Health Perspectives* 124.10 (2016): 1600.

[36] Rattan, Saniya, et al. "Exposure to endocrine disruptors during adulthood: consequences for female fertility." *Journal of Endocrinology* 233.3 (2017): R109-R129.

[37] Frazier, Linda M. "Reproductive disorders associated with pesticide exposure." *Journal of agromedicine* 12.1 (2007): 27-37.

[38] Koifman, Sergio, Rosalina Jorge Koifman, and Armando Meyer. "Human reproductive system disturbances and pesticide exposure in Brazil." *Cadernos de Saúde Pública* 18.2 (2002): 435-445.

[39] Fernandez, Mariana F., et al. "Human exposure to endocrine-disrupting chemicals and prenatal risk factors for cryptorchidism and hypospadias: a nested case-control study." (2007).

[40] Fernandez, Mariana F., et al. "Human exposure to endocrine-disrupting chemicals and prenatal risk factors for cryptorchidism and hypospadias: a nested case-control study." (2007).

[41] Andersen, Helle R., et al. "Impaired reproductive development in sons of women occupationally exposed to pesticides during pregnancy." *Environmental health perspectives* 116.4 (2008): 566.

[42] Jurewicz, Joanna, and Wojciech Hanke. "Prenatal and childhood exposure to pesticides and neurobehavioral development: review of epidemiological studies." *International journal of occupational medicine and environmental health* 21.2 (2008): 121-132.

[43] Brucker-Davis, F. "Effects of environmental synthetic chemicals on thyroid function." *Thyroid: Official Journal of the American Thyroid Association* 8.9 (1998): 827.

[44] Colborn, Theo. "A case for revisiting the safety of pesticides: a closer look at neurodevelopment." *Environmental health perspectives* (2006): 10-17.

[45] Toft, Gunnar, et al. "Fetal loss and maternal serum levels of 2, 2', 4, 4', 5, 5'-hexachlorbiphenyl (CB-153) and 1, 1-dichloro-2, 2-bis (p-chlorophenyl) ethylene (p, p'-DDE) exposure: a cohort study in Greenland and two European populations." *Environmental Health* 9.1 (2010): 22.

[46] Toft, Gunnar, et al. "Fetal loss and maternal serum levels of 2, 2', 4, 4', 5, 5'-hexachlorbiphenyl (CB-153) and 1, 1-dichloro-2, 2-bis (p-chlorophenyl) ethylene (p, p'-DDE) exposure: a cohort study in Greenland and two European populations." *Environmental Health* 9.1 (2010): 22.

[47] Guyton, Kathryn Z., et al. "Carcinogenicity of tetrachlorvinphos, parathion, malathion, diazinon, and glyphosate." *Lancet Oncology* 16.5 (2015): 490.

[48] Vandenberg, Laura N., et al. "Is it time to reassess current safety standards for glyphosate-based herbicides?." *J Epidemiol Community Health* 71.6 (2017): 613-618.

[49] Cuhra, Marek. "Review of GMO safety assessment studies: glyphosate residues in Roundup Ready crops is an ignored issue." *Environmental Sciences Europe* 27.1 (2015): 20.

[50] Samsel, A., and Seneff, S. "Glyphosate's suppression of cytochrome P450 enzymes and amino acid biosynthesis by the gut microbiome: pathways to modern diseases." *Entropy* 15.4 (2013): 1416-1463.

[51] Samsel, A., and Seneff, S. "Glyphosate's suppression of cytochrome P450 enzymes and amino acid biosynthesis by the gut microbiome: pathways to modern diseases." *Entropy* 15.4 (2013): 1416-1463.

[52] Samsel, A., and Seneff, S. "Glyphosate's suppression of cytochrome P450 enzymes and amino acid biosynthesis by the gut microbiome: pathways to modern diseases." *Entropy* 15.4 (2013): 1416-1463.

[53] Schimpf, Marlise Guerrero, et al. "Neonatal exposure to a glyphosate based herbicide alters the development of the rat uterus." *Toxicology* 376 (2017): 2-14.

[54] Richard, Sophie, et al. "Differential effects of glyphosate and roundup on human placental cells and aromatase." *Environmental health perspectives* (2005): 716-720.

[55] Nicolopoulou-Stamati, Polyxeni, et al. "Chemical Pesticides and Human Health: The Urgent Need for a New Concept in Agriculture." *Frontiers in Public Health* 4 (2016).

[56] Barański, Marcin, et al. "Higher antioxidant and lower cadmium concentrations and lower incidence of pesticide residues in organically grown crops: a systematic literature review and meta-analyses." *British Journal of Nutrition* 112.05 (2014): 794-811.

[57] "Oates, Liza, and Marc Cohen. "Assessing diet as a modifiable risk factor for pesticide exposure." *International journal of environmental research and public health* 8.6 (2011): 1792-1804.

[58] Krüger, Monika, et al. "Detection of glyphosate residues in animals and humans." *Journal of Environmental & Analytical Toxicology* 4.2 (2014): 1.

[59] Keikotlhaile, Boitshepo Miriam, Pieter Spanoghe, and Walter Steurbaut. "Effects of food processing on pesticide residues in fruits and vegetables: a meta-analysis approach." *Food and Chemical Toxicology* 48.1 (2010): 1-6.

[60] "eCFR — Code of Federal Regulations - acamedia.info." 2 Sep. 2016, http://www.acamedia.info/sciences/sciliterature/globalw/reference/glyphosate/US_eCFR.pdf. Accessed 19 May. 2017.

[61] Canadian Food Inspection Agency: Science Branch Survey Report. *"Safeguarding with Science: Glyphosate Testing in 2015-2016."* Ottawa, Ontario Canada.

[62] Krüger, Monika, et al. "Detection of glyphosate residues in animals and humans." *Journal of Environmental & Analytical Toxicology* 4.2 (2014): 1.

[63] "Strawberries | EWG's 2017 Shopper's Guide to Pesticides in Produce." https://www.ewg.org/foodnews/strawberries.php. Accessed 2 Jun. 2017.

[64] Colborn, Theo. "A case for revisiting the safety of pesticides: a closer look at neurodevelopment." *Environmental health perspectives* (2006): 10-17.

[65] Relea, AL, and Oking Tempera. "Teflon can't stand the heat." *Environmental Working Group.* 2013.

[66] Olsen, Geary W., et al. "Half-life of serum elimination of perfluorooctanesulfonate, perfluorohexanesulfonate, and perfluorooctanoate in retired fluorochemical production workers." *Environmental health perspectives* (2007): 1298-1305.

[67] Mitro, Susanna D., Tyiesha Johnson, and Ami R. Zota. "Cumulative chemical exposures during pregnancy and early development." *Current environmental health reports* 2.4 (2015): 367-378.

[68] Fei, Chunyuan, et al. "Perfluorinated chemicals and fetal growth: a study within the Danish National Birth Cohort." Environmental health perspectives (2007): 1677-1682.

[69] Washino, Noriaki, et al. "Correlations between prenatal exposure to perfluorinated chemicals and reduced fetal growth." *Environmental Health Perspectives* 117.4 (2009): 660.

[70] Fei, Chunyuan, et al. "Fetal growth indicators and perfluorinated chemicals: a study in the Danish National Birth Cohort." *American journal of epidemiology* 168.1 (2008): 66-72.

[71] Savitz, David A., et al. "Perfluorooctanoic acid exposure and pregnancy outcome in a highly exposed community." *Epidemiology (Cambridge, Mass.)* 23.3 (2012): 386.

[72] Fei, Chunyuan, Clarice R. Weinberg, and Jørn Olsen. "Commentary: perfluorinated chemicals and time to pregnancy: a link based on reverse causation?." *Epidemiology* 23.2 (2012): 264-266.

[73] Inoue, Koichi, et al. "Perfluorooctane sulfonate (PFOS) and related perfluorinated compounds in human maternal and cord blood samples: assessment of PFOS exposure in a susceptible population during pregnancy." *Environmental health perspectives* (2004): 1204-1207.

[74] Melzer, David, et al. "Association between serum perfluorooctanoic acid (PFOA) and thyroid disease in the US National Health and Nutrition Examination Survey." (2010).

[75] Wang, Yan, et al. "Association between maternal serum perfluoroalkyl substances during pregnancy and maternal and cord thyroid hormones: Taiwan maternal and infant cohort study." *Environmental Health Perspectives (Online)* 122.5 (2014): 529.

[76] Dallaire, Renée, et al. "Thyroid hormone levels of pregnant Inuit women and their infants exposed to environmental contaminants." *Environmental health perspectives* 117.6 (2009): 1014.

[77] Shah-Kulkarni, Surabhi, et al. "Prenatal exposure to perfluorinated compounds affects thyroid hormone levels in newborn girls." *Environment International* 94 (2016): 607-613.

[78] Melzer, David, et al. "Association between serum perfluorooctanoic acid (PFOA) and thyroid disease in the US National Health and Nutrition Examination Survey." (2010).

[79] "Strawberries | EWG's 2017 Shopper's Guide to Pesticides in Produce." https://www.ewg.org/foodnews/strawberries.php. Accessed 5 Jun. 2017.

[80] Iheozor-Ejiofor, Zipporah, et al. "Water fluoridation for the prevention of dental caries." *The Cochrane Library* (2015).

[81] Caldera, R., et al. "Maternal-fetal transfer of fluoride in pregnant women." *Neonatology* 54.5 (1988): 263-269.

[82] Chen, Y. X., et al. "Research on the intellectual development of children in high fluoride areas." *Fluoride* 41.2 (2008): 120-124.

[83] Zhao, L. B., et al. "Effect of a high fluoride water supply on children's intelligence." *Fluoride* 29.4 (1996): 190-192.

[84] Bashash, Morteza, et al. "Prenatal Fluoride Exposure and Cognitive Outcomes in Children at 4 and 6–12 Years of Age in Mexico." *Environmental Health Perspectives* 87008: 1 (2017).

[85] Jiménez, L. Valdez, et al. "In utero exposure to fluoride and cognitive development delay in infants." *Neurotoxicology* 59 (2017): 65-70.

[86] Yanni, Y. U. "Effects of fluoride on the ultrastructure of glandular epithelial cells of human fetuses." *Chinese Journal of Endemiology* 19.2 (2000): 81-83.

[87] Dong, Zhong, et al. "Determina on of the Contents of Amino Acid and Monoamine Neurotransmitters in Fetal Brains from a Fluorosis Endemic Area." Journal of Guiyang Medical College 18.4 (1997): 241-245.

[88] He, Han, Zaishe Cheng, and WeiQun Liu. "Effects of fluorine on the human fetus." *Fluoride* 41.4 (2008): 321-6.

[89] Du, Li, et al. "The effect of fluorine on the developing human brain." *Fluoride* 41.4 (2008): 327-30.

[90] Yu, Yanni, et al. "Neurotransmitter and receptor changes in the brains of fetuses from areas of endemic fluorosis." *Fluoride* 41.2 (2008): 134-138.

[91] Yu, Yanni, et al. "Neurotransmitter and receptor changes in the brains of fetuses from areas of endemic fluorosis." *Fluoride* 41.2 (2008): 134-138.

[92] Li, Jing, et al. "Effects of high fluoride level on neonatal neurobehavioral development." *Fluoride* 41.2 (2008): 165-70.

[93] Wang, J. D., et al. "Effects of high fluoride and low iodine on oxidative stress and antioxidant defense of the brain in offspring rats." *Fluoride* 37.4 (2004): 264-270.

[94] Christie, David P. "The spectrum of radiographic bone changes in children with fluorosis." *Radiology* 136.1 (1980): 85-90.

[95] "Fluoride Action Network | Dental Products." http://fluoridealert.org/issues/sources/f-toothpaste/. Accessed 13 Jun. 2017.

[96] Lu, Y. I., Wen-Fei Guo, and Xian-Qiang Yang. "Fluoride content in tea and its relationship with tea quality." *Journal of agricultural and food chemistry* 52.14 (2004): 4472-4476.

[97] Whyte, Michael P., et al. "Skeletal fluorosis from instant tea." *Journal of Bone and Mineral Research* 23.5 (2008): 759-769.

[98] Malinowska, E., et al. "Assessment of fluoride concentration and daily intake by human from tea and herbal infusions." *Food and Chemical Toxicology* 46.3 (2008): 1055-1061.

[99] Nayak, Prasunpriya. "Aluminum: impacts and disease." *Environmental research* 89.2 (2002): 101-115.

[100] Karimour, A., et al. "Toxicity Effects of Aluminum Chloride on Uterus and Placenta of Pregnant Mice." *JBUMS*, (2005): 22-27.

[101] Nayak, Prasunpriya. "Aluminum: impacts and disease." *Environmental research* 89.2 (2002): 101-115.

[102] Reinke, Claudia M., Jörg Breitkreutz, and Hans Leuenberger. "Aluminium in over-the-counter drugs." *Drug Safety* 26.14 (2003): 1011-1025.

[103] Abu-Taweel, Gasem M., Jamaan S. Ajarem, and Mohammad Ahmad. "Neurobehavioral toxic effects of perinatal oral exposure to aluminum on the developmental motor reflexes, learning, memory and brain neurotransmitters of mice offspring." *Pharmacology Biochemistry and Behavior* 101.1 (2012): 49-56.

[104] Fanni, Daniela, et al. "Aluminum exposure and toxicity in neonates: a practical guide to halt aluminum overload in the prenatal and perinatal periods." *World J Pediatr* 10.2 (2014): 101-107.

[105] Dórea, José G. "Exposure to mercury and aluminum in early life: developmental vulnerability as a modifying factor in neurologic and immunologic effects." *International journal of environmental research and public health* 12.2 (2015): 1295-1313.

[106] Fanni, Daniela, et al. "Aluminum exposure and toxicity in neonates: a practical guide to halt aluminum overload in the prenatal and perinatal periods." *World Journal of Pediatrics* 10.2 (2014): 101-107.

[107] Exley, Christopher. "Human exposure to aluminium." *Environmental Science: Processes & Impacts* 15.10 (2013): 1807-1816.

[108] Reinke, Claudia M., Jörg Breitkreutz, and Hans Leuenberger. "Aluminium in over-the-counter drugs." *Drug Safety* 26.14 (2003): 1011-1025.

[109] Fanni, Daniela, et al. "Aluminum exposure and toxicity in neonates: a practical guide to halt aluminum overload in the prenatal and perinatal periods." *World Journal of Pediatrics* 10.2 (2014): 101-107.

[110] Exley, Christopher. "Human exposure to aluminium." *Environmental Science: Processes & Impacts* 15.10 (2013): 1807-1816.

[111] Dórea, José G. "Exposure to mercury and aluminum in early life: developmental vulnerability as a modifying factor in neurologic and immunologic effects." *International journal of environmental research and public health* 12.2 (2015): 1295-1313.

[112] Shaw, C. A., and L. Tomljenovic. "Aluminum in the central nervous system (CNS): toxicity in humans and animals, vaccine adjuvants, and autoimmunity." *Immunologic research* 56.2-3 (2013): 304.

[113] Crépeaux, Guillemette, et al. "Non-linear dose-response of aluminium hydroxide adjuvant particles: Selective low dose neurotoxicity." *Toxicology* 375 (2017): 48-57.

[114] Crépeaux, Guillemette, et al. "Non-linear dose-response of aluminium hydroxide adjuvant particles: Selective low dose neurotoxicity." *Toxicology* 375 (2017): 48-57.

[115] Inbar, Rotem, et al. "Behavioral abnormalities in female mice following administration of aluminum adjuvants and the human papillomavirus (HPV) vaccine Gardasil." *Immunologic Research* 65.1 (2017): 136-149.

[116] "Ranau, R., J. Oehlenschläger, and H. Steinhart. "Aluminium levels of fish fillets baked and grilled in aluminium foil." *Food Chemistry* 73.1 (2001): 1-6.

Real Food for Pregnancy

[117] Bassioni, Ghada, et al. "Risk assessment of using aluminum foil in food preparation." *Int. J. Electrochem. Sci* 7.5 (2012): 4498-4509.

[118] Cardenas, Andres, et al. "Persistent DNA methylation changes associated with prenatal mercury exposure and cognitive performance during childhood." *Scientific Reports* 7 (2017).

[119] Cardenas, Andres, et al. "Persistent DNA methylation changes associated with prenatal mercury exposure and cognitive performance during childhood." *Scientific Reports* 7 (2017).

[120] Oken, Emily, et al. "Maternal fish intake during pregnancy, blood mercury levels, and child cognition at age 3 years in a US cohort." *American Journal of Epidemiology* 167.10 (2008): 1171-1181.

[121] Hibbeln, Joseph R., et al. "Maternal seafood consumption in pregnancy and neurodevelopmental outcomes in childhood (ALSPAC study): an observational cohort study." *The Lancet* 369.9561 (2007): 578-585.

[122] Björnberg, K. Ask, et al. "Methyl mercury and inorganic mercury in Swedish pregnant women and in cord blood: influence of fish consumption." *Environmental Health Perspectives* 111.4 (2003): 637.

[123] Palkovicova, Lubica, et al. "Maternal amalgam dental fillings as the source of mercury exposure in developing fetus and newborn." *Journal of Exposure Science and Environmental Epidemiology* 18.3 (2008): 326-331.

[124] Anderson BA, Arenholt-Bindslev D, Cooper IR, et al. Dental amalgam—a report with reference to the medical devices directive 93/42/EEC from an Ad Hoc Working Group mandated by DGIII of the European Commission. Angelholm, Sweden: Nordiska Dental AB, 1998.

[125] Mahboubi, Arash, et al. "Evaluation of thimerosal removal on immunogenicity of aluminum salts adjuvanted recombinant hepatitis B vaccine." *Iranian journal of pharmaceutical research: IJPR* 11.1 (2012): 39.

[126] Pletz, Julia, Francisco Sánchez-Bayo, and Henk A. Tennekes. "Dose-response analysis indicating time-dependent neurotoxicity caused by organic and inorganic mercury—Implications for toxic effects in the developing brain." *Toxicology* 347 (2016): 1-5.

[127] Rattan, Saniya, et al. "Exposure to endocrine disruptors during adulthood: consequences for female fertility." *Journal of Endocrinology* 233.3 (2017): R109-R129.

[128] Mitro, Susanna D., Tyiesha Johnson, and Ami R. Zota. "Cumulative chemical exposures during pregnancy and early development." *Current environmental health reports* 2.4 (2015): 367-378.

[129] Hu, Jianzhong, et al. "Effect of postnatal low-dose exposure to environmental chemicals on the gut microbiome in a rodent model." *Microbiome* 4.1 (2016): 26.

[130] Philippat, Claire, et al. "Prenatal exposure to phenols and growth in boys." *Epidemiology (Cambridge, Mass.)* 25.5 (2014): 625.

[131] "Hu, Jianzhong, et al. "Effect of postnatal low-dose exposure to environmental chemicals on the gut microbiome in a rodent model." *Microbiome* 4.1 (2016): 26.

[132] Geer, Laura A., et al. "Association of birth outcomes with fetal exposure to parabens, triclosan and triclocarban in an immigrant population in Brooklyn, New York." *Journal of hazardous materials* 323 (2017): 177-183.

[133] Marcus, Donald M., and Arthur P. Grollman. "Botanical medicines—the need for new regulations." *The New England Journal of Medicine* 347.25 (2002): 2073.

[134] "Metals > Questions and Answers on Lead-Glazed Traditional ... - FDA." 9 May. 2017, https://www.fda.gov/food/foodborneillnesscontaminants/metals/ucm233281.htm. Accessed 15 Jun. 2017.

[135] Morita, K., T. Matsueda, and T. Iida. "Effect of green vegetable on digestive tract absorption of polychlorinated dibenzo-p-dioxins and polychlorinated dibenzofurans in rats." *Fukuoka igaku zasshi= Hukuoka acta medica* 90.5 (1999): 171-183.

[136] Navarro, Sandi L., et al. "Modulation of human serum glutathione S-transferase A1/2 concentration by cruciferous vegetables in a controlled feeding study is influenced by GSTM1 and GSTT1 genotypes." *Cancer Epidemiology and Prevention Biomarkers* 18.11 (2009): 2974-2978.

[137] Sears, Margaret E. "Chelation: harnessing and enhancing heavy metal detoxification—a review." *The Scientific World Journal* 2013 (2013).

[138] Morita, Kunimasa, Masahiro Ogata, and Takashi Hasegawa. "Chlorophyll derived from Chlorella inhibits dioxin absorption from the gastrointestinal tract and accelerates dioxin excretion in rats." *Environmental Health Perspectives* 109.3 (2001): 289.

[139] Nakano, Shiro, Hideo Takekoshi, and Masuo Nakano. "Chlorella (Chlorella pyrenoidosa) supplementation decreases dioxin and increases immunoglobulin a concentrations in breast milk." *Journal of medicinal food* 10.1 (2007): 134-142.

[140] Uchikawa, Takuya, et al. "The enhanced elimination of tissue methylmercury in Parachlorella beijerinckii-fed mice." *The Journal of toxicological sciences* 36.1 (2011): 121-126.

[141] Banji, David, et al. "Investigation on the role of Spirulina platensis in ameliorating behavioural changes, thyroid dysfunction and oxidative stress in offspring of pregnant rats exposed to fluoride." *Food chemistry* 140.1 (2013): 321-331.

[142] Gargouri, M., et al. "Toxicity of Lead on Femoral Bone in Suckling Rats: Alleviation by Spirulina." *Research & Reviews in BioSciences* 11.3 (2016).

[143] Niang, Khadim, et al. "Spirulina Supplementation in Pregnant Women in the Dakar Region (Senegal)." *Open Journal of Obstetrics and Gynecology* 7.01 (2016): 147.

[144] Whanger, P. D. "Selenium in the treatment of heavy metal poisoning and chemical carcinogenesis." *Journal of trace elements and electrolytes in health and disease* 6.4 (1992): 209-221.

145 Lundebye, Anne-Katrine, et al. "Lower levels of persistent organic pollutants, metals and the marine omega 3-fatty acid DHA in farmed compared to wild Atlantic salmon (Salmo salar)." *Environmental research* 155 (2017): 49-59.

146 Verma, R. J., and DM Guna Sherlin. "Vitamin C ameliorates fluoride-induced embryotoxicity in pregnant rats." *Human & experimental toxicology* 20.12 (2001): 619-623.

147 Karthikeyan, Subramanian, et al. "Polychlorinated biphenyl (PCBs)-induced oxidative stress plays a role on vertebral antioxidant system: Ameliorative role of vitamin C and E in male Wistar rats." *Biomedicine & Preventive Nutrition* 4.3 (2014): 411-416.

148 Lee, Jun-Ho, et al. "Dietary vitamin C reduced mercury contents in the tissues of juvenile olive flounder (Paralichthys olivaceus) exposed with and without mercury." *Environmental toxicology and pharmacology* 45 (2016): 8-14.

Chapter 11

1 Shahhosseini, Zohreh, et al. "A Review of the Effects of Anxiety During Pregnancy on Children's Health." *Materia socio-medica* 27.3 (2015): 200.

2 Field, Tiffany, Miguel Diego, and Maria Hernandez-Reif. "Prenatal depression effects on the fetus and newborn: a review." *Infant Behavior and Development* 29.3 (2006): 445-455.

3 Wadhwa, Pathik D., et al. "The contribution of maternal stress to preterm birth: issues and considerations." *Clinics in Perinatology* 38.3 (2011): 351-384.

4 Vianna, Priscila, et al. "Distress conditions during pregnancy may lead to pre-eclampsia by increasing cortisol levels and altering lymphocyte sensitivity to glucocorticoids." *Medical hypotheses* 77.2 (2011): 188-191.

5 Shahhosseini, Zohreh, et al. "A Review of the Effects of Anxiety During Pregnancy on Children's Health." *Materia socio-medica* 27.3 (2015): 200.

6 Fowden AL, Forhead AJ, Coan PM, Burton GJ. The placenta and intrauterine programming. *J Neuroendocrinol.* 2008;20(4):439-450.

7 Scheinost, Dustin, et al. "Does prenatal stress alter the developing connectome?." *Pediatric research* 81.1-2 (2017): 214-226.

8 Baibazarova, Eugenia, et al. "Influence of prenatal maternal stress, maternal plasma cortisol and cortisol in the amniotic fluid on birth outcomes and child temperament at 3 months." *Psychoneuroendocrinology* 38.6 (2013): 907-915.

9 Qiu, A., et al. "Maternal anxiety and infants' hippocampal development: timing matters." *Translational psychiatry* 3.9 (2013): e306.

10 Field, Tiffany, Miguel Diego, and Maria Hernandez-Reif. "Prenatal depression effects on the fetus and newborn: a review." *Infant Behavior and Development* 29.3 (2006): 445-455.

11 Urizar, Guido G., et al. "Impact of stress reduction instructions on stress and cortisol levels during pregnancy." *Biological Psychology* 67.3 (2004): 275-282.

12 Goodman, Janice H., et al. "CALM Pregnancy: results of a pilot study of mindfulness-based cognitive therapy for perinatal anxiety." *Archives of women's mental health* 17.5 (2014): 373-387.

13 Ahmadi, Zohre, et al. "Effect of breathing technique of blowing on the extent of damage to the perineum at the moment of delivery: A randomized clinical trial." *Iranian journal of nursing and midwifery research* 22.1 (2017): 62.

14 Haseeb, Yasmeen A., et al. "The impact of valsalva's versus spontaneous pushing techniques during second stage of labor on postpartum maternal fatigue and neonatal outcome." *Saudi Journal of Medicine and Medical Sciences* 2.2 (2014): 101.

15 Church, Dawson, Garret Yount, and Audrey J. Brooks. "The effect of emotional freedom techniques on stress biochemistry: a randomized controlled trial." *The Journal of nervous and mental disease* 200.10 (2012): 891-896.

16 Field, Tiffany, Miguel Diego, and Maria Hernandez-Reif. "Prenatal depression effects on the fetus and newborn: a review." *Infant Behavior and Development* 29.3 (2006): 445-455.

17 Errington-Evans, Nick. "Acupuncture for anxiety." *CNS neuroscience & therapeutics* 18.4 (2012): 277-284.

18 Manber, Rachel, et al. "Acupuncture: a promising treatment for depression during pregnancy." *Journal of affective disorders* 83.1 (2004): 89-95.

19 Leung, Brenda MY, and Bonnie J. Kaplan. "Perinatal depression: prevalence, risks, and the nutrition link—a review of the literature." *Journal of the American Dietetic Association* 109.9 (2009): 1566-1575.

20 DiGirolamo, Ann M., and Manuel Ramirez-Zea. "Role of zinc in maternal and child mental health." *The American journal of clinical nutrition* 89.3 (2009): 940S-945S.

21 Ramakrishnan, Usha. "Fatty acid status and maternal mental health." *Maternal & Child Nutrition* 7.s2 (2011): 99-111.

22 Beard, John L., et al. "Maternal iron deficiency anemia affects postpartum emotions and cognition." *The Journal of Nutrition* 135.2 (2005): 267-272.

23 Lin, Pao-Yen, et al. "Polyunsaturated Fatty Acids in Perinatal Depression: A Systematic Review and Meta-analysis." *Biological Psychiatry* (2017).

24 Rios, Adiel C., et al. "Microbiota abnormalities and the therapeutic potential of probiotics in the treatment of mood disorders." *Reviews in the Neurosciences* (2017).

Real Food for Pregnancy

[25] Foster, Jane A., and Karen-Anne McVey Neufeld. "Gut–brain axis: how the microbiome influences anxiety and depression." *Trends in neurosciences* 36.5 (2013): 305-312.

Chapter 12

[1] Campbell, Olivia. "Unprepared and unsupported, I fell through the cracks as a new mom." Quartz. 15 May. 2017, https://qz.com/959420/unprepared-and-unsupported-i-fell-through-the-cracks-as-a-new-mom/. Accessed 12 Sept. 2017.

[2] Kim-Godwin, Yeoun Soo. "Postpartum beliefs and practices among non-Western cultures." *MCN: The American Journal of Maternal/Child Nursing* 28.2 (2003): 74-78.

[3] Piperata, Barbara Ann. "Forty days and forty nights: a biocultural perspective on postpartum practices in the Amazon." *Social Science & Medicine* 67.7 (2008): 1094-1103.

[4] Dennis, Cindy-Lee, et al. "Traditional postpartum practices and rituals: a qualitative systematic review." *Women's Health* 3.4 (2007): 487-502.

[5] Kim-Godwin, Yeoun Soo. "Postpartum beliefs and practices among non-Western cultures." *MCN: The American Journal of Maternal/Child Nursing* 28.2 (2003): 74-78.

[6] "Secrets Of Breast-Feeding From Global Moms In The Know - NPR." 26 Jun. 2017, http://www.npr.org/sections/goatsandsoda/2017/06/26/534021439/secrets-of-breast-feeding-from-global-moms-in-the-know. Accessed 6 Jul. 2017.

[7] Dennis, Cindy-Lee, et al. "Traditional postpartum practices and rituals: a qualitative systematic review." *Women's Health* 3.4 (2007): 487-502.

[8] White, Patrice. "Heat, balance, humors, and ghosts: postpartum in Cambodia." *Health care for women international* 25.2 (2004): 179-194.

[9] Waugh, Lisa Johnson. "Beliefs associated with Mexican immigrant families' practice of la cuarentena during postpartum recovery." *Journal of Obstetric, Gynecologic, & Neonatal Nursing* 40.6 (2011): 732-741.

[10] Freeman, Marci. "Postpartum care from ancient India." *Midwifery Today* 61 (2002): 23-4.

[11] Lennox, Jessica, Pammla Petrucka, and Sandra Bassendowski. "Eating practices during pregnancy: perceptions of select Maasai women in Northern Tanzania." *Global Health Research and Policy* 2.1 (2017): 9.

[12] Piperata, Barbara Ann. "Forty days and forty nights: a biocultural perspective on postpartum practices in the Amazon." *Social Science & Medicine* 67.7 (2008): 1094-1103.

[13] Dennis, Cindy-Lee, et al. "Traditional postpartum practices and rituals: a qualitative systematic review." *Women's Health* 3.4 (2007): 487-502.

[14] Kim-Godwin, Yeoun Soo. "Postpartum beliefs and practices among non-Western cultures." *MCN: The American Journal of Maternal/Child Nursing* 28.2 (2003): 74-78.

[15] Dennis, Cindy-Lee, et al. "Traditional postpartum practices and rituals: a qualitative systematic review." *Women's Health* 3.4 (2007): 487-502.

[16] Poh, Bee Koon, Yuen Peng Wong, and Norimah A. Karim. "Postpartum dietary intakes and food taboos among Chinese women attending maternal and child health clinics and maternity hospital, Kuala Lumpur." *Malaysian Journal of Nutrition* 11.1 (2005): 1-21.

[17] Poh, Bee Koon, Yuen Peng Wong, and Norimah A. Karim. "Postpartum dietary intakes and food taboos among Chinese women attending maternal and child health clinics and maternity hospital, Kuala Lumpur." *Malaysian Journal of Nutrition* 11.1 (2005): 1-21.

[18] Ou, Heng, et al. *The First Forty Days.* Abrams. New York, 2016.

[19] Poh, Bee Koon, Yuen Peng Wong, and Norimah A. Karim. "Postpartum dietary intakes and food taboos among Chinese women attending maternal and child health clinics and maternity hospital, Kuala Lumpur." *Malaysian Journal of Nutrition* 11.1 (2005): 1-21.

[20] Dennis, Cindy-Lee, et al. "Traditional postpartum practices and rituals: a qualitative systematic review." *Women's Health* 3.4 (2007): 487-502.

[21] Poh, Bee Koon, Yuen Peng Wong, and Norimah A. Karim. "Postpartum dietary intakes and food taboos among Chinese women attending maternal and child health clinics and maternity hospital, Kuala Lumpur." *Malaysian Journal of Nutrition* 11.1 (2005): 1-21.

[22] Waugh, Lisa Johnson. "Beliefs associated with Mexican immigrant families' practice of la cuarentena during postpartum recovery." *Journal of Obstetric, Gynecologic, & Neonatal Nursing* 40.6 (2011): 732-741.

[23] Piperata, Barbara Ann. "Forty days and forty nights: a biocultural perspective on postpartum practices in the Amazon." *Social Science & Medicine* 67.7 (2008): 1094-1103.

[24] "Kim-Godwin, Yeoun Soo. "Postpartum beliefs and practices among non-Western cultures." *MCN: The American Journal of Maternal/Child Nursing* 28.2 (2003): 74-78.

[25] White, Patrice. "Heat, balance, humors, and ghosts: postpartum in Cambodia." *Health care for women international* 25.2 (2004): 179-194.

[26] Iliyasu, Z., et al. "Postpartum beliefs and practices in Danbare village, Northern Nigeria." *Journal of obstetrics and gynaecology* 26.3 (2006): 211-215.

[27] Ngunyulu, Roinah N., Fhumulani M. Mulaudzi, and Mmapheko D. Peu. "Comparison between indigenous and Western postnatal care practices in Mopani District, Limpopo Province, South Africa." *Curationis* 38.1 (2015): 1-9.

[28] Duffield, Todd. "Subclinical ketosis in lactating dairy cattle." *Veterinary clinics of north america: Food Animal Practice* 16.2 (2000): 231-253.

29 Feldman, Anna Z., and Florence M. Brown. "Management of type 1 diabetes in pregnancy." *Current diabetes reports* 16.8 (2016): 1-13.

30 Mohammad, Mahmoud A., Agneta L. Sunehag, and Morey W. Haymond. "Effect of dietary macronutrient composition under moderate hypocaloric intake on maternal adaptation during lactation." *The American journal of clinical nutrition* 89.6 (2009): 1821-1827.

31 Allen, Lindsay H. "B vitamins in breast milk: relative importance of maternal status and intake, and effects on infant status and function." *Advances in Nutrition: An International Review Journal* 3.3 (2012): 362-369.

32 Valentine, Christina J., and Carol L. Wagner. "Nutritional management of the breastfeeding dyad." *Pediatric clinics of North America* 60.1 (2013): 261-274.

33 Emmett, Pauline M., and Imogen S. Rogers. "Properties of human milk and their relationship with maternal nutrition." *Early human development* 49 (1997): S7-S28.

34 Allen, Lindsay H. "B vitamins in breast milk: relative importance of maternal status and intake, and effects on infant status and function." *Advances in Nutrition: An International Review Journal* 3.3 (2012): 362-369.

35 Greer, Frank R., et al. "Improving the vitamin K status of breastfeeding infants with maternal vitamin K supplements." *Pediatrics* 99.1 (1997): 88-92.

36 "Gilmore JH, Lin W, Prasatwa MW, et al. Regional gray matter growth, sexual dimorphism, and cerebral asymmetry in the neonatal brain. Journal of Neuroscience. 2007;27(6):1255-1260

37 Allen, Lindsay H. "B vitamins in breast milk: relative importance of maternal status and intake, and effects on infant status and function." *Advances in Nutrition: An International Review Journal* 3.3 (2012): 362-369.

38 Valentine, Christina J., and Carol L. Wagner. "Nutritional management of the breastfeeding dyad." *Pediatric clinics of North America* 60.1 (2013): 261-274.

39 Graham, Stephen M., Otto M. Arvela, and Graham A. Wise. "Long-term neurologic consequences of nutritional vitamin B 12 deficiency in infants." *The Journal of pediatrics* 121.5 (1992): 710-714.

40 Kühne, T., R. Bubl, and R. Baumgartner. "Maternal vegan diet causing a serious infantile neurological disorder due to vitamin B 12 deficiency." *European journal of pediatrics* 150.3 (1991): 205-208.

41 Weiss, Rachel, Yacov Fogelman, and Michael Bennett. "Severe vitamin B12 deficiency in an infant associated with a maternal deficiency and a strict vegetarian diet." *Journal of pediatric hematology/oncology* 26.4 (2004): 270-271.

42 Sklar, Ronald. "Nutritional vitamin B12 deficiency in a breast-fed infant of a vegan-diet mother." *Clinical pediatrics* 25.4 (1986): 219-221.

43 Allen, Lindsay H. "B vitamins in breast milk: relative importance of maternal status and intake, and effects on infant status and function." *Advances in Nutrition: An International Review Journal* 3.3 (2012): 362-369.

44 Kühne, T., R. Bubl, and R. Baumgartner. "Maternal vegan diet causing a serious infantile neurological disorder due to vitamin B 12 deficiency." *European journal of pediatrics* 150.3 (1991): 205-208.

45 Herrmann, Wolfgang, et al. "Vitamin B-12 status, particularly holotranscobalamin II and methylmalonic acid concentrations, and hyperhomocysteinemia in vegetarians." *The American journal of clinical nutrition* 78.1 (2003): 131-136.

46 Davenport, Crystal, et al. "Choline intakes exceeding recommendations during human lactation improve breast milk choline content by increasing PEMT pathway metabolites." *The Journal of nutritional biochemistry* 26.9 (2015): 903-911.

47 Meck, Warren H., and Christina L. Williams. "Metabolic imprinting of choline by its availability during gestation: implications for memory and attentional processing across the lifespan." *Neuroscience & Biobehavioral Reviews* 27.4 (2003): 385-399.

48 U.S. National Library of Medicine. *"LACTMED: Lecithin"* TOXNET. https://toxnet.nlm.nih.gov/. Accessed 14 Nov. 2017.

49 Kim, Hyesook, et al. "Breast milk fatty acid composition and fatty acid intake of lactating mothers in South Korea." *British Journal of Nutrition* 117.4 (2017): 556-561.

50 Ratnayake, WM Nimal, et al. "Mandatory trans fat labeling regulations and nationwide product reformulations to reduce trans fatty acid content in foods contributed to lowered concentrations of trans fat in Canadian women's breast milk samples collected in 2009–2011." *The American journal of clinical nutrition* 100.4 (2014): 1036-1040.

51 Mohammad, Mahmoud A., Agneta L. Sunehag, and Morey W. Haymond. "Effect of dietary macronutrient composition under moderate hypocaloric intake on maternal adaptation during lactation." *The American journal of clinical nutrition* 89.6 (2009): 1821-1827.

52 Innis, Sheila M., Judith Gilley, and Janet Werker. "Are human milk long-chain polyunsaturated fatty acids related to visual and neural development in breast-fed term infants?" *The Journal of pediatrics* 139.4 (2001): 532-538.

53 Innis, Sheila M., Judith Gilley, and Janet Werker. "Are human milk long-chain polyunsaturated fatty acids related to visual and neural development in breast-fed term infants?." *The Journal of pediatrics* 139.4 (2001): 532-538.

54 Carlson, Susan E. "Docosahexaenoic acid supplementation in pregnancy and lactation." *The American journal of clinical nutrition* 89.2 (2009): 678S-684S.

[55] Francois, Cindy A., et al. "Supplementing lactating women with flaxseed oil does not increase docosahexaenoic acid in their milk." *The American journal of clinical nutrition* 77.1 (2003): 226-233.

[56] Finley, Dorothy Ann, et al. "Breast milk composition: fat content and fatty acid composition in vegetarians and non-vegetarians." *The American journal of clinical nutrition* 41.4 (1985): 787-800.

[57] Chang, Pishan, et al. "Seizure control by ketogenic diet-associated medium chain fatty acids." *Neuropharmacology* 69 (2013): 105-114.

[58] Muneta, Tetsuo, et al. "Ketone body elevation in placenta, umbilical cord, newborn and mother in normal delivery." *Glycative Stress Research* 3.3 (2016): 133-140.

[59] Desbois, Andrew P., and Valerie J. Smith. "Antibacterial free fatty acids: activities, mechanisms of action and biotechnological potential." *Applied microbiology and biotechnology* 85.6 (2010): 1629-1642.

[60] Rist, Lukas, et al. "Influence of organic diet on the amount of conjugated linoleic acids in breast milk of lactating women in the Netherlands." *British journal of Nutrition* 97.4 (2007): 735-743.

[61] Thijs, C., et al. "Fatty acids in breast milk and development of atopic eczema and allergic sensitisation in infancy." *Allergy* 66.1 (2011): 58-67.

[62] Helland, Ingrid B., et al. "Similar effects on infants of n-3 and n-6 fatty acids supplementation to pregnant and lactating women." *Pediatrics* 108.5 (2001): e82-e82.

[63] Friesen, Russell, and Sheila M. Innis. "Trans fatty acids in human milk in Canada declined with the introduction of trans fat food labeling." *The Journal of nutrition* 136.10 (2006): 2558-2561.

[64] Innis, Sheila M. "Trans fatty intakes during pregnancy, infancy and early childhood." *Atherosclerosis Supplements* 7.2 (2006): 17-20.

[65] Albuquerque, KT, Sardinha, FL, Telles, MM, Watanabe, RL, Nascimento, CM, Tavares do Carmo, MG et al. Intake of trans fatty acid-rich hydrogenated fat during pregnancy and lactation inhibits the hypophagic effect of central insulin in the adult offspring. *Nutrition.* 2006; 22: 820–829.

[66] Pimentel, GD, Lira, FS, Rosa, JC, Oliveira, JL, Losinskas-Hachul, AC, Souza, GI et al. Intake of trans fatty acids during gestation and lactation leads to hypothalamic inflammation via TLR4/NFκBp65 signaling in adult offspring. *J Nutr Biochem.* 2012; 23: 265–271.

[67] Elias, Sandra L., and Sheila M. Innis. "Bakery foods are the major dietary source of trans-fatty acids among pregnant women with diets providing 30 percent energy from fat." *Journal of the American Dietetic Association* 102.1 (2002): 46-51.

[68] Valentine, Christina J., and Carol L. Wagner. "Nutritional management of the breastfeeding dyad." *Pediatric clinics of North America* 60.1 (2013): 261-274.

[69] Bahl, Rajiv, et al. "Vitamin A supplementation of women postpartum and of their infants at immunization alters breast milk retinol and infant vitamin A status." *The Journal of nutrition* 132.11 (2002): 3243-3248.

[70] Gurgel, Cristiane Santos Sânzio, et al. "Effect of routine prenatal supplementation on vitamin concentrations in maternal serum and breast milk." *Nutrition* 33 (2017): 261-265.

[71] Hollis, Bruce W., et al. "Maternal versus infant vitamin D supplementation during lactation: a randomized controlled trial." *Pediatrics* 136.4 (2015): 625-634.

[72] Hollis, Bruce W., et al. "Maternal versus infant vitamin D supplementation during lactation: a randomized controlled trial." *Pediatrics* 136.4 (2015): 625-634.

[73] Mulrine, Hannah M., et al. "Breast-milk iodine concentration declines over the first 6 mo postpartum in iodine-deficient women." *The American journal of clinical nutrition* 92.4 (2010): 849-856.

[74] Azizi, Fereidoun, and Peter Smyth. "Breastfeeding and maternal and infant iodine nutrition." *Clinical endocrinology* 70.5 (2009): 803-809.

[75] Azizi, Fereidoun, and Peter Smyth. "Breastfeeding and maternal and infant iodine nutrition." *Clinical endocrinology* 70.5 (2009): 803-809.

[76] Leung, Angela M., Elizabeth N. Pearce, and Lewis E. Braverman. "Iodine nutrition in pregnancy and lactation." *Endocrinology and metabolism clinics of North America* 40.4 (2011): 765-777.

[77] Dasgupta, Purnendu K., et al. "Intake of iodine and perchlorate and excretion in human milk." *Environmental science & technology* 42.21 (2008): 8115-8121.

[78] Levant, Beth, Jeffery D. Radel, and Susan E. Carlson. "Reduced brain DHA content after a single reproductive cycle in female rats fed a diet deficient in N-3 polyunsaturated fatty acids." *Biological psychiatry* 60.9 (2006): 987-990.

[79] Veugelers, Paul J., and John Paul Ekwaru. "A statistical error in the estimation of the recommended dietary allowance for vitamin D." *Nutrients* 6.10 (2014): 4472-4475.

[80] Papadimitriou, Dimitrios T. "The big Vitamin D mistake." *Journal of Preventive Medicine and Public Health* (2017).

[81] Heaney, Robert P., et al. "Vitamin D3 is more potent than vitamin D2 in humans." *The Journal of Clinical Endocrinology & Metabolism* 96.3 (2011): E447-E452.

[82] Alexander, Erik K., et al. "2017 Guidelines of the American Thyroid Association for the diagnosis and management of thyroid disease during pregnancy and the postpartum." *Thyroid* 27.3 (2017): 315-389.

[83] Aceves, Carmen, Brenda Anguiano, and Guadalupe Delgado. "Is iodine a gatekeeper of the integrity of the mammary gland?." *Journal of mammary gland biology and neoplasia* 10.2 (2005): 189-196.

[84] Soto, Ana, et al. "Lactobacilli and bifidobacteria in human breast milk: influence of antibiotherapy and other host and clinical factors." *Journal of pediatric gastroenterology and nutrition* 59.1 (2014): 78.

[85] Rautava, Samuli, Marko Kalliomäki, and Erika Isolauri. "Probiotics during pregnancy and breast-feeding might confer immunomodulatory protection against atopic disease in the infant." *Journal of Allergy and Clinical Immunology* 109.1 (2002): 119-121.

[86] Baldassarre, Maria Elisabetta, et al. "Administration of a multi-strain probiotic product to women in the perinatal period differentially affects the breast milk cytokine profile and may have beneficial effects on neonatal gastrointestinal functional symptoms. A randomized clinical trial." *Nutrients* 8.11 (2016): 677.

[87] Young, Sharon Marie, "Effects of Human Maternal Placentophagy on Postpartum Maternal Affect, Health, and Recovery" (2016). *UNLV Theses, Dissertations, Professional Papers, and Capstones*. 2818.

[88] Young, Sharon M., et al. "Human placenta processed for encapsulation contains modest concentrations of fourteen trace minerals and elements." *Nutr Res* (2016).

[89] Abascal, Kathy, and Eric Yarnell. "Botanical galactagogues." *Alternative and Complementary Therapies* 14.6 (2008): 288-294.

[90] Silva, Fernando V., et al. "Chamomile reveals to be a potent galactogogue: the unexpected effect." *The Journal of Maternal-Fetal & Neonatal Medicine* (2017): 1-3.

[91] Chang, Shao-Min, and Chung-Hey Chen. "Effects of an intervention with drinking chamomile tea on sleep quality and depression in sleep disturbed postnatal women: a randomized controlled trial." *Journal of advanced nursing* 72.2 (2016): 306-315.

[92] Klier, C. M., et al. "St. John's Wort (Hypericum Perforatum)-Is it Safe during Breastfeeding?." *Pharmacopsychiatry* 35.01 (2002): 29-30.

[93] Palacios, Cristina, and Lilliana Gonzalez. "Is vitamin D deficiency a major global public health problem?." *The Journal of steroid biochemistry and molecular biology* 144 (2014): 138-145.

[94] Murphy, Pamela K., et al. "An exploratory study of postpartum depression and vitamin D." *Journal of the American Psychiatric Nurses Association* 16.3 (2010): 170-177.

[95] "Vitamin D Council | Testing for vitamin D." https://www.vitamindcouncil.org/about-vitamin-d/testing-for-vitamin-d/. Accessed 8 May. 2017.

[96] Le Donne, Maria, et al. "Postpartum mood disorders and thyroid autoimmunity." *Frontiers in endocrinology* 8 (2017).

[97] Stagnaro-Green, Alex. "Postpartum management of women begun on levothyroxine during pregnancy." *Frontiers in endocrinology* 6 (2015).

[98] Le Donne, Maria, et al. "Postpartum mood disorders and thyroid autoimmunity." *Frontiers in endocrinology* 8 (2017).

[99] Le Donne, Maria, et al. "Postpartum mood disorders and thyroid autoimmunity." *Frontiers in endocrinology* 8 (2017).

[100] Le Donne, Maria, et al. "Postpartum mood disorders and thyroid autoimmunity." *Frontiers in endocrinology* 8 (2017).

[101] Stagnaro-Green, Alex. "Postpartum management of women begun on levothyroxine during pregnancy." *Frontiers in endocrinology* 6 (2015).

[102] Krysiak, R., K. Kowalcze, and B. Okopien. "The effect of vitamin D on thyroid autoimmunity in non-lactating women with postpartum thyroiditis." *European journal of clinical nutrition* (2016).

[103] Jeffcoat, Heather. "Postpartum Recovery After Vaginal Birth: The First 6 Weeks." *International Journal of Childbirth Education* 24.3 (2009): 32.

[104] Reimers, C., et al. "Change in pelvic organ support during pregnancy and the first year postpartum: a longitudinal study." *BJOG: An International Journal of Obstetrics & Gynaecology* 123.5 (2016): 821-829.

[105] Dennis, Cindy-Lee, et al. "Traditional postpartum practices and rituals: a qualitative systematic review." *Women's Health* 3.4 (2007): 487-502.

[106] Gyhagen, M. 1., et al. "Prevalence and risk factors for pelvic organ prolapse 20 years after childbirth: a national cohort study in singleton primiparae after vaginal or caesarean delivery." *BJOG: An International Journal of Obstetrics & Gynaecology* 120.2 (2013): 152-160.

[107] Wu, Jennifer M., et al. "Lifetime risk of stress incontinence or pelvic organ prolapse surgery." *Obstetrics and gynecology* 123.6 (2014): 1201.

[108] Kandadai, Padma, Katharine O'Dell, and Jyot Saini. "Correct performance of pelvic muscle exercises in women reporting prior knowledge." *Female pelvic medicine & reconstructive surgery* 21.3 (2015): 135-140.

[109] Price, Natalia, Rehana Dawood, and Simon R. Jackson. "Pelvic floor exercise for urinary incontinence: a systematic literature review." *Maturitas* 67.4 (2010): 309-315.

[110] Strang, Victoria R., and Patricia L. Sullivan. "Body image attitudes during pregnancy and the postpartum period." *Journal of Obstetric, Gynecologic, & Neonatal Nursing* 14.4 (1985): 332-337.

[111] Leahy, Katie, et al. "The Relationship between Intuitive Eating and Postpartum Weight Loss." *Maternal and Child Health Journal* (2017): 1-7.

[112] Fergerson SS, Jamieson DJ, Lindsay M. "Diagnosing postpartum depression: can we do better?" *Am J Obstet Gynecol* 2002 May; 186(5):899-902.

[113] Leung, Brenda MY, and Bonnie J. Kaplan. "Perinatal depression: prevalence, risks, and the nutrition link—a review of the literature." *Journal of the American Dietetic Association* 109.9 (2009): 1566-1575.

[114] Candela, C. Gómez, LMa Bermejo López, and V. Loria Kohen. "Importance of a balanced omega 6/omega 3 ratio for the maintenance of health. Nutritional recommendations." *Nutricion hospitalaria* 26.2 (2011): 323-329.

[115] Le Donne, Maria, et al. "Postpartum mood disorders and thyroid autoimmunity." *Frontiers in endocrinology* 8 (2017).

[116] Smits, Luc JM, and Gerard GM Essed. "Short interpregnancy intervals and unfavourable pregnancy outcome: role of folate depletion." *The Lancet* 358.9298 (2001): 2074-2077.

[117] Conde-Agudelo, Agustín, Anyeli Rosas-Bermudez, and Maureen H. Norton. "Birth spacing and risk of autism and other neurodevelopmental disabilities: a systematic review." *Pediatrics* (2016): e20153482.

[118] DaVanzo, Julie, et al. "Effects of interpregnancy interval and outcome of the preceding pregnancy on pregnancy outcomes in Matlab, Bangladesh." *BJOG: An International Journal of Obstetrics & Gynaecology* 114.9 (2007): 1079-1087.

[119] Conde-Agudelo, Agustín, et al. "Effects of birth spacing on maternal, perinatal, infant, and child health: a systematic review of causal mechanisms." *Studies in family planning* 43.2 (2012): 93-114.

[120] Conde-Agudelo, Agustín, et al. "Effects of birth spacing on maternal, perinatal, infant, and child health: a systematic review of causal mechanisms." *Studies in family planning* 43.2 (2012): 93-114.

[121] Conde-Agudelo, Agustín, Anyeli Rosas-Bermudez, and Maureen H. Norton. "Birth spacing and risk of autism and other neurodevelopmental disabilities: a systematic review." *Pediatrics* (2016): e20153482.

[122] DaVanzo, Julie, et al. "Effects of interpregnancy interval and outcome of the preceding pregnancy on pregnancy outcomes in Matlab, Bangladesh." *BJOG: An International Journal of Obstetrics & Gynaecology* 114.9 (2007): 1079-1087.

[123] Price, Weston A. *Nutrition and Physical Degeneration A Comparison of Primitive and Modern Diets and Their Effects.* New York: Hoeber. 1939. Print.

About the Author

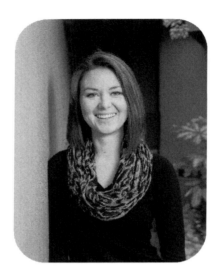

Lily Nichols is a Registered Dietitian/Nutritionist, Certified Diabetes Educator, researcher, and author with a passion for evidence-based prenatal nutrition. Drawing from the current scientific literature and the wisdom of traditional cultures, her work is known for being research-focused, thorough, and sensible. Her bestselling book, *Real Food for Gestational Diabetes* (and online course of the same name), presents a revolutionary nutrient-dense, lower carb approach for managing gestational diabetes. Her work has not only helped tens of thousands of women manage their gestational diabetes (most without the need for blood sugar-lowering medication), but has also influenced nutrition policies internationally. Lily's clinical expertise and extensive background in prenatal nutrition have made her a highly sought after consultant and speaker in the field. When she's not writing and researching, you can find Lily hiking, gardening, cooking, and eating real food with her husband and son.

To learn more, visit www.LilyNicholsRDN.com

Real Food for Pregnancy

Printed in Poland
by Amazon Fulfillment
Poland Sp. z o.o., Wrocław